# Diets and Dieting

## A Cultural Encyclopedia

# Diets and Dieting

## A Cultural Encyclopedia

Sander L. Gilman

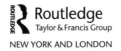
Routledge
Taylor & Francis Group

NEW YORK AND LONDON

First published 2008
by Routledge
270 Madison Ave, New York, NY 10016

Simultaneously published in the UK
by Routledge
2 Park Square, Milton Park, Abingdon, Oxon OX14 4RN

*Routledge is an imprint of the Taylor & Francis Group, an informa business*

© 2008 Taylor & Francis

Typeset in Sabon by RefineCatch Limited, Bungay, Suffolk
Printed and bound in the United States of America on acid-free paper by Sheridan Books, Inc., MI

*Library of Congress Cataloging in Publication Data*
Gilman, Sander L.
    Diets and dieting : a cultural encyclopedia / Sander L. Gilman.
        p. ; cm.
    Includes bibliographical references and index.
    ISBN-13: 978–0–415–97420–2 (hardback)
    ISBN-10: 0–415–97420–8 (hardback)
 1. Diets—History—Encyclopedias.    2. Dieting—History—Encyclopedias.    3. Diet therapy—History—Encyclopedias.    I. Title.
    [DNLM: 1. Diet Therapy—history—Encyclopedias—English.    2. Diet—history—Encyclopedias—English.    3. Famous
Persons—Encyclopedias—English.    4. History, Modern 1601—Encyclopedias—English.    5. Nutrition Disorders—diet therapy—
Encyclopedias—English.    6. Nutrition Disorders—history—Encyclopedias—English.    WB 13 G487d 2008]
    RM214.5.G55 2008
    613.2′503—dc22
2007027896

ISBN10: 0–415–97420–8 (hbk)
ISBN10: 0–203–93550–0 (ebk)

ISBN13: 978–0–415–97420–2 (hbk)
ISBN13: 978–0–203–93550–7 (ebk)

# CONTENTS

# LIST OF ENTRIES

# INTRODUCTION

## Some Weighty Thoughts on Dieting and Epidemics

In July 2004, the then-American Health and Human Services Secretary Tommy G. Thompson announced that Medicare was abandoning a long-held policy that said obesity was not a disease, opening the way for the Government to pay for a whole range of possible treatments. Soon after Thompson's decision, a cartoon by Dick Locher of Tribune Media Services appeared. A portly little boy having read the newspaper with the headline "Obesity Now Considered a Disease" announces into the telephone, "Hello, Principal's office? This is Tommy Frobish . . . I won't be in school today, I got a disease."

We know what type of disease Tommy Frobish had. As early as 1987, the media began to evoke the specter of a forthcoming epidemic of obesity: "Childhood obesity is epidemic in the United States," stated Dr. William H. Dietz Jr. of New England Medical Center. The World Health Organization declared obesity the new "global epidemic" in 1998. By 2004, headlines such as "Obesity Epidemic Raises Risk of Children Developing Diabetes" grabbed (and continue to grab) the attention of readers. Scientists at the American Association for the Advancement of Science annual meeting in February 2002 had already warned the Government that obesity was now a "global epidemic"—no longer confined to Western, industrialized societies. This reflected a growing consensus in the 1990s that obesity (not smoking) was going to be the major public health issue of the new millennium.

Parallel to the seemingly unstoppable spread of this new epidemic was the development of new, radical cures: Would it be surgical (stomach stapling), genetic (the "ob [esity]-gene") or would it be the old, tried and true "cure" of dieting? In the twenty-first century, dieting has come to mean the control of the intake of nutrients and the use of parallel interventions such as exercise, psycho-logical therapy, surgery, or pharmaceuticals to control (increase or decrease) body weight, strength, health, and/or shape. From the mid-nineteenth century to today, medical specialists and lay practitioners have tried to claim too fat or too thin people (however defined) as their patients. Fat and thinness is truly in the eye of the beholder. Each age, culture, and tradition defines unacceptable weight for itself: Yet, all do have a point beyond which excess or inadequate weight is unacceptable—unhealthy, ugly, or corrupt. Today, we call this "morbid obesity or anorexia," and both are always seen as an issue of health. Thus, dieting today may also limit the intake of foods, such as salt or transfats, that are labeled unhealthy.

Yet health, as we well know, is a code word for a positive range of qualities that any given society wishes to see in its citizens: From beauty to loyalty to responsibility to fecundity (and the list marches on). Thus, today, the very opposite illness, anorexia nervosa, it would seem, has become what George Devereux in the 1950s called a pre-scribed template for mental illness: "Don't go crazy, but if you do, do it this way." Obesity has precisely the opposite quality. The morbidly obese do not figure in society as a socially acceptable form of mental illness in any way. The asymmetry between today's image of obesity and of anorexia points to the complex meanings given to weight and body shape over history. All of these impact and are impacted by the culture of diet and dieting in which individuals find themselves.

From the 1860s, it was the diet culture that dominated the market even as biomedical science developed tools to understand the biochemical nature of metabolism, endrocrinological imbalance, and, more recently, genetics. Dieting was the tool of the physician, but it was also the means by which lay practitioners of the modern "health culture" were able to claim the too fat and the very thin as their clients. Dieting, or (more recently) "lifestyle change," became a way to halt the obesity epidemic, to intervene to improve the private life of the individual and, thus, the health of the nation.

These two qualities were regularly linked. Whether through claims that morbid obesity impacted on the health of the mother and child and thus weakened the state or whether the fat man and the thin man could not fulfill their civic and military duty and became a drain on the state, the obese, from at least mid-nineteenth century, were seen as a danger to themselves as well as others. When it was clear that too many men had failed the draft physical in World War II because of malnutrition, Harry S Truman created the school lunch program in 1946, which stood accused in the 1990s of being one of the causes of obesity. The general stigma associated with a potentially unhealthy body that stood out because of its size made it imperative that the fat and the thin seek or be forced to treatment. Thus, there were financial incentives to seek this group out and rehabilitate them. Too fat and too skinny people could be made productive and healthy people through the interventions of medical professionals but also lay specialists. In France, the modern food culture, without its sauces and exotic ingredients, was created in the 1820s by Jean Anthelme Brillat-Savarin, whose *The Physiology of Taste or, Meditations on Transcendental Gastronomy* was a fat man's confession about how he tried to lose weight. It was a self-help book that created the French cult of modern food. "Obesity," as Brillat-Savarin states, "is not actually a disease, it is at least a most unpleasant state of ill health, and one into which we almost always fall because of our own fault." It was a change in the way one ate that could control one's weight.

The American food faddists of the late nineteenth century, who produced "modern" machine-made foods such as "corn flakes," sought to reform the body politic; today we hear their heirs advocate "natural" or "organic" food. Their argument is that unprocessed food is close to nature and, thus, healthier. In 1894, Will Keith Kellogg was trying to improve the vegetarian diet of sanatorium patients when he invented Corn Flakes; one of them, Charles William Post invented Postum cereal beverage in 1895. Two years later, Post developed Grape-Nuts cereal, part of the new health-industrial complex. They followed the lead of those who first canned milk at mid-century;

they saw in the modern manufacture of food the introduction of the principles of hygiene. And they were certainly right—boiled, condensed milk was certainly healthier than milk from tuberculosis-infected cows. Well, if you discounted the lead that leached into the milk in the early containers.

All aimed and aim at healthier, better citizens. And all succeed in making a profit doing it. The cereal manufacturers of the nineteenth century, like Post and Kellogg, moved from fringe-food-fad operations in "Wellville" (read T. Coraghessan Boyle's 1993 novel *The Road to Wellville*, the title of which is taken from a pamphlet by C. W. Post) to dominate the food market; "organic" food today may well rescue the small farm as it returns much greater profit than "traditional" food. Health and wealth are linked by more than a rhyme.

Dieting aims at both cure and profit. It is, thus, very modern. Certainly, fasting as a religious observance was part and parcel of Western Christianity, beginning with Paul. (It also became part of both rabbinic Judaism and Islam.) But religious fasting is not dieting. It was (and is) a sign of man's relationship to God and to God's complex world. Ironically, this is not much different from the ancient Greeks who saw food (and food reduction) as part of a complex web that spanned human beings and the gods through the humors. Dieting arises in the post-Copernican world when scientists and lay people from the late seventeenth to early nineteenth century began to think of the human body more as a machine and then as a collection of chemical processes. The dieting body is not necessarily an extension of the divine. Here we can evoke Zygmunt Bauman's distinction in his 1998 *Globalization: The Human Consequences* between "pilgrims" and "tourists." In a real sense, fasters are pilgrims who believe that their world is bounded by God (or the gods) and fasting will bind them to that world. Dieters are tourists in the new economy of the body.

The rise of the modern dieting culture comes to hold powerful metaphoric implications for all bodies, including, as Thomas Hobbes observes in *The Leviathan* (1651), the body politic. Hobbes observes that (like human beings) "Commonwealths can endure no diet: for seeing their expense is not limited by their own appetite but by external accidents, and the appetites of their neighbours, the public riches cannot be limited by other limits than those which the emergent occasions shall require." Here is perhaps the best sense of the conflict between the desire for food and the difficulty (if not

Reid, Thomas (1854) "Essay II, Chapter 1," in *Works*, edited by William Hamilton, Edinburgh: Maclachan and Stewart.

Wilson, G. Terence and Brownell, Kelly D. (2002) "Behavioral Treatment for Obesity," in Christopher G. Fairburn and Kelly D. Brownell (eds), *Eating Disorders and Obesity: A Comprehensive Handbook*, New York: Guilford Press, pp. 524–8.

# Advertising

## Regulation

Advertising is a staple of modern, capitalist societies. Arising in the course of the nineteenth century, its goal was to encourage the consumption of specific objects. Celebrity advertising, begun in late-nineteenth-century Britain, used glamour to sell things. Few or no questions were asked about the safety or efficacy of the things sold. It has become the way that producers communicate with their consumers. However, today, many pose the question of where the line should be drawn in regard to potentially dangerous advertisements. In recent decades, the nation witnessed the battle between antismoking lobbyists advocating the censorship of tobacco ads and the tobacco industry's marketing platform. This came as a result of research regarding the links between cancer and smoking cigarettes.

Similarly, some people are up in arms at the "irresponsible behavior" of the food industry in relation to its advertisements of junk food. The basis of their argument is that "advertising of food products alters consumers' preferences for foods so that they consume more of the advertised foods than they would have absent the advertising" (Zywicki et al. 2004). Thus, advertising is theorized to play a powerful role in shaping the behavior of denizens of society. Advertisers, as a result, are charged with the responsibility of ensuring morality in what they endorse. When they fail at this, the American Federal Trade Commission (FTC) gets involved in regulating what the public sees.

In light of the obesity epidemic that is claimed to be sweeping the nation, there has been fierce controversy regarding whether or not the Government should intervene to curb advertising of "junk food" to children. Junk food can be understood as snacks, candy, and breakfast food that have little to no nutritional value. Of the over-10,000 food and beverage commercials children see a year, less than 2 percent are for "foods that promote a balanced diet such as fruits, milk, vegetables, and cheese" (Sommer 2006). However, more than two-thirds of these television commercials are for junk food. The U.S. Government claims that "an estimated 10% of America's preschoolers are dangerously overweight and that obesity rates for elementary school students have tripled in the last three decades" (Anon. 2005). Thus, some argue that the Government should get involved in censoring television ads for specific foods aimed at children.

The traditional food logos and icons aimed at children, such as "Ronald McDonald" and "Captain Crunch," designed to persuade children to demand certain foods, have become "one of the most contentious aspects of the nation's struggle with obesity" (Mishra 2005). Similar to the controversy that raged regarding the use of the "Joe Camel" cartoon as a marketing ploy of Camel cigarettes from 1987 to 1997 aimed at younger smokers, the food industry creates "cool" "pop" culture icons aimed at children which are viewed as causing them to make poor food choices. (Like many of the "junk food" manufacturers, the R.J. Reynolds Company, which manufactures Camels, denied any intention in appealing to the youngest members of their audience.)

The food industry spends over 10 billion dollars a year trying to shape the appetite of children (Mishra 2005). However, parallel to the claims of the tobacco companies in denying the relationship between tobacco and lung cancer (Brandt 2007), the food industry insists that there is no direct linkage between junk-food marketing and childhood obesity.

Yet, some companies are taking responsibility for the effect of their marketing campaigns. For example, Lance Friedmann, Senior Vice President at Kraft, admits that "advertising plays a role" in influencing children's eating habits (Mishra 2005). Thus, Kraft—as well as Coca-Cola—is voluntarily limiting its advertisements aimed at children (especially those aimed at kids younger than twelve years of age). Kraft now "only runs commercials featuring healthy foods such as sugar-free drinks, low-fat meat products, and whole-grain products" (Mishra 2005) aimed at children. This is a drastic change from their traditional advertising campaigns, which gained success through products like Oreos (with excess saturated fats) and Kool-Aid (with excess sugar).

Additionally, McDonald's, the home of Ronald McDonald, has altered its advertising, and even its menu. In 2004, McDonald's announced its program committed to "balanced lifestyles." The fast-food franchises added healthy options, such as salads and fruit, to its menu in order to afford its customers more options. However, it may be the case that McDonald's adopted healthy alternatives in order to avoid class-action law suits. In 2002, McDonald's faced a landmark lawsuit, in which the teenage plaintiffs accused the restaurant of fraud. They claimed that McDonald's failure to "disclose clearly and conspicuously the ingredients" (Wald 2003) of its hamburgers was a violation of New York state's consumer fraud statutes. They, therefore, claimed that the restaurant should be liable for their health conditions: obesity, heart disease, high blood pressure, and elevated cholesterol. Although the case was thrown out by the judge, it still set a precedent in regard to responsibility of food distributors and advertisers. The teens' lawyer, Samuel Hirsch, made an interesting point that, "young individuals are not in a position to make a choice after the onslaught of advertising and promotions" (Wald 2003). Another possible reason for McDonald's menu change is Morgan Spurlock's documentary, *Super Size Me*, which demonstrated the health damage that a McDonald's-only diet could do. After the film's release, McDonald's dropped the "super size" option from their menu. Therefore, it is not accurate to say that McDonald's voluntarily made their menu and advertisements more health-minded. Rather, the company was forced to respond to public pressure to reform.

On the other hand, there are those that promote weight-loss methods to excess. In fact, diet advertisements are ubiquitous in magazines, television, and the media at large. However, fast-fix diet promotions that promise impossible results are becoming more and more common. For example, diet pills are the new miracle weight-loss solution, or at least this is what their commercials guarantee. On December 9, 2003, the FTC announced its "Red Flag" education campaign "to assist media outlets voluntarily to screen out weight-loss product ads containing claims that are too good to be true" (Cleland and Mack 2003). The FTC's primary goal is to weed out false advertisements from those that promise realistic weight-loss products. The weight-loss industry earns 30 billion dollars in its products and services. Thus, there exists a huge incentive to come up with products that appeal to the consumer—especially those that are supposedly quicker, easier, and more effective than the competition.

The problem is that what many of these companies claim is simply not true. The proliferation of ads that offer false promises have "proceeded in the face of, and in spite of, an unprecedented level of FTC enforcement activity, including the filing of more than 80 cases during the last decade" (Cleland et al. 2002: 2). This poses a huge problem in terms of both ethical advertising and, more importantly, public health. The existence of "miracle drugs" gives people hope that they can shed the necessary pounds to get to a healthy weight. However, when these drugs fail to work, people are left with hopelessness and may give up on weight loss entirely.

Government interventions of any kind in the commercial sector of society raise questions and debates regarding laissez-faire, the notion of a free economy, and the free market. However, in this case, because censorship is also being instituted to some degree, some challenge that their First Amendment rights are being violated as well. In early 2005, a group called the Alliance for American Advertising—consisting of the American Advertising Federation, the American Association of Advertising Agencies, the Association of National Advertising and the Grocery Manufacturers Association—was created in order to persuade legislators not to introduce bills that would restrict food ads targeted to children (Anon. 2005). Moreover, networks, advertisers, ad agencies, and their trade associations vigorously opposed the FTC proposals, "claiming that the FTC had no authority to ban truthful advertising for lawful products" (Sommer 2006).

SLG/Jessica Rissman

*See also* Celebrities; Children; Diet Pills; Obesity Epidemic; Smoking; Spurlock

### References and Further Reading

Anon. (2005) "Food Fight: Obesity Raises Difficult Marketing Questions," *Knowledge @ Wharton*. Available online at <http://knowledge.wharton.upenn.edu/index.cfm-?fa=viewfeature&id=1149> (accessed May 5, 2006).

Brandt, Alan (2007) *The Cigarette Century: The Rise, Fall, and Deadly Persistence of the Product That Defined America*, New York: Basic Books.

Cleland, Richard L., Gross, Walter C., Koss, Laura D., Daynard, Matthew, and Muoio, Karen M. (2002) "Weight-Loss Advertising: An Analysis of Current Trends. A Report of the Staff of the Federal Trade Commission." Available online at <http://files.findlaw.com/news.findlaw.com/hdocs/docs/ftc/902weightlossadsrpt.pdf> (accessed May 6, 2006).

Cleland, Richard and Mack, Brenda (2003) "FTC Releases Guidance to Media on False Weight-Loss Claims," Federal Trade Commission for the Consumer. Available online at <http://www.ftc.gov/opa/2003/12/weightlossrpt.htm> (accessed May 6, 2006).

Mishra, Raja (2005) "Push Grows to Limit Food Ads to Children," Campaign for a Commercial-Free Childhood. Available online at <http://www.commercialexploitation.org/news/articles/push-tolimitfoodads.htm> (accessed May 6, 2006).

Sommer, Ralph (2006) "TV Food Messages and Children's Diets," Center for Media Literacy. Available online at <http://www.medialit.org/reading_room/article145.html> (accessed May 4, 2006).

Wald, Jonathan (2003) "McDonald's Obesity Suit Tossed," Cable News Network. Available online at <http://money.cnn.com/2003/01/22/news/companies/mcdonalds/index.htm> (accessed May 6, 2006).

Zywicki, Todd J., Holt, Debra, and Ohlhausen, Maureen (2004) "Obesity and Advertising Policy," *George Mason Law Review* 12 (4): 979–1011. Available online at <http://ssrn.com/abstract = 604781> (accessed May 4, 2006).

# Alternative Medicine

Alternative and complementary medicine (CAM) are two different but interrelated approaches to health. Alternative medicine refers to those therapeutic practices, systems, and products that are employed instead of conventional or allopathic "medical" means, while complementary medicine refers to those practices used in conjunction with allopathic ("medical") treatment. "Conventional or allopathic" medicine is practiced by MDs (doctors of medicine) or DOs (doctors of osteopathy) and their allied health professionals. Ayurveda, acupuncture, and homeopathy fall into the category of alternative medicine, as they are based on systems of medicine radically different to the allopathic approach. Yoga and meditation, for example, would be characterized as "complementary" therapies in that many hospitals and medical centers incorporate them into their treatment programs.

According to the National Center for Complementary and Alternative Medicine (NCCAM), diets such as the Atkins, Zone and Ornish diets fall into the category of CAM, though they form only 3.5 percent of the totality of CAM. This is, nevertheless, a reflection on the interconnections between CAM and dieting culture and a demonstration of how various complementary and alternative therapies have been mobilized toward weight loss, their texts and practitioners forming an integral part of the contemporary dieting milieu.

The immensely popular Deepak Chopra (1947–), an allopath by training, is now a widely read proponent of contemporary versions of the Indian Ayurvedic systems of healing in books such as *Perfect Weight: The Complete Mind/Body Program for Achieving and Maintaining Your Perfect Weight* (2004). Chopra draws on what is also referred to as the "holistic health" model, where there is a strong emphasis on the relationship between one's mind, body, and lifestyle practices in general. He advocates diets and yogic exercises based on the type of constitution or "dosha" one has; dosha theory is similar to the Western therapeutic model of "humors" popular before the advent of biomedicine. Chopra recommends other holistic lifestyle changes in conjunction with changes in diet, including: sleeping and waking early, doing deep breathing and other gentle yogic exercises, avoiding alcohol and caffeine and eating freshly prepared food in accordance with one's dosha requirements.

One can also note that there are a number of alternative approaches to weight loss that stress exercise as the central means for weight loss. These approaches are "anti-dieting" in their assumptions and, as with many of the alternative approaches, assume that all allopathic medical interventions are faulty and are in many ways part of a behavioral endorsement of the cultural norms that stress thinness over a "healthy," if larger body. Indeed, such approaches see dieting as harmful, as ineffective, and as rooted in a set of false assumptions, such as the corollary between pathological medical conditions and overweight (Foster 2002).

Such Western appropriations of "Eastern" medicine, whether from India or China or Japan, ignore the fact that the systematization of such approaches was and is in the light of responding to the dominance of allopathic medicine and the marginalization of "traditional forms" of treatment. The importation and refashioning of Ayurvedic medicine from India in the seventeenth century, following Sir Thomas Roe's mission to the Mughal Court, created a powerful association between such "alternative" forms of dieting and mystical vegetarianism, which linked health and ethics.

Ironically, the vegetarianism of Mahatma Gandhi (1869–1948), which is one of the most powerful representations of an authentic "Indian" link between health and morality for alternative medicine has, according to Gandhi, its origins in his reading of Percy Bysshe Shelley's (1792–1822) advocacy of a "bloodless regimen" in 1812 (Stuart 2006). While virtually all of these traditional systems recognized massive weight loss as a pathological sign, most were highly ambivalent about the meanings of weight gain. Thus, approaches such as acupuncture for the treatment of obesity come to represent a merging of CAM and allopathic goals in seeing obesity as clearly defined and inherently dangerous. Only the approaches vary, and the appropriateness of complementary treatments in allopathic medicine illus-

trates how close to Western ideals such approaches actually are.

Other CAM approaches abound as the claim of "placing one's own weight in one's own hands" recognizes the anxiety about weight gain (or loss) as a sign of a weakness of will, as a highly stigmatized form of mental illness. Andrew Weil (1942–), a popular health guru, also trained as an allopathic physician, writes books dedicated to holistic ways of maintaining the perfect body weight. Weil sees alternative approaches as preventative but also advocates the use of allopathic medicine for treatment of pathologies. In 1994, he created the Program in Integrative Medicine in Tucson, Arizona, which focuses on nutrition, "natural" medicine, and "mind–body interventions" (Weil 2004: 4).

Paul Ernsberger and Richard Koletsky from the Case Western Reserve School of Medicine argue that the negative impacts of obesity, "though real, are overstated" (1999: 222). They also posit that many of the negative side effects can be attributed to "weight-cycling"—the tendency of dieters to repeatedly put on and lose weight. Other problems, such as heart disease, may be the result of obesity treatments, such as diet pills, rather than obesity itself. As an alternative, Ernsberger and Koletsky suggest a "wellness approach" to health. According to them, weight loss itself is often not the best way to deal with health issues such as hypertension, type-2 diabetes, hyperlipidemia and sleep apnea because, "although many diseases are more chronic in obese patients, in many cases a direct causal link cannot be made" (1999: 222). Health can best be improved though "lifestyle enhancement [which] can improve health independent of loss of body fat" (1999: 222). There is a gendered dimension to this phenomenon as well. According to a 2002 survey conducted by the National Institute for Health Statistics (NIHS), more women than men make use of CAM (Anon. 2004).

SLG/Shruthi Vissa

See also China in the Early Twentieth Century; Gandhi; Greek Medicine and Dieting; Vegetarianism

## References and Further Reading

Anon. (2004) "The Use of Complementary and Alternative Medicine in the United States," Bethesda, Md.: National Center for Complementary and Alternative Medicine, National Institutes of Health,

U.S. Department of Health and Human Services. GPO item number: 0507. Available online at <http://purl.access.gpo.gov/GPO/LPS58156> (accessed May 7, 2006).

Chopra, Deepak (2004) *Perfect Weight: The Complete Mind/Body Program for Achieving and Maintaining Your Perfect Weight*, New York: Rider & Co.

Ernsberger, Paul and Koletsky, Richard J. (1999) "Biomedical Rationale for a Wellness Approach to Obesity," *Journal of Social Issues* 55 (2): 221–59.

Foster, Gary D. (2002) "Nondieting Approaches," in

Christopher G. Fairburn and Kelly D. Brownell (eds), *Eating Disorders and Obesity: A Comprehensive Handbook*, 2nd edn, New York: Guilford Press, pp. 604–8.

Stuart, Tristram (2006) *The Bloodless Revolution: Radical Vegetarianism and the Discovery of India*, New York: HarperCollins.

Weil, Andrew (2004) *Natural Health, Natural Medicine: The Complete Guide to Wellness and Self-Care for Optimum Health*, New York: Houghton Mifflin Company.

# Anorexia

The medicalization of disorders of eating begins in the seventeenth century. The Christian tradition of self-abnegation meant that fasting became a common form of religious practice in the Middle Ages with spiritual rather than pathological implications (Ove 2002). In the course of the nineteenth century, self-imposed starvation came to be a syndrome clearly delineated by physical signs and symptoms and which was understood to have a psychogenic origin. This idea that food had a special status was uncontested. Some theoreticians saw the manipulation of the middle-class family by their daughters as the place where rebellion could most meaningfully take place (Brumberg 1988). Yet anorexia nervosa, a name coined by William Gull in 1868, was still a rare and therefore clinically fascinating aberration. In the 1920s, the view of Morris Simmonds dominated: Anorexia was the result of a lesion of the pituitary gland. This endocrinological definition of radical thinness fitted well with the redefinition of obesity as the result of metabolic imbalance. It was only after World War II that Hilde Bruch began to speak of the lack of self-esteem and a distorted body image caused by maternal rejection in such patients. By the mid-1970s, "anorexia" had become a household word through her popular writings. During the 1980s, it was "widely publicized, glamorized, and to some extent romanticized" (Gordon 2000: 3). In 1979, the diagnostic category of "bulimia nervosa," binge-eating and purging, was coined by the British psychiatrist Gerald Russell and

was added to the mix of eating disorders, having a similar tangled history (Russell 1997). Certainly, the use of purges and emetics in this context has its origin in ancient medicine and cultural practices concerning excessive eating. By this point, eating disorders such as anorexia and bulimia had become acceptable vehicles for the expression of mental illness in Western, industrialized culture, what George Devereux calls a prescribed template for mental illness: "Don't go crazy, but if you, do it this way" (Devereux 1980).

Today, if one were to play a word-association game, anorexia would be linked to words like: starved, skinny, malnourished, or excessive self-control. While the term "anorexia" technically refers only to low body weight or lack of appetite, anorexia nervosa is a syndrome with both psychological and physical aspects. The latter is a relatively rare illness, as it occurs, even in high-risk groups such as middle-class adolescent girls and young women, in only about 0.05 percent of that population. Considerably more, however, suffer from the broader definition. In contemporary culture, the term "anorexia" is generally used interchangeably with anorexia nervosa. The importance of this is that the frequency (or at least the perceived frequency) of the disorder has increased significantly during the past fifty years (Walsh 2003). The creation of the EAT scale (Eating Attitudes Test) by Garner, Olmstead and Polivy in 1983, provided a scale for evaluating specific (culture-bound) actions from "cutting one's food up into small pieces" to believing that "food controls my life." The score on the EAT seemed to provide documentation for the existence of a specific eating disorder.

In the twenty-first century, it is seen as a "mental disease." The standard American presentation of mental illnesses, the *Diagnostic and Statistical Manual of Mental Disorders* (DSM; American Psychiatric Association 2000) defines anorexia nervosa as:

1. "Refusal to maintain body weight at or above a minimally normal weight for age and height." Specifically, a person with a body weight less than 85 percent of what is expected.
2. "An intense fear of gaining weight or becoming fat, even though underweight."
3. "Disturbance in the way in which one's body weight is experienced, undue influence of body weight or shape on self-evaluation, or denial of the seriousness of the current low body weight."
4. "In post-menarcheal females, amenorrhea, i.e., the absence of at least three consecutive menstrual cycles. A woman is considered to have amenorrhea if her periods occur only following hormone, e.g., estrogen administration."

(American Psychiatric Association 2000: 583–9)

While the DSM requires all four of these for a clinical diagnosis of anorexia nervosa, individuals suffering from only some of these symptoms are still at serious mental and physical risk.

Following the DSM-IV-TR criteria, anorexia nervosa and bulimia can be seen as "addictive behaviors," in analogy to other psychological states such as chemical dependence, compulsive gambling, sex addiction, workaholism, and compulsive buying (Coombs 2004). As such, it is seen to have a multifactorial cause. The environment factors are the sociocultural emphasis on thinness, the association between dieting and self-control and self-discipline, participation in sports emphasizing thinness, sexual or physical abuse, and the need for attention from others. The individual risk factors include genetic vulnerability; depression; obsessive-compulsive traits; a cognitive style preferring order, exactness, precision, and sameness; impulse control problems; low self-esteem; extreme need for approval; perfectionism; early onset of puberty; sexual maturation; restrictive dieting; fear of psychosocial maturity; extreme need for control; harm and risk avoidance; pursuit of an eating-disorder

identity (Garner and Gerborg 2004). While many of these factors are truly suspect as "causal," even in the broadest sense of the word, an addictive model needs to have a set of primary causes, which are amenable to therapeutic interventions. To simply label such addictions as "genetic," following the older model for the medicalization of alcoholism, leaves little space for psychological intervention. The newer model of addiction now does. The treatment of such an addiction to dieting/starvation is "interpersonal therapy," emphasizing the "inner world and dynamics of the patient" (Petrucelli 2004: 312). The irony, of course, is that as obesity is not listed in the DSM-IV-TR, an addiction to food rather than its avoidance is missing in such approaches.

Such a narrow scope constructs the illness in a way that can limit the patients' understanding of their own condition. Anorexia, like other eating disorders, can, and does, vary greatly between individuals. A person may exhibit eating-disordered behavior or emotions without meeting the DSM definition. This has led to questioning of the criteria's absolute nature. Therefore, we must ask where the line should be drawn—and how to go about drawing it—between dieting behavior and anorexia. In light of these difficulties, encapsulating all aspects of eating-disordered behavior into a working definition is problematic.

Anorexia nervosa is often claimed to overlap with clinical depression. It is not clear, however, what is causative: Is the depression the cause of the eating disorder or is it the eating disorder that is the result of the depression, or do they merely share a common cause? Depression is commonly cited as one of the psychological symptoms that can coexist with anorexia. Additionally, the obsession with thinness is a defining aspect of this illness, and it is possible to exhibit eating-disordered behavior without actually being underweight or taking extreme weight-loss measures. Psychiatrist Hilde Bruch, who in the 1970s popularized modern notions of anorexia in her book *Eating Disorders*, states that its core elements are:

A distorted body image, which consists of the virtually delusional misperception of the body as fat;

An inability to identify internal feelings and need states, particularly hunger, but more generally the whole range of emotions; and

An all-pervasive sense of ineffectiveness, a feeling that one's actions, thoughts, and feelings do not actively originate within the self but rather are passive reflections of external expectations and demands.

(Gordon 2000: 18–19)

Bruch has analyzed the emotional side of anorexia via her psychological training. Specifically, she claims that childhood experiences and problems in psychological maturation can foster eating disorders, which often manifest in adolescence. Psychiatrist Richard Gordon reinforces Bruch's limited time scope in his argument about why teenagers are most vulnerable to a "deficient sense of self" (Gordon 2000: 19). Adolescence is the time period where self-autonomy is usually developed. Thus, refusal to become an active agent in this process can result in an identity centered on control of one's environment, specifically eating. While there is certainly a prevalence of anorexia in teenagers, the illness can present itself at any stage of life.

A possible explanation of anorexia offered in our age that desires to reduce mental illness to physiological causes is that it is caused by serotonin imbalance in the brain. Here, the notion of the common cause of depression and eating disorders is located in brain chemistry. This theory implies that anorexia can be remedied through pharmacological means, specifically selective serotonin reuptake inhibitors (SSRIs) (Hoek et al. 1998). If a lack of serotonin has a causal effect on the existence of anorexia, then the increase in serotonin should eliminate all side effects, including the eating disorder. Another school of thought is more multifaceted than this cause-and-effect relationship. Patient advocates, such as Mary Ann Marrazzi, believe that those suffering from anorexia are "predisposed to an addiction cycle that is set into motion by chronic dieting [. . . whereupon] the brain releases opioids, known to cause a 'high' " (Psychology Today Staff 1995). They claim that although such an addiction can be offset by SSRIs, psychological therapy is a crucial phase of the treatment of anorexia.

Yet another view sees a person suffering from anorexia as having an obsessive need to be thin stemming from the need for control (Kalodner 2000: 12–13). Eating often can seem to be more easily controlled than many other aspects of a person's life. Food and body become obsessions that permeate every facet of a person's life, sometimes even intruding into dreams. Karen Way's book *Anorexia Nervosa and Recovery*, explains,

thinness is the obsession and losing weight is the fix. When you're anorexic, watching the numbers

go down on the scale is the only thing in the world that matters to you. It's the center of your life, the only meaning to your existence. Pursuing it takes all your time, and energy.

(Way 1996: 21)

The excessive need to shed pounds at an ever-increasing rate is the result of a desire to a gain control over life. Ironically, this obsession with weight loss becomes life and spirals out of control.

It is further noted in the DSM-IV-TR that a dieting culture is where "being considered attractive is linked with being thin" (American Psychiatric Association 2000: 587). In these circumstances, "weight loss is viewed as an impressive achievement and a sign of extraordinary self-discipline, whereas weight gain is perceived as an unacceptable failure of self-control" (American Psychiatric Association 2000: 584). This seems simply a misplaced extension of the underlying claims of twentieth-century (Western, industrialized) diet culture: that thin is beautiful, that thin is good. If some self-control, even in starvation, is a sign of control, total self-control must be better.

Interestingly, a group known as "pro-ana" (pro-anorexia) resonates with this tenet of the illness in their belief system. This small faction of people believes that excessive thinness is a "lifestyle choice" (Shafran 2002; Ana's Underground Grotto 2005). In short, one who lives a pro-ana lifestyle is someone who has purposely chosen to adopt permanently an extremely limited, low-calorie diet. Pro-ana followers commonly feel that thinness should take precedence above all else and will voluntarily make sacrifices to that end.

Cultural pressures foster both dieting and anorexia. Contrary to popular opinion, anorexia is not *only* a disease that affects the very young, the very rich, the very white. It is true, however, that anorexia is more common among cultures that value thinness as beautiful (Kalodner 2000: 55). One can add that it appears in those subcultures that acquire such ideals in their integration into a majority view of the body. Thus, the shift in body image and the sudden appearance of anorexia in the African American community at the end of the twentieth century follows African American women entering more and more into the mainstream image of what an appropriate body must be. In 1960, Hilde Bruch found a "conspicuous absence of Negro patients" (Bruch 1966). By the mid-1990s, the rates had begun to approach the numbers in white middle-class (Pumariega et al. 1994). Anorexia does not discriminate, and many groups within modern Western culture are affected by it. Indeed, some groups, such as Jews and Italians in America, living in traditions where food is a major ethnic marker, seem to actually have higher rates of the syndrome (Rowland 1970). The attraction of thinness as a body type has not been prevalent throughout history. Throughout the twentieth century, an ideal of thinness has been constantly evolving throughout the West (Gordon 2000: 135). The incidence of anorexia in non-Western cultures has increased in recent years. As globalization has caused popular culture to infiltrate non-Western cultures, thinness as a necessity of beauty is further popularized, and the attractiveness of anorexia as a "prescribed template for mental illness" also is available. The question of whether there are cultural "pathofacilitative effects" that underlie the appearance of eating disorders has been the subject of studies in India and China. In India at least, while the EAT (Eating Attitudes Test) labeled "cutting one's food into small pieces" as pathological behavior, it was clear that this was understood as appropriate etiquette among those questioned and was in no way a sign of pathology. Likewise, the category of "food controlling one's life" was read in terms of Hindu religious fasting practices, rather than individual anxiety about dieting and body appearance (Tseng 2003: 183–9).

In addition to cultural biases, anorexia has been gender biased as well. While the prevalence among men is much lower than women, it is still evident amongst a faction of the male population. Anorexia and other eating disorders in men have often been neglected by society as well as clinical researchers. Arnold Anderson explains that, "Males with eating disorders may have sought professional help so infrequently that they have become a statistical rarity" (Anderson 1999: 73). Moreover, typical symptoms of anorexia that are present in females are usually correctly identified, whilst the same indicators in males are overlooked. This is due, in part, to the sociocultural beliefs held in the Western world about men and the assumption that extreme thinness is only a feminine desire. Similarly, dieting culture sidelines men, while it focuses primarily on women.

Thus, men imagine themselves thin, while women imagine themselves fat. By interviewing a selected group of undergraduates at comparable American and Australian universities, Marika Tiggemann and Esther Rothblum tested the "social consequences of perceived weight" (Tiggemann and Rothblum 1988: 76). When asked about their ideal weight, the women on average wanted to be 9 pounds thinner, while the men wanted to be 1 pound heavier. While only 20 percent of the participants actually were overweight, 50 percent felt themselves to be so, and women comprised the majority of this percentage. The second part of the project examined to what extent stereotypes about the obese are prevalent in Western society. On average, fat men and women were perceived by all participants as being warm, friendly, lazy, less self-confident and not as attractive as their thinner counterparts. The authors concluded that women have "higher public body consciousness" (Tiggemann and Rothblum 1988: 85) than men and that stereotyping persists, leading possibly to social adjustment problems.

Anorexia is often viewed as a diet gone too far, resulting in virtual starvation. The boundary between anorexia and dieting is hazy. Dieting is comparable to anorexia in the strict sense that it is, by nature, a controlling act. When one is dieting, food is being restricted in a variety of different ways, and, if followed, the diet is controlling a facet of life. While dieting does play a large part in life, there is a difference between dieting and an irrational obsession with food. A nonobsessive average dieter's personality and lifestyle are not affected by their dieting regimen. However, someone with anorexia undergoes a radical change in lifestyle. This is due to the controlling nature of the illness. For instance, people with anorexia often plan out their meals when they wake up for the day and cannot waver at all from this schedule. By contrast, an average dieter's daily routine does not solely revolve around food.

Another important difference between anorexia and dieting is that most people with anorexia must receive treatment in order to recover. Eating disorders are seen today as psychological problems that often require the intervention of mental-health professionals and physicians. In general, a combination of treatments—such as individual psychotherapy, group therapy, family therapy, medication, nutritional counseling, support groups, self-help groups, and classes—may be used (Ellis-Ordway 1999: 189). Treatment of the problem has to start with addressing the underlying emotional and mental states. Physicians provide instructions that are necessary to remedy physical consequences.

SLG/LAURA GOLDSTEIN AND JESSICA RISSMAN

*See also* Aboulia; Binge-Eating; Bruch; China Today; Globalization; Gull; Marcé; Morton

## References and Further Reading

American Psychiatric Association (2000) "Eating Disorders: Anorexia Nervosa," in *Diagnostic and Statistical Manual of Mental Disorders*, 4th edn, Text Revision IV-R, Washington, DC: American Psychiatric Association, pp. 583–9.

Ana's Underground Grotto (2005). Available online at <http://www.plagueangel.org/grotto/id1.html> (accessed April 17, 2006).

Anderson, Arnold E. (1999) "Eating Disorders in Males: Critical Questions," in Raymond Lemberg (ed.), *Eating Disorders: A Reference Sourcebook*, Phoenix, Ariz.: Oryx Press, pp. 189–92.

Bruch, Hilde (1966) "Anorexia Nervosa and Its Differential Diagnosis," *Journal of Nervous and Mental Diseases* 141: 555–66.

Brumberg, Joan (1988) *Fasting Girls: The History of Anorexia Nervosa*, Cambridge, Mass.: Harvard University Press.

Coombs, Robert Holman (ed.) (2004) *Handbook of Addictive Disorders*, New York: John Wiley.

Devereux, George (1980) "Normal and Abnormal," in his *Basic Problems of Ethnopsychiatry*, trans. Basia Miller Gulati and George Devereux, Chicago, Ill.: University of Chicago Press, pp. 3–71.

Ellis-Ordway, Nancy (1999) "How To Find Treatment for an Eating Disorder," in Raymond Lemberg (ed.), *Eating Disorders: A Reference Sourcebook*, Phoenix, Ariz.: Oryx Press, pp. 189–92.

Garner, David M. and Gerborg, Anna (2004) "Understanding and Diagnosing Eating Disorders," in Robert Holman Coombs (ed.) *Handbook of Addictive Disorders*, New York: John Wiley, pp. 275–311.

Garner, David M., Olmstead, M.P., and Polivy, J. (1983) "Development and Validation of a Multidimensional Eating Disorder Inventory for Anorexia Nervosa and Bulimia," *International Journal of Eating Disorders* 2: 15–34.

Gordon, Richard A. (2000) *Eating Disorders: Anatomy of a Social Epidemic*, Oxford: Blackwell Publishers.

Heywood, Leslie (1996) *Dedication to Hunger: The Anorexic Aesthetic in Modern Culture*, Berkeley, Calif.: University of California Press.

Hoek, H.W., Treasure, J.L., and Katzman, M.A. (eds) (1998) *Neurobiology in the Treatment of Eating Disorders*, New York: John Wiley & Sons.

Hsu, George L.K. (1990) *Eating Disorders*, New York: The Guilford Press.

Kalodner, Cynthia R. (2000) *Too Fat or Too Thin?* Westport, Conn.: Greenwood Press.

Ove, Marcia K. (2002) "The Evolution of Self-Starvation Behaviors into the Present-Day Diagnosis of Anorexia Nervosa: A Critical Literature Review," Dissertation, California School of Professional Psychology.

Petrucelli, Jean (2004) "Treating Eating Disorders," in Robert Holman Coombs (ed.) *Handbook of Addictive Disorders*, New York: John Wiley, pp. 312–52.

Psychology Today Staff (1995) "Treating Anorexia Like Addiction," *Psychology Today*. March/April. Available online at <http://www.psychologytoday.com/ articles/ pto-19950301-000008.html> (accessed April 30, 2004).

Pumariega, A., Gustavson, C.R., Gustavson, J.C., Stone Motes, P. and Ayers, S. (1994) "Eating Attitudes in African-American Women: The *Essence* Eating Disorders Survey," *Eating Disorders* 2 (1): 5–16.

Rowland, C.V. (1970) "Anorexia and Obesity," *International Psychiatry Clinics* 7 (1): 37–137.

Russell, Gerald F.M. (1997) "The History of Bulimia Nervosa," in David M. Garner and Paul E. Garfinkel (eds), *Handbook of Treatment for Eating Disorders*, New York: Guilford Press, pp. 11–24.

Russell, Sherman Apt (2005) *Hunger: An Unnatural History*, New York: Basic Books.

Shafran, Roz (2002) "Eating Disorders and the Internet," in Christopher G. Fairburn and Kelly D. Brownell (eds), *Eating Disorders and Obesity: A Comprehensive Handbook*, 2nd edn, New York: Guilford Press, pp. 362–6.

Tiggemann, Marika and Esther Rothblum (1988) "Gender Differences in Social Consequences of Perceived Overweight in the United States and Australia," *Sex Roles* 18 (1/2): 75–86.

Tseng, Wen-Shing (2003) *Clinician's Guide to Cultural Psychiatry*, Amsterdam: Academic Press.

Walsh, B. Timothy (2003) "Eating Disorders," in Allan Tasman, Jerald Kay, and Jeffrey A. Lieberman (eds), *Psychiatry*, 2nd edn, New York: John Wiley, Vol. II, pp. 1501–18.

Way, Karen (1996) *Anorexia Nervosa and Recovery: A Hunger for Meaning*, Binghamton, NY: Haworth Press.

# Atkins, Robert, MD (1930–2003)

## American doctor and cardiologist, best known for his unconventional and controversial Atkins Nutritional Approach diet

Atkins first proposed his high-protein, high-fat, low-carbohydrate diet in 1972 in his book, *Dr. Atkin's Diet Revolution: The High Calorie Way to Stay Thin Forever*. This radical approach in the 1970s told dieters they could eat as much red meat, eggs, cheese, and other high-fat foods as they desired but not eat pasta, cereal, bread or other carbohydrates. The diet was relatively popular as a fad diet, but "low-carb" would not become a buzz word for several decades. Even though it was originally designed as a diet to maintain blood-sugar levels for diabetics, it became a popular weight-loss strategy that started the "low-carb" movement.

Over the next twenty years, Atkins founded the Atkins Center for Complementary Medicine and continued to write new books. However, it was the revised versions of his original book that he published in 1992 and 1999, respectively, that brought the diet guru back into the public eye (*Dr. Atkins' New Diet Revolution, Dr. Atkins' New Diet Revolution: Revised and Updated*). Atkins faced intense criticism about the updated books, with many health organizations, doctors, and dieticians attacking the lack of balance prescribed in his diet. Major critics included the American Medical Association, the American Dietetic Association, and the American Heart Association. Despite these various denunciations of the diet, the book was wildly popular: its various versions spent five years on the *New York Times*'s bestseller list and earned a place among the top fifty bestselling books in history (Womble and Wadden 2002).

Even in the face of such controversy and criticism, according to the *British Medical Journal*'s obituary of Atkins, the various editions of his *New Diet Revolution* book sold 12 million copies, making it the bestselling fad-diet book ever written. In addition to the success of his books, Atkins saw more than 600,000 patients since receiving his medical degree in 1955; he also had his own syndicated radio program, *Your Health Choices*, and his own monthly newsletter, *Dr. Atkins' New Diet Revolution*.

Atkins' death in 2003, attributed to a heart attack, was used by many critics of his diet as evidence of the danger of high-fat, high-protein diets. While there has been much controversy over the true cause of his death, as well as the report that Atkins weighed 258 pounds at his death, no consensus has been reached about the effects of his diet on his own health.

SLG/SARAH GARDINER

*See also* Banting; Sugar Busters; Zone Diet

## References and Further Reading

McConnell, Tandy (ed.) (2001) "Robert C. Atkins," *American Decades 1990–1999*, Detroit, Mich.: Manly.

Anon. (2000) "Robert C. Atkins," *Biography resource center online*. Detroit: Gale Group. Available online at <http://www.galenet.com.proxy.library.emory.edu/servlet/BioRC?vrsn=149&OP=contains&locID=emory&srchtp=name&ca=5&c=3&AI=U13424901&NA=atkins+robert&ste=12&tbst=prp&tab=1&docNum=K1650000877&bConts=47> (accessed June 23, 2007)

Anon. (2003) "Robert Coleman Atkins: Obituary," *British Medical Journal* 326 (5): 1090.

Anon. (2004) "The Diet Fad of the 21st Century." Available online at <http://www.atkinsexposed.org/atkins/11/The_Diet_Fad_of_the_21st_Century.htm> (accessed March 12, 2007).

Womble, Leslie G. and Wadden, Thomas (2002) "Commercial and Self-Help Weight Loss Programs," in Christopher G. Fairburn and Kelly D. Brownell (eds), *Eating Disorders and Obesity: A Comprehensive Handbook*, 2nd edn, New York: Guilford Press, pp. 546–50.

# Atlas, Charles (1893–1972)

Born Angelo Siciliano in Calabria, Italy, Atlas came to the U.S.A. in 1903 and was raised by his mother in Brooklyn, New York. According to Atlas's own promotional literature, as a teenager he was a "98 pound weakling," who was the favorite pick of many bullies in the neighborhood ("98 pound" may well be a free adaptation of the British "7 stone [= 98 pound] weakling"). Those who towered over him more and more often bullied the young Atlas. He repeatedly swore that he would build muscles. One day, he toured the Brooklyn Museum and carefully studied the muscular bodies of Roman and Greek gods. He claims that he learned thereafter how they attained their strength through exercise.

Even as he used the statues of the gods for inspiration and began to lift weights, Atlas still did not build the muscle he desired. On a trip to the Prospect Park Zoo, Atlas came across a rather large lion and stopped in awe to admire the lion's behavior. Atlas rationalized that lions' strength was achieved in a more natural way. From that point on, Atlas began to use a system of isotonic exercise, which worked one muscle against a fixed point rather than trying to exercise the entire body at once. The use of barbells and Indian clubs had been a feature of late-nineteenth- and early twentieth-century bodybuilding courses, such as those sold to eager young men through the mail by the first, modern bodybuilder Eugene Sandow (1867–1925). This worked not only to transform his body but his life as well. Within a year he perfected his system and, supposedly, doubled his body weight. Actually, a similar system had been earlier developed by strong man Alois P. Swoboda (1873–1938), whose widely sold "Conscious Evolution" course featured isotonic exercise.

By age nineteen, Atlas earned a living by demonstrating a chest developer in a storefront on Broadway. It was there that his peers began calling him "Atlas," because of his growing resemblance to a statue of the mythical Titan holding up the world. He legally took the name Charles Atlas in 1922. His physique became widely recognized by many artists, and they modeled many statues after him, including Alexander Stirling Calder's 1916 sculpture of George Washington in Peacetime in Washington Square Park (New York). In 1921, he won 1,000 dollars as the winner of Bernarr Macfadden's contest for the "World's Most Perfectly Developed Man."

In late 1922, Atlas used his prize money to start a mail-order bodybuilding business to market his exercise methods. Atlas himself was a poor businessman and unable to turn his company into a success. However, after he hired Charles P. Roman, a young advertising director, and eventually sold the business to him in 1928, the company began to prosper. Illustrated advertisements about the "98 pound weakling" getting sand tossed in his face on the beach became ubiquitous from comic books to men's magazines. Indeed, the power of this approach allowed the company to survive and, indeed, flourish during the Great Depression. After his death in 1972, Charles Atlas Ltd, continued to sell Atlas's original "Dynamic Tension" program, a term Roman coined, and eventually expanded onto the Internet.

SLG/LAURA K. GOLDSTEIN

*See also* Bodybuilding; Macfadden

## References and Further Reading

Anon. (1994) "Charles S. Atlas," *Dictionary of American Biography*, New York: Charles Scribner's Sons. Supplement 9, pp. 1971–5.

Anon. (2001) "Charles Atlas," *Encyclopedia of World Biography*, supplement. Detroit: Gale Group. Vol. 21. Available online at <http://www.galenet.com.proxy.library.emory.edu/servlet/BioRC?vrsn=149&OP=contains&locID=emory&srchtp=name&ca=1&AI=U13638419&NA=atlas+charles&ste=4&tbst=prp&n=10> (accessed June 23, 2007).

Pendergast, Tom, and Pendergast, Sara (eds) (2000) "Charles Atlas," *St. James Encyclopedia of Popular Culture*, 5 vols, Detroit, Mich.: St. James Press.

# Atwater, Wilbur Olin (1844–1907)

## American agricultural chemist whose studies on respiration and metabolism contributed greatly to the science of human nutrition and exercise

After receiving his Ph.D. from Yale in 1869 studying the chemical composition of corn, Atwater studied with German chemists and physiologists such as Nathan Zuntz (1847–1920), who developed the first portable apparatus to measure metabolism, Carl von Voit (1831–1908), who established the study of the physiology of metabolism in mammals, and his student, Max Rubner (1854–1932) who proved that the energy released by food was the same if digested or burned. When he returned to the U.S.A., he directed extensive studies on food analysis, dietary evaluations, energy requirements for work, digestibility of foods, and the economics of food production. He was Professor of Chemistry at Wesleyan College in Connecticut and established the first agricultural experimental station in the U.S.A. at Wesleyan in 1875. Atwater went on to become first the director of the Office of Experiment Stations for the U.S. Department of Agriculture in 1888 (to 1891), and later the Chief of Nutrition Investigations (1894–1903).

Atwater collaborated with Edward Bennett Rosa to develop a respiration calorimeter, which very accurately measured the practical energy values of various foods. This allowed them to create calorie-conversion tables that are still widely used today.

SLG/Sarah Gardiner

*See also* Metabolism

## References and Further Reading

Anon. (1928) "Wilbur Olin Atwater," *Dictionary of American Biography* Base Set. American Council of Learned Societies, 1928–36. Available online at <http://www.galenet.com/servlet/BioRC?locID=emory&srchtp=person&AI=1150850&c=1&DO=is&BA=a.d.&docNum=BT2310018566&bConts=35&vrsn=149&OP=contains&BO=is&ca=1&ste=12&NA=wilbur+atwater&tab=1&tbst=prp&n=10&DA=AD> (accessed April 18, 2006).

Anon. (2001) "Biography of Wilbur Olin Atwater," *GeneaBios: Biographies for Genealogy*. Available online at <http://www.geneabios.com/wesleyan/atwater.htm> (accessed April 18, 2006).

Anon. (2005) "Atwater, Wilber Olin," *The Columbia Electronic Encyclopedia*, New York: Columbia University Press. Available online at <http://columbia.thefreedictionary.com/Atwater,+Wilbur+Olin> (accessed April 18, 2006).

Katch, Frank L. (1999) "Wilbur Olin Atwater," *Sports Science History Makers*. Available online at <http://sportsci.org/news/history/atwater/atwater.html> (accessed April 18, 2006).

# B

## Banting, William (1796–1878)

### English undertaker, best known as the "Father of the Low-Carbohydrate Diet"

Banting, who was 5 foot 5 inches, first became overweight in his thirties, and by the age of sixty-five weighed over 200 pounds, despite great efforts to lose and keep off excess weight. At this point, Banting consulted Dr. William Harvey, an ear, nose, and throat specialist, for his hearing loss. The doctor believed his obesity to be the cause of his increasing deafness, and Harvey put him on an experimental low-carbohydrate diet. The diet resulted in him losing 46 pounds over the next year and a great increase in his overall health, including the restoration of his hearing.

Banting's "Letter on Corpulence Addressed to the Public" was an account of how a successful, middle-class undertaker and coffinmaker (he had actually supplied the coffin for the Duke of Wellington) overcame his fat (Huff 2001). He was not fat because of inaction or lassitude:

> Few men have led a more active life—bodily or mentally—from a constitutional anxiety for regularity, precision, and order, during fifty years' business career . . . so that my corpulence and subsequent obesity was not through neglect of necessary bodily activity, nor from excessive eating, drinking, or self-indulgence of any kind.
>
> (Banting 1864: 10–11)

And yet, at the age of sixty-six, he stood at about 5 feet 5 inches tall and weighed 202 pounds. He sensed that he had stopped being corpulent and had become obese. A "corpulent man eats, drinks, and sleeps well, has not pain to complain of, and no particular organic disease"

(Banting 1864: 13). But obesity was now a source of illness. He developed "obnoxious boils" (Banting 1864: 15), failing sight and hearing, and a "slight umbilical rupture" (1864: 16). He could neither stoop to tie his shoes "nor attend to the little offices humanity requires without considerable pain and difficulty." Indeed, he was "compelled to go down stairs slowly backward" (Banting 1864: 14). All of these pathologies were seen by Banting (and his physicians agreed) as the direct result of his obesity rather than his aging. In the appendix to the second edition, still distributed for free, Banting states that,

> I am told by all who know me that my personal appearance is greatly improved, and that I seem to bear the stamp of good health; this may be a matter of opinion or a friendly remark, but I can honestly assert that I feel restored in health, "bodily and mentally," appear to have more muscular power and vigour, eat and drink with a good appetite, and sleep well.
>
> (Banting 1863: 28)

Health is beauty.

Most galling for Banting, however, was the social stigma:

> no man labouring under obesity can be quite insensible to the sneers and remarks of the cruel and injudicious in public assemblies, public vehicles, or the ordinary street traffic. . . . He naturally keeps away as much as possible from places where he is

likely to be made the object of the taunts and remarks of others.

(Banting 1864: 14)

Underlying Banting's desire to lose weight is the fact that he was seen as a fat man and his body was perceived as useless and parasitic. One of his critics saw this as the core of Banting's personal dilemma. It was not fat but a "morbid horror of corpulence" and an "extreme dislike to be twitted on the subject of paunchiness" that is at the core of Banting's anxiety about his body (Aytoun 1864: 609). But he was certainly not alone. Brillat-Savarin tells the story of Edward of New York, who was

a minimum of eight feet in circumference. . . . Such an amazing figure could not help but be stared at, but as soon as he felt himself watched by the passersby Edward did not wait long to send them packing, by saying to them in a sepulchral voice: WHAT HAVE YOU TO STARE LIKE WILD CATS? . . . GO YOU WAY YOU LAZY BODY . . . BE GONE YOU FOR NOTHING DOGS . . . and other similarly charming phrases.

(Brillat-Savarin 1999: 245)

Stigma, as much as physical disability, accounted for Banting's sense of his own illness.

Having been unable to achieve weight loss through the intervention of physicians, Banting was desperate. One physician urged him to exercise, and he rowed daily, which gave him only a great appetite. One physician told him that weight gain was a natural result of aging and that he had gained a pound for every year since he had attained manhood (Banting 1864: 13). Indeed, the medical literature of the mid-nineteenth century had come to consider obesity a problem of medical therapy; it condemned self-help: "Domestic medicine is fraught with innumerable evils—it is false economy to practice physic upon yourselves, when a little judicious guidance would obviate all difficulties" (Banting 1864: 20). He took the waters at Leamington, Cheltenham and Harrogate; he took Turkish baths at a rate of up to three a week for a year but lost only 6 pounds in all that time and had less and less energy. Nothing helped.

Failing a treatment for his weakened hearing, he turned to William Harvey, an ear, nose, and throat specialist and a fellow of the Royal College of Surgeons in August 1862. Harvey had heard Claude Bernard lecture

in Paris on the role that the liver had in diabetes (Harvey 1872: 69). Bernard believed that in addition to secreting bile, the liver also secreted something that aided in the metabolism of sugars. Harvey began to examine the role that the various types of foods, specifically starches and sugars, had in the diseases such as diabetes. He urged Banting to reduce the amount of these in his diet, arguing "that certain articles of ordinary diet, however beneficial in youth, are prejudicial in advanced life, like beans to a horse, whose common food is hay and corn" (Banting 1864: 17). The aging body could not use the common diet and needed much less sugar and starch.

Banting's body finally began to shed its excess weight. He lost 35 pounds, could walk down stairs "naturally," take ordinary exercise, and could "perform every necessary office for himself," his rupture was better, and he could hear and see (Banting 1864: 22–3). But, equally important, his "dietary table was far superior to the former—more luxurious and liberal, independent of its blessed effect" (Banting 1864: 21). He remained at a normal weight until his death in London in 1878 at the age of eighty-one. Not quite 100, but not bad either.

Banting's pamphlet became a bestseller and started a serious, scientific concern as to the meaning of obesity. It was actually one of a number of such pamphlets of the day. One, by A.W. Moore in 1857, cited Cornaro as the prime case of one who was able to lose weight and become healthy (Moore 1857: 12–13). Watson Bradshaw, a physician who had written on dyspepsia before Banting's pamphlet appeared, countered it in 1864 with his own work on obesity warning against "rash experiment upon themselves in furtherance of that object" (Bradshaw 1864: iii). For Watson Bradshaw, the ideal of the fat body in cultures such as China and Turkey, where the "ultima thule of human beauty is to possess a face with a triple chin, and a huge abdomen" had become impossible in the West. It was impossible because the "assimilative function has changed its character—the absorbents have varied their duties—fat forsakes the lower extremities and other parts of the body; and persists in concentrating itself in the abdomen, giving rise to what is called 'Corpulence'" (Bradshaw 1864: 6). Corpulence is a condition of the modern, Western age, and, concentrated as it is in the gut, a quality of men. It is clear that this is a pathological state for Bradshaw, but it is only the extreme cases that he sees as diseased. In a pamphlet of 1865, "A London Physician" wrote about "How to Get Fat or the Means of Preserving the Medium between Leanness and

Obesity." He begins by saying that the one question that everyone asks is "Have you read Banting?" and this has "invaded all classes, and doubtless, will descend to posterity" ("A London Physician" 1865: 7). "Corpulence is a parasite, that the parasite is a disease, and the close ally of a disease, and the said parasite has been exposed and his very existence threatened" by writers such as Banting and William Harvey. This pamphlet then turned to the emaciated body, which is seen as equally at risk and in need of diet and reform.

But it was Banting's text that became most popular because it was sold as autobiographical. People spoke of "banting" when they tried to shed weight. Even today, the term in Swedish to diet is "bantning." The obese patient was the subject of reform, and for a rather long time, the patient was seen as a European one. Banting's mentor, William Harvey, turned to this topic in 1872, spurred on, he wrote, by Banting's success. Harvey stressed that the new scientific advances in "physiology and animal chemistry" (1872: vi) have meant that one could treat obesity as a disease. Banting began his pamphlet with the argument that obesity was a "parasite affecting humanity" (Harvey 1872: 7). Suddenly, sufferer and physician saw it alone as the product of forces beyond the will. But Harvey agreed with Banting that until this stage of pathology is reached, "persons rarely become objects of attention; many have even congratulated themselves on their comely appearance, not seeking advice or a remedy for that which they did not consider an evil" (Harvey 1872: ix). One of Banting's severest contemporary critics, William E. Aytoun, observed that:

We are acquainted with many estimable persons of both sexes, turning considerably more than fifteen stone in the scales—a heavier weight than Mr. Banting ever attained—whose health is unexceptionable, and who would laugh to scorn the idea of applying to a doctor for recipe or regimen which might have the effect of marring their developed comeliness.

(Aytoun 1864: 609)

Is fat a definitive sign of disease? Even Daniel Lambert was seen as healthy until his death.

Banting and Harvey redefined obesity as a physiological disease rather than as a fashion or a moral failing.

Yet Harvey could not make a sufficient leap between his knowledge and the actual mechanism by which "respiratory foods" (carbohydrates) caused obesity and then other ailments. It was Felix Niemeyer from Stuttgart who later argued that it was the ingestion of more or less pure protein that would reduce the toxic effects of sugars and starches (Harvey 1872: 129–48). All believed that the body was a collection of chemical processes. Questions of will and its attendant diseases are eliminated.

SLG

*See also* Atkins; Brillat-Savarin; Cornaro; Lambert; Sugar Busters; Zone Diet

## References and Further Reading

"A London Physician" (1865) *How to Get Fat or the Means of Preserving the Medium Between Leanness and Obesity*, London: John Smith.

Aytoun, William E. (1864) "Banting on Corpulence," *Blackwood's Edinburgh Magazine* 96 (November): 607–17.

Banting, William (1863) *Letter on Corpulence, Addressed to the Public*, London: Harrison.

—— (1864) *Letter on Corpulence, Addressed to the Public*, 3rd edn, London: Harrison.

Bradshaw, Watson (1864) *On Corpulence*, London: Philip & Son.

Brillat-Savarin, Jean-Anthelme (1999) *The Physiology of Taste or, Meditations on Transcendental Gastronomy*, trans. M.F.K. Fisher, Washington, DC: Counterpoint.

Harvey, William (1872) *On Corpulence in Relation to Disease: with Some Remarks on Diet*, London: Henry Renshaw.

Huff, Joyce L. (2001) "A 'Horror of Corpulence': Interrogating Bantingism and Mid-Nineteenth-Century Fat-Phobia," in Jana Evans Braziel and Kathleen LeBesco (eds), *Bodies Out of Bounds: Fatness and Transgression*, Berkeley, Calif.: University of California Press, pp. 39–59.

Moore, A.W. (1857) *Corpulency, i.e., Fat, or Emponpoint, in Excess*, London: For the Author by Frederick William Ruston.

Weir Mitchell, S. (1877) *Fat and Blood and How to Make Them*, Philadelphia, Pa.: Lippincott.

# Bariatric Surgery

Bariatric surgery is the practice of bypassing parts of the digestive tract to allow a morbidly obese patient (BMI > 40) to lose weight either through consuming less food or through malabsorption. Malabsorption refers to food passing directly through the digestive tract without the nutrients being absorbed by the body. This practice is only recommended for patients for whom other weight-loss options, including medical diets, have failed, and if the patient has a serious condition assumed to be caused by the weight, such as diabetes or sleep apnea. They are usually at least 100 pounds overweight. These patients must have failed earlier psychological attempts at changing behavior, such as Weight Watchers or Jenny Craig. There can be no uncorrected metabolic diseases that may be responsible for the obesity, such as low thyroid function. Most importantly, the patients are screened (and most eliminated) for any psychological imbalance or unrealistic expectations of surgery and of weight loss.

The first surgeries, jejunoileal bypasses, were performed in the 1950s at the University of Minnesota, in order to cause malabsorption by bypassing most of the intestines and result in weight loss. This uncontrolled malabsorption almost always led to severe negative consequences, and the procedure is no longer considered safe. Drs. Edward Mason and Chikashi Ito developed the gastric bypass in the late 1960s at the University of Iowa.

In the late 1970s, Dr. Ward Griffin refined the gastric bypass into its currently most popular form, the Roux-En-Y (RYGBP). The RYGBP surgically bypasses most of the stomach and a small amount of the small intestine. Theoretically, patients with reduced stomach size feel full more quickly, rather than losing weight due to intentional malabsorption. This procedure is widely agreed to be fairly safe as the mortality risk is less than 0.5 percent. There is still considerable controversy over the procedure because it can have severe complications. If patients do not follow the correct diet, they can easily reverse the effectiveness of the surgeries that reduce the volume of the stomach or rupture the staples, and malabsorption can lead to severe diarrhea, bloating, cramping, and various diseases caused by vitamin deficiency.

Bariatric surgery can now be done using the minimally invasive laparoscopic technique (which depends on long tiny cameras and instruments inserted through tubes called trocars), rather than the traditional open approach. More controversial procedures include the biliopancreatic diversion and duodenal switch, which both cause controlled malabsorption. The adjustable gastric band (lap-band), which controls the volume of the stomach by physically encircling it, is currently being developed. Bariatric surgery leads to long-term lifestyle changes (patients have to eat less and may be able to consume fewer sweets, for example), and frequently requires either surgical revision of the original procedure because the stomach stretches or cosmetic surgery to remove excess skin.

In a complex way, this surgery is a type of placebo or behavior modification through the radical procedure of surgery. Such procedures are well known in the history of aesthetic surgery. Thus, when this patient population was given the standard Minnesota Multiphasic Personality Inventory (MMPI) before and after surgery, they showed marked psychological improvement even if they did not show significant weight loss. There was a clear distinction between the psychological profile of obese men and women independent of the procedure. This is a strong indicator that obese men and obese women responded differently to their obesity and to the surgery. In general, there was a change in self-assessment concerning their physical appearance and reports that the patients experienced an improvement in current relationships and sexual functioning. And yet, while there was little change in eating habits, there was some minor behavioral change subsequent to weight loss.

SLG/Kathy Mancuso

*See also* Craig; Hormones used in Dieting; Metabolism; Nidetch

## References and Further Reading

American Society for Bariatric Surgery (2006) "Story of Surgery for Obesity." Available online at <http://www.asbs.org/patients/story.html> (accessed January 30, 2006).

Pories, Walter and Beshay, Joseph E. (2002) "Surgery for Obesity: Procedures and Weight Loss," in Christopher G. Fairburn and Kelly D. Brownell (eds), *Eating Disorders and Obesity: A Comprehensive Handbook*, 2nd edn, New York: Guilford Press, pp. 562–7.

Pories, Walter and Beshay, Joseph E., Togerson, Jarl, and Sjöström, Lars (2002), "Surgery for Obesity: Psychosocial and Medical Outcomes," in Christopher G. Fairburn and Kelly D. Brownell (eds), *Eating Disorders and Obesity: A Comprehensive Handbook*, 2nd edn, New York: Guilford Press, pp. 658–72.

Zingmond, David S., McGory, Marcia L., Ko, and Clifford Y. (2005) "Hospitalization Before and After Gastric Bypass Surgery," *Journal of the American Medical Association* (special issue), 294: 1918–24.

# Barr, Roseanne (1952–)

## Comedian and star of the hit television series *Roseanne* (1988–97)

Roseanne's years in the limelight have been rife with controversy over her life and work. She is a woman of size who has been hated for her weight, celebrated for her success "in spite of it," claimed as a role model for fat women, and criticized for her eventual decision to have bariatric surgery. She is a tough, gritty actress who appears not to care what the critics think. She is known for being unpredictable, performing such acts as "grabbing her crotch and spitting" after an off-key rendition of the "Star Spangled Banner" at a 1990 San Diego Padres game. Behaviors such as these combined with her weight, fueled media mockery of her femininity.

The show, and much of Roseanne's comedy, is about working-class culture. In part because of her weight, "Roseanne's body . . . can perhaps be read as an expression of gender-specific class culture" (Bettie 1995: 138). In the show, Roseanne plays a hard-working, no-nonsense mother, who bounces from job to job in an effort to make enough money to pay the bills. She is quite the opposite of the "domestic goddess" image common to many other sit-com mothers. Her husband, played by John Goodman, is also an overweight/obese man who passes in and out of various blue-collar jobs. All three of the children are thin, reinforcing the contemporary image in the 1990s of working-class families.

Despite being considered by some as a fat-positive icon, Roseanne has been fairly public about her struggles with dieting and her weight obsession. In her autobiographies, her issues with weight are linked to childhood sexual assault. More recently, she has been very open about her gastric bypass surgery and weight-loss success, serving as a sort of unofficial spokesperson for weight-loss surgeries.

SLG/Angie Wiley

*See also* Bariatric Surgery; Fat-Positive; Sex; Socioeconomic Status

## References and Further Reading

Anon. "Celebrities Increase Popularity of Gastric Bypass Surgery." Available online at <http://ezinearticles.com/?Celebrities-Increase-Popularity-of-Gastric-Bypass-Surgery&id=94828> (accessed March 18, 2007).

Barr, Roseanne (1991) *Roseanne: My Life as a Woman*, New York: Random House.

Bettie, Julie (1995) "Class Dismissed? Roseanne and the Changing Face of Working-Class Iconography," *Social Text* 45 (14): 125–49.

Tomasson, Robert E. (1990) "Boos for Roseanne Barr," *New York Times*, July 27, B4.

# Beaumont, William, MD (1785–1853)

## American doctor and physiologist, best known for conducting a series of experiments on the trapper Alexis St. Martin that produced significant findings about the chemistry of digestion

Beaumont, educated through the old apprenticeship system, was an army surgeon during and after the war of 1812. On June 6, 1822, while stationed at Fort Mackinac (Michigan) he treated Alexis St. Martin, a French Canadian *voyageur* (an intermediary between Indian trappers and a fur company). St. Martin had been wounded in the side with duck shot, severely injuring his lower ribs, left lung, diaphragm, and stomach. He survived but was left with a permanent fistula, or opening, in his stomach.

Taking advantage of the perforation, which allowed him to see into the stomach, Beaumont performed a series of experiments on St. Martin. In 1825, Beaumont became the first to see the process of digestion as it occurred in the stomach. He dangled pieces of food on a string, removed and then replaced them. He was able to observe the process of digestion through the hole in St. Martin's stomach. He then compared this process to the chemical process of digestion by gastric juice in test tubes. With the aid of the chemist Benjamin Silliman at Yale, it was determined that free hydrochloric acid formed the basis for the digestive juices. In 1829–31, when stationed at Fort Crawford (in Prairie du Chien, Wisconsin), St. Martin rejoined Beaumont for a second set of experiments. In addition to his general observation of St. Martin's digestion, Beaumont studied the correlation between digestion and weather, proving that temperature and humidity have a direct impact on digestion. His laboratory work on digestion showed that gastric juices need heat to break down food. A side effect of the uncomfortable experiments was a high level of stress, which led to Beaumont's unanticipated observation that anger can hinder digestion.

Beaumont published his *Experiments and Observations on the Gastric Juice and the Physiology of Digestion* in 1833. This widely cited book made Beaumont one of America's scientific heroes. It provided practical dietary advice and offered evidence for a new chemical theory of the stomach's function. It was previously believed that the stomach served a mechanical digestive function as a grinding organ or was involved in chemical digestion only as a fermentation vat. While earlier physiologists had speculated that the process was more complex, it was Beaumont who was able to prove this. By observing the digestion of a wide range of foods, he determined how they were processed. Thus, a bit of raw potato took many hours to even be slightly "processed," while fish "may be regarded as easily susceptible of digestion" (Beaumont 1833: 48). He provided a detailed table of the digestive times for a wide range of foods. Beaumont's observation of hunger and thirst provided some of the first pragmatic insights into the relationship between satiety and the actual process of digestion. He was able to show that hunger "is the effect of distention of the vessels that secrete the gastric juice" (Beaumont 1833: 276). The book contained 238 experiments and fifty-one conclusions, surprisingly few of which have been shown to be flawed.

Beaumont and St. Martin never met again. Beaumont, who subsequently had a lucrative private practice, died in St. Louis in 1853 of a head injury from falling on an icy step. St. Martin, although he had been paid rather well by both Beaumont and the U.S. Government, was frustrated with the experiments. Prior to his death in 1880, it was rumored that St. Martin had requested that his body be allowed to decompose for days to prevent it from being used for experiment before burial in an unmarked grave. Certainly, when the great Canadian physician and teacher William Osler requested that he be permitted to undertake an autopsy, he was informed by the local priest that "the body was in such an advanced stage of decomposition that it could not be admitted into the Church . . . the family resisted all requests . . . for an autopsy" (Myer 1912: xvii). He was warned by a local physician, "Don't come for autopsy; will be killed." In 1962, a plaque was erected at the Church at St. Thomas de Joliette in Quebec commemorating St. Martin's services to science. It reads: "Through his Affliction he served all Humanity."

SLG

## References and Further Reading

Beaumont, William (1833) *Experiments and Observations on the Gastric Juice and the Physiology of Digestion*, introduction by William Osler, New York: Dover.

Myer, Jesse S. (1912) *Life and Letters of Dr. William Beaumont*. St. Louis, Miss.: C.V. Mosby.

Nelson, Rodney B. (1990) *Beaumont: America's First Physiologist*. Geneva, Ill.: Grant House Press.

# Beecher, Catharine (1800–78)

## Early promoter of health, physical education, and higher learning for middle-class women and girls in America

Beecher came from a large family of thirteen children and was home-schooled while helping care for her large family. At the age of ten, Beecher began education at a private school. She noticed the limited resources and curriculum available to young women and began teaching herself subjects not offered in school. Beecher convinced herself that her mission in life was to "find happiness in living to do good," (Anon. "American Family") and decided that there was a need for higher-education schools for women. In 1823, Beecher founded the Hartford Female Seminary, where her sister Harriet Beecher studied. The school began with only seven students, and in three years grew to nearly 100 students. Beecher went west with her father, Lyman Beecher, the controversial Calvinist preacher, and organized the Western Female Institute in Cincinnati, which prospered until 1837.

In 1841, Beecher published *A Treatise on Domestic Economy for the Use of Young Ladies at Home and at School*, which emphasized the value of women's role in society. Her ideal reader is certainly middle class, as she stresses the importance of learning to deal with "domestics." She is an advocate of reform within the model of the Christian family. She centers its claims for social reform on the newest findings of "Physiology and Hygiene" (Beecher 1841: ix). One chapter is devoted to the role of the woman as "the person who decides what shall be the food and drink of a family" (Beecher 1841: 70). Here, she begins with a detailed account of the digestive system influenced by the recent work of William Beaumont on digestion, referring to his experiments with Alexis St. Martin (Beecher 1841: 82). But her model for eating is that of self-control. "When a tempting article is presented every person should exercise sufficient self-denial to wait until the proper time for eating arrives" (Beecher 1841: 73). Regular meals, no snacks is the rule. The portion size is dependent on the amount of work undertaken by the individual. What can occur is that "a student . . . or a lady who spends the day in her parlor or chamber" loses any senses of the meaning of hunger and overeats (Beecher 1841: 75). They will "load the stomach with a supply, which a stout farmer could scarcely digest" (Beecher 1841: 75). But some foods are also naturally "stimulating" and make one "live faster than Nature designed, and soon his constitution is worn out" (Beecher 1841: 76). Eat "meat but once a day and in small quantities, compared with the vegetables taken" (Beecher 1841: 77). Avoid tea and coffee, the "most extensive cause of much of the nervous debility and suffering endured by American women" (Beecher 1841: 87). In addition to her comments on diet, she provided a model for calisthenics to provide further training for the female body (Beecher 1841: 34). After returning east, she helped organize "The Ladies Society for Promoting Education in the West," and in 1850 the "American Women's Education Association." She also played an important role in founding women's colleges in Burlington, Iowa, Quincy, Illinois, Milwaukee, and Wisconsin. Beecher taught, lectured, and wrote on the subjects of physical education, domestic economy, women's health and nutrition, and her system of calisthenics to make women's bodies stronger and healthier.

"Poor health" stands as much at the center of her system of education as any other failure. As she writes in the preface to the third edition of 1846:

The number of young women whose health is crushed, ere the first few years of married life are past, would seem incredible to one who has not investigated this subject, and it would be vain to attempt to depict the sorrow, discouragement, and distress experienced in most families where the wife and mother is a perpetual invalid.

(Beecher 1846: 5)

One of the causes of this "debilitated constitution" is: "Eating too much, eating *too often*, eating *too fast*, eating food and condiments that are *too stimulating*, eating food that is *too warm* or *too cold*, eating food that is *highly-concentrated*, without a proper admixture of less nourishing matter, and eating food that is *difficult of digestion*" (Beecher 1846: 106). Dieting would be the reform of such bad eating habits. Indeed, she stresses in the third edition of 1846 that the "health of the mind" demands the limitation of the "excessive exercise of the intellect or feelings" (Beecher 1846: 197). If too rich foods are to be avoided, then too is "novel reading" which "wastes time and energies, [and] undermines the vigor of the nervous system" (Beecher 1846: 199).

In 1869, she wrote *The American Woman's Home*, together with her much younger sister Harriet Beecher Stowe, the author of *Uncle Tom's Cabin*. This was a systematic guide for the middle-class homemaker "to the formation and maintenance of economical, healthful, beautiful and Christian homes" (Beecher and Stowe 1869: 10). Their discussion of food, certainly written by Catharine Beecher, as it draws heavily on her earlier work, was putatively rooted in the biochemistry of the time, but it also has a strong moral tone. She advocates for a "healthy diet" and stresses that it is fashion which leads to obesity and illness. It is the "customs of society, which present incessant change, and a great variety of food" which "lead almost every person very frequently to eat merely to gratify the palate" (Beecher and Stowe 1869: 127). Such excesses shorten the life and weaken the constitution. The diet she proposes is to limit the amounts and types of foods, "eat only one or two articles of simple food, such as bread or milk, and at the same time eat less than the appetite demands" (Beecher and Stowe 1869: 131). Such a diet leads to a retraining of the body's expectation for excessive amounts and varieties of food. Bread is a better food than meat and contains "more nourishment" (Beecher and Stowe 1869: 133). The simpler the food the better: "The fewer mixtures there are in cooking, the more healthful is the food to be" (Beecher and Stowe 1869: 133). She notes the bad manners of Americans at the table and urges that food "be well chewed and taken slowly" (Beecher and Stowe 1869: 134). Moderation is, thus, a social goal; the alteration of the American diet to include snacks between meals and meals eaten in great haste is seen by her as unhealthful. Her ideas and doctrines of education were implemented in some of the schools she helped to found. Beecher also spoke out against women wearing corsets, believing they were hazardous to the internal organs of women, making exercise impossible and actually deforming women's bodies.

SLG/RAKHI PATEL

*See also* Beaumont

## References and Further Reading

Anon. *Schoolhouse Pioneers: Catharine Beecher* (2006) Public Broadcasting System. Available online at <http://www.pbs.org/onlyateacher/beecher.html> (accessed April 11, 2006).

Anon. "The American Family: The Beecher Tradition—Catharine Beecher." Available online at <http://newman.baruch.cuny.edu/digital/2001/beecher/catherine.htm> (accessed March 6, 2007).

Beecher, Catharine E. (1841) *A Treatise on Domestic Economy for the Use of Young Ladies at Home and at School*, Boston, Mass.: Marsh, Capen, Lyon, & Webb.

—— (1846) *A Treatise on Domestic Economy for the Use of Young Ladies at Home and at School*, New York: Harper & Brothers.

Beecher, Catharine E. and Harriet Beecher Stowe (1869) *The American Woman's Home*, New York: J.B. Ford.

# Behavior

At the dinner table, your mother has probably told you to eat your fish to become smarter or to finish your spinach so that you, like Popeye, can defend yourself against those bullies who keep shoving you in lockers at school. In fact, maybe she still controls your diet and has told you to lay off the carbs with the hope that you'll finally move out of the house and get married. Regardless, the belief that diet or dieting can control and modify such behaviors as criminality, alcoholism, and performance in school, or can even enhance one's chances at marriage, has become part of the mantra of professional nutritionists. The use of dieting as a "correction tool" draws on scientific evidence, but within the scientific community, there are still serious doubts as to its effectiveness, with some dismissing it as "food faddism."

Some researchers believe that poor diet, or, more specifically, food allergies, malnutrition, and hypoglycemia, can provoke criminal behaviors. Food allergies and malnutrition in particular have been linked to mental imbalances, such as abnormal serotonin activity, which have been linked to violent behavior. Examples of this include a twelve-year-old who, after eating a banana, tried to hit another patient with a stick and a fifty-two-year-old woman who, after having wheat, said she wanted to punch someone (Schellhardt 1977: 1). Hypoglycemia, or having low blood sugar, has also been linked to irrational behavior that is controllable through diet.

The penal system has been one area of focus of such dietary interventions. In the 1970s, new procedures were implemented in Cuyahoga Falls, Ohio, based on the link between hypoglycemia and criminal behavior. Probation Officer Barbara Reed tested the blood-sugar level of all criminals, and if the level was too low, lawbreakers were required to change to a more nutritious diet at the risk of losing probation. The link between diet and criminal behavior was supported by a study that provided vitamin supplements to half of a group of prisoners and gave a placebo to the other half. It was found that prisoners who took the vitamins reduced their "antisocial behavior," which included violence and rule-breaking (Gesch et al. 2002: 24). Commenting on his findings, Gesch says, "What would have happened to these young men had they been properly nourished all their lives? Would they have been in prison? We don't know but I think it's about time we started looking into it" (quoted in Anon. "Crime Diet").

Modification of young people's behavior has also been a subject of particular interest. Findings have suggested that binge-drinking, poor academic performance, and disobedience can be cured through an improved diet, but such claims are generally not the basis of today's school cafeteria reforms.

One study found that rats that were on a typical nutrient-deficient "teenage diet" of pastries, hot dogs, carbonated beverages, spaghetti, salad, and candy drank more 20-proof alcohol (as opposed to water) when compared with rats that ate fruits, vegetables, nuts, legumes, whole-wheat flour, and whole-milk powder. Switching to the healthier diet or taking vitamin supplements reduced alcohol intake while the addition of coffee or caffeine increased it. This suggests that the nutrient content of one's diet affects "the 'biological thirst' of animals to drink alcohol" (Register et al. 1972: 162).

Another study found that children who were put on an enrichment program for nutrition, education, and physical exercise had fewer cases of schizotypal personality and antisocial and criminal behavior than control subjects (Raine et al. 2003). Although the most dramatic change in behavior was found among children who were initially malnourished, Raine believes that the fatty acid supplements were responsible for this difference (Arehart-Treichel 2003: 43). However, another study reinforces the possibility that malnourishment versus proper nourishment is the key difference in behavior modification, suggesting that vitamin-mineral supplementation only increases the nonverbal intelligence of Western schoolchildren if they were inadequately nourished (Schoenthaler et al. 2000).

In 1998, Appleton Central Alternative High School of Wisconsin began a new food program based on this belief. The high school collaborated with Natural Ovens Bakery in an attempt to redress their students' antisocial and violent behaviors. The program replaced the junk food available at the school with healthier alternatives, like fruits, vegetables, and low-fat/low-salt/low-sugar foods without additives. In the period following this change, grades improved while incidences of misconduct, vandalism, and littering decreased. The idea for the program began with cofounder Barbara Stitt's experiences as a probation officer.

After this program was featured in *Super Size Me* and

on *Good Morning America*, the U.S. Department of Justice filed a lawsuit against Natural Ovens Bakery, Inc. The company was charged with mislabeling ingredients and making misleading health claims without the approval of the Federal Drug Administration. The National Council Against Health Fraud (NCAHF) also believes that there is not enough evidence to support the link between improper diet and criminal behavior.

While ongoing research continues to suggest that diet can control behavior, many in the Government and scientific community are still skeptical of the validity of such claims. On the other hand, if these claims are true, then it looks like the solution to improving humanity is not found in rehab but in the kitchen.

SLG/DOROTHY CHYUNG

*See also* Children; Spurlock

**References and Further Reading**

Anon. (2003) "Crime Diet," *ACF Newsource*. Available online at <http://www.acfnewsource.org/science/crime_diet.html> (accessed April 12, 2006).

Arehart-Treichel, Joan (2003) "Can Better Diet Prevent Antisocial Behavior?" *Psychiatric News* 38 (9): 43.

Denison, Niki (2006) "Flour Power," *CPI's Crisis Response Newsletter*. Available online at <http://www.crisisprevention.com/whatsnew/CRNews/CRNews_Dec2005/CRN_12-4_NDenison.html> (accessed April 12, 2006).

Gesch, C.B., Hammond, S.M., Hampson, S.E., Eves, A., and Crowder, M.J. (2002) "Influence of Supplementary Vitamins, Minerals and Essential Fatty Acids on the Antisocial Behaviour of Young Adult Prisoners," *The British Journal of Psychiatry* 181 (19): 22–8.

Hajewski, Doris (2006) "Bakery Resolves Suit over Labeling: Natural Ovens Brand Was Accused of Making Misleading Health Claims," *Milwaukee Journal Sentinal*, February 7: D1.

National Council Against Health Fraud (1983) "NCAHF Position Paper on Diet and Criminal Behavior," April 17. Available online at <http://www.ncahf.org/pp/diet.html> (accessed April 11, 2006).

Natural Ovens Bakery. Available online at <http://www.naturalovens.com> (accessed April 12, 2006).

Raine A., Mellingen, K., Liu, J., Venables, P., and Mednick, S.A. (2003) "Effects of Environmental Enrichment at Ages 3–5 Years on Schizotypal Personality and Antisocial Behavior at Ages 17 and 23 Years," *The American Journal of Psychiatry* 160 (9): 1627–35.

Register, U.D., Marsh, S.R., Thurston, C.T., Fields, B.J., Horning, M.C., Hardinge, M.G. and Sanchez, A. (1972) "Influence of Nutrients on Intake of Alcohol," *Journal of the American Dietetic Association* 61 (2): 59–62.

Schellhardt, Timothy D. (1977) "Chocolate Turn You into a Criminal? Some Experts Say So; Food Allergies, Malnutrition Are Tied to Violent Acts; A Banana Leads to Blows; Can Chocolate Turn You to Crime? Food-Aggression Link Is Studied," *Wall Street Journal*, June 2: 1, 23.

Schoenthaler S.J., Bier, I.D., Young, K., Nichols, D., and Jansenns, S. (2000) "The Effect of Vitamin-Mineral Supplementation on the Intelligence of American Schoolchildren: A Randomized, Double-Blind Placebo-Controlled Trial," *Journal of Alternative Complementary Medicine* 6 (1): 19–29.

# Benedict, Francis Gano (1870–1957)

At age thirteen, Benedict's interest in chemistry was sparked by attending a lecture in Boston by chemist and assayer James Francis Babcock (1844–94) who wrote widely on the hygiene and chemistry of food. While studying at Harvard, he took courses from chemist Josiah Parsons Cooke (1827–94), who in 1850, founded the Harvard Chemistry Department. After completing his graduate study at Heidelberg University in Germany,

Benedict returned to the U.S.A. to work with Wilbur Olin Atwater. Following on his work with Atwater in chemistry and nutrition, Benedict soon became involved with physiology. The two scientists began studies of metabolism in humans, by means of a respiration calorimeter, a piece of equipment created by Benedict to measure oxygen consumption and heat in the body. The machine was able to provide exact measurements of heat production and loss in animals and humans.

Benedict published his results in his *An Experimental Inquiry Regarding the Nutritive Value of Alcohol*. In 1907, after the publishing of his findings, Benedict was appointed Director of the newly established Carnegie Nutrition Laboratory in Boston, Massachusetts. At the laboratory, Benedict developed new equipment, which including a smaller instrument for measuring oxygen consumption in humans. Using the machine, Benedict, and fellow colleagues, studied the production of heat, changing the conditions of working, exercising, and eating or fasting on his subjects. From his studies, he determined a basal metabolism in humans, then wrote (with James Arthur Harris [1880–1930]) *A Biometric Study of Basal Metabolism in Man* (1919), which remains a classic in the field. Benedict's studies on metabolism extended to animals as well as humans. The equipment that Benedict developed as well as his research on basal metabolism in humans became standards in the medical profession and enabled future work in the field.

SLG/Laura K. Goldstein

*See also* Atwater; Metabolism

## References and Further Reading

Anon. (2004) "Benedict, Francis Gano," *American National Biography, New York*: American Council of Learned Societies and Oxford University Press. Available online at <http://www.anb.org> (accessed June 23, 2007).

Benedict, Francis Gano and Wilbur Olin Atwater (1902) *An Experimental Inquiry Regarding the Nutritive Value of Alcohol*, Washington: Government Printing Office.

Benedict, Francis Gano and James Arthur Harris (1919) *A Biometric Study of Basal Metabolism in Man*, Washington: Carnegie Institution of Washington.

Shor, Elizabeth Noble (2000) "Benedict, Francis Gano," *American National Biography Online*. Available online at <http://www.anb.org/login.html?url=%2Farticles%2Fhome.html&ip=68.219.108.222&nocookie=0> (accessed March 6, 2007).

# Binge-Eating

With the problems of obesity and disordered eating growing in the United States and around the world public health professionals have focused research efforts on identifying potential causes and treatments for these related problems. The most obvious advancement made by this work has been the introduction of a diagnostic category for binge-eating disorder (BED) in the fourth edition of the *Diagnostic and Statistical Manual of Mental Disorders* (DSM-IV-R). In addition, there is a growing body of literature on binge-eating and obesity that has attempted to define the prevalence, causes, effects, and treatment options for this relatively new disorder. Dieting, in particular, has been implicated as a possible causal factor in the development of both BED and related obesity.

Binge-eating was first identified in 1959 by Albert Stunkard as a distinctive pattern of eating observable in some obese persons (Stunkard 1959: 588–91; Spitzer 1991; Devlin et al. 2003: 627). In the following decades, there was much debate amongst clinicians about how to differentiate BED from already diagnosed "non-purging" forms of bulimia nervosa; it was not clear to many researchers that BED should be a separate diagnostic category (Spitzer 1991; Devlin et al. 2003: 627; Yanovski 1995: 403–4). Nevertheless, in 1991, a core group of eating-disorder clinicians and researchers recommended that BED be entered into the DSM-IV as a diagnosable eating disorder (Spitzer 1991; Devlin et al. 2003: 628). Today, BED is part of the Eating Disorder Not Otherwise Specified (EDNOS) category and appears in Appendix B of the DSM-IV, among the "Criteria Sets and Axes Provided for Further Study" with roughly the same criteria recommended by Robert Spitzer and his colleagues in 1991. The DSM-IV research criteria for BED are (American Psychiatric Association; Grilo 2002: 178–9; Spitzer 1991; Yanovski et al. 1995: 139):

- Recurrent episodes of binge-eating, characterized by both eating an amount of food in a discrete period of time (two hours) that is definitely larger than most people would eat and a sense of lack of control over eating during the episodes.
- The binge-eating episodes are associated with three (or more) or the following: eating much more rapidly than normal, eating until uncomfortably full, eating large amounts of food when not physically hungry, eating alone because of embarrassment about the amount of food eaten, and feeling disgusted with oneself, depressed, or very guilty after overeating.
- Marked distress about binge-eating is present.
- Binge-eating occurs at least twice a week during a six-month period.
- The binge-eating is not associated with regular use of inappropriate compensatory behaviors (purging, fasting, excessive exercise) and does not occur exclusively during the course of anorexia nervosa or bulimia nervosa.

Yet, while BED is now recognized as a category distinct from bulimia nervosa (BN), researchers have struggled since the mid-1990s to sort out how to diagnose and treat this disorder, which overlaps and is frequently confused with BN and behavior subtypes of obesity (Devlin et al. 2003).

In addition, even though binge-eating is the central diagnostic criterion of BED and is generally considered to be a pathological form of eating, it is also present in non-clinical male and female populations (Waller 2002: 98), and many non-eating-disordered individuals may engage in some form of binge-eating at various times in their lives. In fact, a significant number of people engage in normative binge behaviors on holidays like Thanksgiving and Christmas, which can be attested to by the proliferation of articles like "Holiday Stress: A Recipe for Overeating?" (MSNBC) and "Your Stay Slim Holiday Survival Plan" (Prevention 2006). However, BED as a diagnosable mental disorder is distinct and affects a much smaller portion of the population than normative and occasional overeating.

Still, the complex overlap between BED and other eating disorders and BED and normative overeating may make it more difficult to exactly describe the prevalence of BED in the general population. Some studies have indicated that as much as 25–30 percent of obese people who enter treatment programs are suffering from BED (Spitzer et al. 1991: 138; Hsu et al. 2002: 1398; Yanovski 2003: S118). The high occurrence of BED in obese people seeking weight-loss treatment has led researchers to investigate the relationship between dieting, psychopathology, and BED in greater depth.

Information disseminated to the public by popular media also suggests that dieting can cause obesity and act as a "trigger for eating disorders" (Hunter 1999: 45; MSNBC; Hill 2004; Cannon and Einzig 1984). Certainly, the popular media has overwhelmingly suggested that overeating is an attempt to assuage emotional distress (Levine 1999; Roth 1982). There is some evidence to suggest that dieting does play a role in onset of binge-eating (Cannon 2005: 569; Wadden et al. 2004: 560). Studies testing restraint theory (the theory that says we are more likely to overeat if we attempt to restrain our eating) have shown that individuals who are currently dieting are more prone to overeat if they feel that they have broken their diets or if they experience disappointment or boredom (Howard and Porzelius 1990: 28; Lowe 1995: 88–9). Obese binge eaters generally report a history of frequent and extensive dieting (Howard and Porzelius 1990: 25; Devlin et al. 2003: S8; Giusti et al. 2004: 47). Yet this dieting history has not been shown definitively to precede or cause BED.

In studies of normal-weight patients with bulimia nervosa, dieting has been shown to nearly always precede binge-eating, and some researchers have suggested that dietary restraint may precipitate binge-eating in the bulimic patient (Devlin et al. 2003: S8; Howard and Porzelius 1990: 26). Furthermore, a 1993 study demonstrated that dietary restraint prescribed by a Very Low Calorie Diet induced binge-eating behaviors in patients who had no prior history of BED (Telch and Agras 1993; Howard and Porzelius 1990: 36; Wadden and Berkowitz 1995: 535). These studies, together with anecdotal evidence, point to the potential of dietary restraint to cause overeating and may implicate dieting in the development of BED; however, not all studies have found such an association (Wadden and Berkowitz 1995: 555–6; Reas and Grilo 2006: 2; Howard and Porzelius 1990: 31; Yanovski 1995: 404).

Even though no direct causal link has been made between dieting and onset of BED, weight status and dieting in childhood or adolescence do appear to be predictive of BED development (Reas and Grilo 2006: 2; Howard and Porzelius 1990: 30; Spitzer et al. 1991: 143 and 146). This evidence suggests that a history of repeated dieting attempts and failures plays an important role in development of BED, which may be a risk factor for extreme obesity (Howard and Porzelius 1990: 31; Hsu et al. 2002; Spitzer et al. 1991: 146). Some researchers have even gone so far as to suggest that treating BED may help to alleviate somewhat the growing obesity epidemic (Yanovski 2003: S117–S118).

Available treatments for BED include cognitive behavioral therapy (CBT), group therapy, and drug therapy (National Institute of Diabetes and Digestive and Kidney Diseases 2004). CBT has been shown to be effective in reducing disordered eating behaviors in BED patients, but it unfortunately has little impact on actual body weight when not combined with surgical or other dietary treatments (Vaidya 2006: 92; Wilfley 1995: 351–2). Similarly, drug therapy appears to alleviate BED in the short term, but medication alone is not effective in the long term for most patients with BED (Devlin 1995: 356). Some people suffering from BED also use self-help methods with varied success, and others join support groups. Overeaters Anonymous (OA) is one of the most well-known support groups for people suffering from BED or compulsive overeating, which is sometimes referred to over-simplistically as an addition to food. While only a few studies have been done on the effectiveness of support groups in treating BED, their findings suggest that, when combined with other methods like CBT, these groups may provide important support for people struggling with compulsive overeating (Ghaderi 2006: 307; Stefano et al. 2006: 457–8; Wilfley 1995: 352).

Now that BED has been identified and studied as a diagnosable eating disorder, the etiology of compulsive overeating and the effects that it has on people's lives are becoming more evident. Research has shown that, while depression and anxiety may be factors in the development of BED, the disorder cannot simply be attributed to emotional overcompensation. Furthermore, restrictive eating may play a role in overeating behaviors, but dieting cannot be said to directly cause BED. Finally, because BED negatively impacts quality of life in substantial ways

(Rieger et al. 2005: 237), we can see that treatment of the underlying causes of BED in obese individuals is just as important as weight loss. Despite all that we have learned since Stunkard first recognized binge-eating in 1959, clinicians are still working on effective methods for diagnosing and treating BED and related obesity, and all agree that more research is necessary.

SLG/C. Melissa Anderson

*See also* Anorexia; Eating Competitions; Obesity Epidemic; Psychotherapy and Weight Change; Religion and Dieting; Very-Low-Calorie Diets

## References and Further Reading

American Psychiatric Association (1994) *Diagnostic and Statistical Manual of Mental Disorders*, 4th edn, Washington, DC: American Psychiatric Association.

Cannon, Geoffrey (2005) "Dieting Makes You Fat?" *British Journal of Nutrition* 93 (4): 569–70.

Cannon G. and Einzig, H. (1984) *Dieting Makes You Fat*, New York: Simon and Schuster.

Devlin, Michael J. (1995) "Pharmacological Treatment of Binge Eating Disorder," in Kelly D. Brownell and Christopher G. Fairburn (eds), *Eating Disorders and Obesity: A Comprehensive Handbook*, New York: Guilford Press, pp. 354–7.

Devlin, Michael J., Goldfein, Juli A., and Dobrow, Ilyse (2003) "What Is This Thing Called BED? Current Status of Binge Eating Disorder Nosology," *International Journal of Eating Disorders* 34: S2–S18.

Ghaderi, Ata (2006) "Attrition and Outcome in Self-Help Treatment for Bulimia Nervosa and Binge Eating Disorder: A Constructive Replication," *Eating Behaviors* 7: 300–8.

Giusti, V., Héraïef, E., Gaillard, R.C. and Burckhardt, P. (2004) "Predictive Factors of Binge Eating Disorders in Women Searching to Lose Weight," *Eating and Weight Disorders* 9: 44–9.

Grilo, Carlos M. (2002) "Binge Eating Disorder," in Christopher G. Fairburn and Kelly D. Brownell (eds), *Eating Disorders and Obesity: A Comprehensive Handbook*, 2nd edn, New York: Guilford Press, pp. 178–82.

Hill, A.J. (2004) "Does Dieting Make You Fat?" *British Journal of Nutrition* 92: S15–S18.

Howard, Christine E. and Porzelius, Linda Krug (1990) "The Role of Dieting in Binge Eating Disorder:

Etiology and Treatment Implications," *Clinical Psychology Review* 19 (1): 25–44.

Hsu, L. K. G., Mulliken, B., McDonagh, B., Krupa Das, S., Rand, W., Fairburn, C. G., Rolls, B., McCrory, M. A., Saltzman, E., Shikora, S., Dwyer, J. and Roberts, S. (2002) "Binge Eating Disorder in Extreme Obesity," *International Journal of Obesity* 26: 1398–1403.

Hunter, Beatric Trum (1999) "Dieting: A Trigger for Eating Disorders," in Myra H. Immell (ed.) *Eating Disorders*, San Diego: Greenhaven, pp. 45–8.

Levine, Michelle Joy (1999) "Why People Overeat," in Myra H. Immell (ed.), *Eating Disorders*, San Diego: Greenhaven, pp. 70–6.

Lowe, Michael R. (1995) "Dietary Restraint and Overeating," in Kelly D. Brownell and Christopher G. Fairburn (eds), *Eating Disorders and Obesity: A Comprehensive Handbook*, New York: Guilford Press, pp. 88–92.

MSNBC (2005) "Holiday Stress—A Recipe for Overeating? Dieting Can Help Make All That Yummy Food Harder to Resist," December 22. Available online at <http://www.msnbc.msn.com/id/10176756> (accessed November 10, 2006).

National Institute of Diabetes and Digestive and Kidney Diseases (2004) "Binge Eating Disorder," September. Available online at <http://win.niddk.nih.gov/publications/binge.htm#treatment> (accessed November 10, 2006).

Reas, Deborah L. and Grilo, Carlos M. (2006) "Timing and Sequence of the Onset of Overweight, Dieting, and Binge Eating in Overweight Patients with Binge Eating Disorder," *International Journal of Eating Disorders* 39: 1–6.

Rieger, E., Wilfley, D. E., Stein, R. I., Marino, V. and J. Crow, S. (2005) "A Comparison of Quality of Life in Obese Individuals and without Binge Eating Disorder," *International Journal of Eating Disorders* 37: 234–40.

Roth, Geneen (1982) *Feeding the Hungry Heart: The Experience of Emotional Overeating*, New York: Penguin Books.

Prevention (2006) Your Stay Slim Holiday Survival Plan: 12 Real-World Tactics for Dealing with the #1 Overeating Season, 58 (12).

Spitzer, Robert L., Stunkard, Albert, Yanovski, Susan, Marcus, Marsha D., Wadden, Thomas, Wing, Rena, Mitchell, James and Hasin, Deborah (1991) "Binge Eating Disorder: To Be or Not to Be in DSM-IV," *International Journal of Eating Disorders* 10 (6): 627–9.

Stefano, S. C., Bacaltchuk, J., Blay, S. L., and Hay, P. (2006) "Self-Help Treatments for Disorders of Recurrent Binge Eating: A Systematic Review," *Acta Psychiatrica Scandinavica* 113: 452–9.

Stunkard, Albert J. (1959) "Eating Patterns and Obesity," *Psychiatric Quarterly* 33: 284–95.

Telch, C.F. and Agras, W.S. (1993) "The Effects of a Very Low Calorie Diet on Binge Eating," *Behavior Therapy* 24: 177–93.

Vaidya, Varsha (2006) "Cognitive Behavior Therapy of Binge Eating Disorder," *Advances in Psychosomatic Medicine* 27: 86–93.

Wadden, Thomas A., Foster, Gary D., Sarwer, David B., Anderson, Drew A., Gladis, Madeline, Sanderson, Rebecca S., Letchak, R.V., Berkowitz, Robert I. and Phelan, Suzanne (2004) "Dieting and the Development of Eating Disorders in Obese Women: Results of a Randomized Controlled Trial," *American Journal of Clinical Nutrition* 80: 560–8.

Wadden, Thomas A. and Berkowitz, Robert I. (1995) "Very-Low-Calorie Diets," in Kelly D. Brownell and Christopher G. Fairburn (eds), *Eating Disorders and Obesity: A Comprehensive Handbook*, New York: Guilford Press, pp. 534–8.

Waller, Glenn (2002) "The Psychology of Binge Eating," in Christopher G. Fairburn and Kelly D. Brownell (eds), *Eating Disorders and Obesity: A Comprehensive Handbook*, 2nd edn, New York: Guilford Press, pp. 98–102.

Wilfley, Denise E. (1995) "Psychological Treatment of Binge Eating Disorder," in Kelly D. Brownell and Christopher G. Fairburn (eds), *Eating Disorders and Obesity: A Comprehensive Handbook*, New York: Guilford Press, pp. 350–3.

Yanovski, Susan (1995) "Binge Eating in Obese Persons," in Kelly D. Brownell and Christopher G. Fairburn (eds), *Eating Disorders and Obesity: A Comprehensive Handbook*, New York: Guilford Press, pp. 403–7.

—— (2003) "Binge Eating Disorder and Obesity in 2003: Could Treating an Eating Disorder Have a Positive Effect on the Obesity Epidemic?" *International Journal of Eating Disorders* 34: S117–20.

# Blood-type diet

In 1996, Peter D'Adamo, ND (Naturopathic Doctorate) (1956–) published a book entitled *Eat Right 4 Your Type* suggesting that people should eat certain foods based on their individual blood types. He recommends that individuals following the diet find out their blood types and then follow the diet for that blood type. There are four blood types: Type A, Type B, Type O, and Type AB. Blood type is determined by proteins on the surface of red blood cells. D'Adamo suggests that the proteins affect blood chemistry, and, therefore, that each blood type has differing nutritional requirements and specific foods which are beneficial and detrimental to the health of the individual. He states that the way to live "disease-free" is to only eat foods prescribed for one's blood type. For example, tomatoes and bananas are not recommended for Type A, whereas they are for Type O blood. He suggests reasons for the dietary requirements by blood type based on the region in the world in which each of the blood types evolved.

This concept of ethnicity influencing diet is not new. In fact, there was early work in nineteenth-century racial "pseudo-science" arguing that blood types were true racial markers and that diet was one predetermined factor (Polsky 2002). In the book, D'Adamo provides anecdotal evidence based on his father's research (he was an ND as well) that eating the proper diet will lead to improved health. Additionally he provides personal testimony from people who have attempted the diet and self-report improvements in health. Since publishing the initial book, he has published twelve supplemental books based on the same premise that blood type should determine dietary practices.

Similar to other popular diets, the blood-type diet is very restrictive, which leads to low compliance rates. To date, there have not been any studies published that support D'Adamo's claims; however, it continues to be a popular diet.

SLG/Suzanne Judd

*See also* Alternative Medicine

### References and Further Reading

D'Adamo, Peter (1996) *Eat Right 4 Your Type: The Individualized Diet Solution to Staying Healthy, Living Longer and Achieving Your Ideal Weight*, New York: C.P. Putnam and Sons.

Polsky, Allyson D. (2002) "Blood, Race, and National Identity: Scientific and Popular Discourses," *Journal of Medical Humanities* 23 (3–4): 171–86.

# Bodybuilding

Bodybuilding includes weight training and increasing caloric intake in order to build muscle mass. Many people compete in bodybuilding competitions, and they are judged on the physical appearance of their muscles. It began as a sport only for men in the 1890s. The first popular bodybuilder was Eugene Sandow (1867–1925), who organized the first bodybuilding contest on September 14, 1901 in London. Sandow and an entire following generation saw bodybuilding as both aesthetic enhancement and body strengthening. What they created was a new masculine ideal: The shaped body rather than the athlete's lithe but strong body. By the 1970s, women began to partake in competition as well. Evidence of the growth in the popularity of bodybuilding for women can be seen in the number of magazines devoted to the subject, such as *Muscle*, *Fitness Hers* and *Oxygen*, on the shelves at bookstores today.

In order to be successful, bodybuilders must closely monitor their nutritional intake. Because bodybuilders exert large amounts of energy, they generally require between 500 and 1,000 more calories per day than the average person. Bodybuilders also need to maintain a low percentage of body fat and a high percentage of muscle to obtain the physical appearance ideal in their sport.

Protein is essential for building muscle mass. Whey protein is the most commonly used protein supplement among bodybuilders because it is absorbed and metabolized by the body at fast rates. Many bodybuilders consume meal replacement products (MRPs) which provide the calories and nutrients that would generally be consumed in a meal. While these are usually powdered drinks mixed with milk, juice, or water, sometimes MRPs come in bar form. MRPs are generally low in fat, have a modest amount of carbohydrates, include vitamins and minerals, and, most importantly, are high in protein.

Many bodybuilders also use thermogenics, another form of dietary supplement. Thermogenics increase metabolism through heat generation, resulting in the loss of fat. Bodybuilders use these in order to reduce their total body fat. Natural products with thermogenic qualities include caffeine and ginger.

Because bodybuilding is a sport in which weight must be controlled, it is considered a "high risk" sport for developing an eating disorder. In addition, the bodybuilding community centers on body image, which can also make bodybuilders more vulnerable to eating disorders. A new study by Amanda Gruber found that female bodybuilders are more likely to suffer from eating disorders and distorted body images than other females. Many male and female bodybuilders have a disorder known as the eating disorder/bodybuilder type (ED/BT), which involves a diet high in protein, calories and low in fat. They also suffer from muscle dysmorphia, a disorder in which they view themselves differently, generally smaller than they really are. Many male athletes, especially bodybuilders, believe that they have smaller muscle mass than they actually do. It is estimated that 10 percent of men in any intense gym setting have muscle dysmorphia.

Bodybuilders are judged on the physical appearance of their muscles, and, therefore, are encouraged to focus on body image. Bodybuilders, as well as other athletes, tend to use dieting to achieve the body type that will help them be effective competitors in their sport. Where that fails, selective silicone or saline implants may be employed.

SLG/MARY STANDEN

*See also* Atlas; Men; Sports

**References and Further Reading**

Anon. (2000–6) "Athletes and Eating Disorders," HealthyPlace.com. Available online at <http://www.healthyplace.com/Communities/Eating_Disorders/athletes.asp> (accessed April 20, 2006).

Anon. (2000–6) "Eating disorders: Bigorexia," HealthyPlace.com. Available online at <http://www.healthyplace.com/Communities/Eating_Disorders/type_bigorexia.asp> (accessed April 22, 2006).

Anon. (2006) "Bodybuilding," *Wikipedia*, available online at <http://en.wikipedia.org/wiki/Bodybuilding#Female_Bodybuilding> (accessed April 20, 2006).

Chapman, David L. (1994) *Sandow the Magnificent: Eugen Sandow and the Beginnings of Bodybuilding*, Urbana, Ill.: University of Illinois Press.

Gruber, Amanda and Harrison G. Pope, Jr. (2000) "Psychiatric and Medical Effects of Anabolic-Androgenic Steroid Use in Women." *Psychotherapy and Psychosomatics* 69: 19–26.

Mann, Denise (2000) "Steroid Use, Eating Disorders Are Common Among Female Bodybuilders." Available online at <http://www.webmd.com/content/article/17/1676_50472.htm> (accessed April 20, 2006).

Porter, Alicia (1996) "Males and Body Image." Available online at <http://www.eatingdisorders.org.nz/Are_Males_Affected_by_Body_Ima.136.0.html> (accessed April 20, 2006).

# Brillat-Savarin, Jean-Anthelme (1755–1826)

Brillat-Savarin's 1825 account of food and its pleasures, *The Physiology of Taste or, Meditations on Transcendental Gastronomy*, was also a study of fat and its dangers and stressed the physiognomy of obesity. The appearance of obesity was a clue to its dangers. A lawyer by trade, Brillat-Savarin had been elected a deputy to the National Assembly in 1789, where he argued for the death penalty. During the Reign of Terror, he was forced to flee France, eventually settling in the U.S.A. He returned to France in 1797, where he became a judge in the Court of Cassation. In 1825, shortly before his death, he wrote his epicurean account of the pleasures (and dangers) of food. He wrote in an autobiographical mode about his sense of his own obese body:

> There is one kind of obesity which centers around the belly; I have never noticed it in women: since they are generally made up of softer tissues, no part of their bodies are spared when obesity attacks them. I call this type of fatness Gastrophoria and its victims Gastrophores. I myself am in their company; but although I carry around with me a fairly prominent stomach, I still have well-formed lower legs, and calves as sinewy as the muscles of an Arabian steed. Nevertheless I have always looked on my paunch as a redoubtable enemy; I have conquered it and limited its outlines to the purely majestic; but in order to win the fight, I have fought hard indeed: whatever is good about the results and my present observations I owe to a thirty-year battle.
>
> (Brillat-Savarin 1999: 186)

Brillat-Savarin was commenting on his struggle with a disease of the will in the form of his own obesity. Yet when he looks to the world of women, he bemoans their thinness as "a terrible misfortune." "Every thin woman wishes to put on weight. This is an ambition that has been confided to us a thousand times" (Brillat-Savarin 1999: 186). For them, he suggests a diet to help them gain weight.

The key was looking and being looked at as too fat or too thin. For men, the potbelly became a major indicator of the potential for illness for the observers of masculine obesity in the late nineteenth century. Indeed, of the 163,567 overweight men in the U.S.A. and Canada identified between 1870 and 1899 (for insurance purposes), abdominal obesity (the waist being of greater circumference than the chest) was present in about 13 percent (Kahn and Williamson 1994). This was taken as an absolute sign of increased morbidity and mortality. The projected deaths of these individuals were almost one-third less than their actual death rate. "Omental fat" in the

disease of Gastrophoria (potbelliedness) comes to represent the bloated and unmasculine over time.

In his chapters on obesity and dieting, Brillat-Savarin positions himself as a "lay expert." For him, obesity is a disease that makes the beautiful ugly, the strong weak, the intelligent dumb. It produces a distaste for dance, that most civilized of social interactions, creates the context for diseases such as apoplexy, dropsy, ulcers in the legs, and makes all diseases difficult to cure. Thus, no obesity is found among that class of persons who eat to live, instead of living to eat. But, "it takes real courage either to lose weight or to keep from gaining it" (Brillat-Savarin 1999: 195). His approach is to avoid excess and the need to balance all qualities of food. "Discretion in eating, moderation in sleeping, and exercise on foot or horseback," is his dieting course (Brillat-Savarin 1999: 195). Yet, he recognizes that such a simple prescription is almost always met with objections by those who need to undertake it. "Diet is the most important, for it acts without cease day and night" (Brillat-Savarin 1999: 196). For him, the reduction of "grains and starches" must be at the center of any weight-loss diet (Brillat-Savarin 1999: 196). The fat man objects: "Here in a single word he forbids us everything we most love, those little white rolls from Limet, and Archard's cakes, and those cookies from. . . ." Yet, Brillat-Savarin is adamant: "Shun anything made with flour . . ., you still have the roast, the salad, the leafy vegetables" (1999: 197). Avoid fad diets, such as the craze for drinking daily a glass of vinegar, which was sweeping the young women at the time and led to dangerous results, including death. The "vinegar cure" has a very long pedigree, going back to humoral medicine. Today, the "Apple Cider Vinegar Diet" has again become a means for weight loss, now as part of a "natural" approach, which also advocates portion control.

Brillat-Savarin, however, also hoped for a quick cure in advocating that a dose of quinine, recently imported, might well be beneficial to weight loss (1999: 199–200). For him, dieting was a neverending challenge, one confronted each day when he sat down to eat. It is to him that we owe our modern fascination with "taste" and the culture of food; but it is to obesity and dieting that he owed his own obsession with both.

SLG

*See also* Byron; Ibn Sina; Medieval Diets

### References and Further Reading
Brillat-Savarin, Jean-Anthelme (1999) *The Physiology of Taste; or, Meditations on Transcendental Gastronomy*, trans. M.F.K. Fisher, Washington, DC: Counterpoint.
Kahn, Henry S. and Williamson, David F. (1994) "Abdominal Obesity and Mortality Risk among Men in Nineteenth-Century North America," *International Journal of Obesity* 18 (10): 686–91.

Krinsky, Alan D. (2001) "Let Them Eat Horsemeat! Science, Philanthropy, State, and the Search for Complete Nutrition in Nineteenth-Century France," Ph.D. dissertation, University of Wisconsin.
MacDonogh, Giles (1992) *Brillat-Savarin: The Judge and His Stomach*, Chicago, Ill.: I.R. Dee.

# Bruch, Hilde (1904–84)

**B**ruch was a German Jewish physician who escaped the Nazis to England and then America and ended her career as Professor of Psychiatry at Baylor Medical School. Her claim to fame is that she popularized the diagnosis of anorexia nervosa and was an often-cited specialist on obesity who revolutionized the debate between those who saw exogenous or endogenous causes for obesity (Heitkamp 1987; Brumberg 1988). She provided the first complex psychological theory of obesity—linking both developmental forces with the external world of the pathological family. Her interest seems to have begun with her arriving in the U.S.A. in 1934, where, according to her own account, she was amazed at the huge number of fat, truly corpulent children, not only in the clinics but also on the street, in the subway and in the schools (Bruch 1957: 5).

Her work on the "psychosomatic aspects of obesity" was funded by the Josiah Macy, Jr. Foundation; the results from this began to appear in the 1940s and were summarized in her 1973 book. She argued that obesity was caused by psychopathological interactions within the family. The core is her view of the child's struggle to develop autonomy in the family setting, a view championed by Theodore Lidz (who created the "schizophrenegenic mother") with whom she had worked in Baltimore between 1941 and 1943. Undergoing a training analysis with Frieda Fromm-Reichmann in Washington at the time, she began to see more complex readings of the work on obesity that had brought her to Fromm-Reichmann's initial attention.

Typical of Bruch's readings of obesity is the case study of a 4½-year-old female child weighing 90 pounds. The child had been accidentally conceived during the war and was initially rejected by the mother (Hilde Bruch 1997: 138). For the mother, "feeding showed love and expiation of guilt" (Hilde Bruch 1997: 140) for rejecting the very idea of bearing the child. The mother is a compulsive fabulator, always embellishing the tales she tells about her daughter's treatments in order to manipulate the physicians. Bruch thus provides obese children with a childhood of rejection that explains their obesity. Now, Bruch's child is female as, following World War I, the exemplary patient in questions of obesity shifts from the male (where it had been since the Ancient Greeks) to the female with the construction of the image of the "New Woman." But this has a special role in Bruch's system. Here, too, it is the mother who is the cause of the obesity. Indeed, the child's obesity is a neurotic response to her mother's "unnatural" rejection of her.

Yet, Bruch's initial work on obesity is little known. In her dissertation of 1928, written under the renowned pediatrician Carl Noeggerath at Freiburg i. Br., she tested the stamina and lung capacity of children with the new instrumentation of the spirometer (Bruch 1928). She traced how their respiration increased with increased work (turning a weighted wheel). One of the children, Maria O., was, according to Bruch, chronically obese, weighing 129 pounds at the age of twelve. She "speaks tiredly and in a monotone, complains about constant tiredness and weakness of memory. There is neither determination nor a joy for work" (Bruch 1928: 10). This case study provides all of the negative images about desire and work and intelligence found in classic images of obese children. But it is also the classic racist image of the nonproductive "fat" Jew that haunts the medical texts of her time.

SLG

See also Jews

### References and Further Reading
Bruch, Hilde (1928) "Gaswechseluntersuchungen über die Erholung nach Arbeit bei einigen gesunden und kranken Kindern [Changes in Blood Gas Levels Following Exercise in Healthy and Ill Children]," Dissertation. (Diss., Freiburg i. Br.). Simultaneously published in the *Jahrbuch für Kinderheilkunde* 121: 7–28.
—— (1957) *The Importance of Overweight*, New York: Norton.
—— (1973) *Eating Disorders*, New York: Norton.
—— (1997) "Obesity in Childhood and Personality Development," *Obesity Research* 5: 157–61. First published 1941.
Bruch, Joanne Hatch (1997) *Unlocking the Golden Cage: An Intimate Biography of Hilde Bruch*, New York: Gurze.
Brumberg, Joan Jacobs (1988) *Fasting Girls: The Emergence of Anorexia Nervosa as a Modern Disease*, Cambridge, Mass.: Harvard University Press.
Heitkamp, Reinhard (1987) "Hilde Bruch (1904–1984): Leben und Werke," Ph.D. dissertation, Cologne University.

# Bulik, Cynthia

Bulik is a clinical psychologist with a specialty in eating disorders based at the University of North Carolina (UNC) at Chapel Hill where she is William R. and Jeanne H. Jordan Distinguished Professor of Eating Disorders, Director of the UNC Eating Disorders program, and a nutrition professor in the School of Public Health. She is well known for her work involving eating disorders. She has won several awards and has the only endowed professorship in eating disorders in the U.S.A. Bulik has been treating and studying eating disorders for the past twenty-four years. She has created two outpatient and inpatient centers for eating disorders both in the U.S.A. and New Zealand.

Bulik's research has focused on twin and molecular genetics, treatment, epidemiology, and laboratory studies on eating disorders. She recently performed a study on genetics and anorexia, which concluded that 56 percent of anorexia nervosa is determined by genetics. Her study involved assessing a large number of twins in order to figure out how great a role genetics plays in anorexia nervosa. Bulik also found that young people who suffer from anxiety and depression are more likely to suffer from anorexia nervosa later in life.

She has written many scientific papers and books on eating disorders. These include: *Eating Disorders: Detection and Treatment* and *Runaway Eating: The 8-Point Plan to Conquer Adult Food and Weight Obsessions*. She also created a CD-ROM called *EMPOWER Solution for Healthy Weight Control*, as well as an internet program called "Food, Fun and Fitness."

SLG/Mary Standen

See also Anorexia; Binge-eating

### References and Further Reading
Bulik, Cynthia M. (1994) *Eating Disorders: Detection and Treatment*, Palmerston North, N.Z.: Dunmore Press.
Bulik, Cynthia M. (2002) "Anxiety, Depression and Eating Disorders," in Christopher G. Fairburn and Kelly D. Brownell (eds), *Eating Disorders and Obesity: A Comprehensive Handbook*, 2nd edn, New York: Guilford Press, pp. 193–98.
Bulik, Cynthia M. and Taylor, Nadine (2005) *Runaway Eating: The 8-Point Plan to Conquer Adult Food and Weight Obsessions*, Emmaus, Pa.: Rodale.

Janelle, Chantelle (2000) "Research Links Anorexia to Genetics." Available online at <http://www.wistv.com/Global/story.asp?S=4592429> (accessed April 11, 2006).

Taylor, Nadine (2005) "The Authors." Available online at <http://www.runawayeating.com/About%20Authors.htm> (accessed March 20, 2006).

The University of North Carolina at Chapel Hill (2006) "Genetics Accounts for More than Half of Anorexia Liability, UNC-Led Study Concludes." Available online at <http://www.sph.unc.edu/news/?fuseaction=press_detail&category=People&subject=events&press_id=29806> (accessed April 19, 2006).

# Butz, Earl (1909–)

Secretary of Agriculture under President Richard Nixon, Butz was a key figure in the lowering of food prices in America, potentially leading to an increase in obesity in Americans. Butz was faced with two problems: (1) falling revenues for farmers and (2) consumers who wanted to lower American food prices which had been rising with inflation. Butz responded by ending restrictions on trade and growing, which led to a domestic corn surplus causing production of a cheaper form of sugar, high-fructose sugar. High-fructose syrup is a liquid sugar produced from cornstarch and is much sweeter than cane sugar. These characteristics matched with manufacturers' needs since they could begin producing less expensive, highly sweetened foods, which could be stored for longer periods as the addition of high-fructose sugar could prevent freezer burn of frozen foods and increase the shelf life of certain foods.

Such foods began to dominate both the soft-drink as well as the fast-food markets. As one critic noted: "The legacy of Earl Butz was that Coca-Cola and Pepsi switched from a 50/50 mix of corn sugar and cane sugar to 100 percent high-fructose corn syrup, enabling them to save 20 per cent costs, boost portion sizes and still make profits" (Critser 2003: 18). In the supermarket, high-calorie foods became even cheaper. "In short, Butz had delivered everything the modern American consumer had wanted. Cheap, abundant and tasty calories had arrived. It was time to eat" (Critser 2003: 19). In addition, Butz arranged with countries such as Malaysia to import palm oil into the U.S.A., also known as "hog's lard" or "tree lard." This heavily saturated, high-calorie oil became a staple of the fast-food industry. The move to cheaper raw materials led consumers to eat cheaper but calorie-dense foods lacking in vitamins and minerals. Recently, some have argued that it was this change in food composition that led to the increase in obesity in the U.S.A. (Critser 2003; Havel 2005; Jurgens et al. 2005).

SLG

## References and Further Reading

Critser, Greg (2003) *Fat Land: How Americans Became the Fattest People in the World*, Boston, Mass.: Houghton Mifflin.

Garner, Lesley (March 2, 2003) "How Americans Became the Fattest People in the World," *The Sunday Mail*. Queensland, Australia.

Havel, P.J. (2005) "Dietary Fructose: Implications for Dysregulation of Energy Homeostasis and Lipid/Carbohydrate Metabolism," *Nutrition Review* 63 (5): 133–57.

Pool, Robert (2001) *Fat: Fighting the Obesity Epidemic*, Oxford: Oxford University Press.

Jurgens H., Haass, W., Castañeda, T., Schürmann, A., Koebnick, C., Dombrowski, F., Otto, B., Nawrocki, A., Scherer, P., Spranger, J., Ristow, M., Joost, H.G., Havel, P.J., and Tschöp, M. (2005) "Consuming Fructose-Sweetened Beverages Increases Body Adiposity in Mice," *Obesity Research* 13: 1146–56.

# Byron, George Gordon Noel, Sixth Baron Byron, a.k.a. Lord Byron (1788–1824)

## British Romantic poet renowned for his prodigious sexual and intellectual appetites

Labeled as "mad, bad and dangerous to know" by embittered ex-lover Lady Caroline Lamb, Byron was also a man preoccupied by his weight. Though the author of *Childe Harold's Pilgrimage* and the *Don Juan* cantos is often portrayed as slender and consumptive, the flesh-and-blood Byron experienced extreme fluctuations in weight throughout his life. In a biography published in 1844, John Cordy Jeafferson warned his public that "readers should be duly mindful of [Byron's] morbid propensity to fatten" (Jeafferson 1883: 69), inadvertently demonstrating that the romantic male ideal of the 1800s was a man possessed of a lean physique. He was, as one writer subsequently noted, "inclined to obesity" (Abeshouse 1965: 13). Jeafferson goes on to speculate that Byron's struggle with his weight was compounded by his "lameness" (he was born with a club foot), which, as another biographer Martin Garrett notes, has also been seen as the root cause of his sexual excess.

By all accounts, Byron worked hard to stay thin. In his early thirties, while traveling and writing poetry in Italy, Byron announced to friends that he was on a claret-and-soda-water diet to help him manage his weight. Indeed, his favorite diet meal consisted of biscuits and soda (Abeshouse 1965: 13). At one point, Byron refused a huge meal set before him and "dined on potatoes sprinkled with vinegar," following one of the fad diets of the time (Abeshouse 1965: 13). He "starved to keep himself thin; then famishing, devoured a heavy meal; then he suffered for it and took overdose of magnesia" for indigestion (Abeshouse 1965: 13). Jeafferson notes that while in Missolonghi in western Greece, Byron "measured himself around wrist and waist and . . . whenever he found these parts, as he thought, enlarged, took a strong dose of medicine" (Garrett 2000: 486). Anecdotes such as these have led biographers like Martin Garrett to claim that Byron had an eating disorder, thus betraying a modern scientific sensibility that subjects changes in body weight to the "gaze" of psychopathology. Yet Byron himself questioned the efficacy of "over-dieting," which he claimed was the "cause of more than half our maladies," through "putting too much oil into the lamp" until "it blazes and burns out" instead of burning "brightly and steadily" (Blessington 1969: 367).

SLG

*See also* Brillat-Savarin

## References and Further Reading

Abeshouse, Benjamin Samuel (1965) *A Medical History of Lord Byron*, Norwich, NY: Eaton Laboratories.

Blessington, Marguerite, Countess of (1969). *Conversations of Lord Byron*. Ed. Ernest James Lovell. Princeton, NJ: Princeton University Press.

Garrett, Martin (2000) *George Gordon, Lord Byron*, New York: Oxford University Press.

Jeafferson, John Cordy (1883) *The Real Lord Byron*, Boston, Mass.: James R. Osgood and Company.

# C

## Cabbage Soup Diet

Cabbage Soup Diet is claimed to be based on a fat-burning soup, low in fat and high in fiber, containing negligible calories (less than 500 if followed exactly). It is part of a longstanding belief that "natural" foods are by definition not only healthful but also health-giving. The diet appeals to most because it is said that the more soup you eat, the more weight is lost. There are no limitations on how much soup one can eat. The diet lasts seven days and is intended for rapid weight loss, usually for a special occasion. People in opposition to the diet suggest that weight loss comes from water weight and muscle tissue and not from fat reserves. In some cases, the diet can be seen as counterproductive if continued for long periods of time or if the body does not feel full. It may force the body into starvation mode, causing metabolism to slow down and hold onto fat. Since the diet is not nutritionally sound, it is not recommended as a long-term weight-loss plan. Although it is unclear where the diet originated, the running myth is that it originated in hospitals for heart patients, but there is no data confirming this, and there have been no medical facilities claiming the diet to be their own.

The seven-day diet plan is as follows:

Day 1: Cabbage soup, plus any fruit (except bananas). Drink unsweetened tea, black coffee, cranberry juice and water.

Day 2: Cabbage soup, plus other vegetables (raw, boiled or steamed) and avoid dry beans, peas and corn. For dinner, eat a baked potato with butter.

Day 3: Cabbage soup, plus other fruits and vegetables (mix of Day 1 and Day 2).

Day 4: Cabbage soup, plus up to eight bananas and fat-free milk.

Day 5: Cabbage soup, plus up to six tomatoes and up to 450 grams of meat or fish.

Day 6: Cabbage soup, plus meat and vegetables.

Day 7: Cabbage soup, plus brown rice, pure fruit juice and vegetables.

SLG/RAKHI PATEL

*See also* Vegetarianism

### References and Further Reading

Anon. "Cabbage Soup Diet information." Available online at <http://www.cabbage-soup-diet.com> (accessed May 2, 2006).

Anon. "Fad Diets." Available online at <http://www.webterrace.com/fad/home.htm> (accessed May 2, 2006).

Anon. (2006) "The Cabbage Soup Diet: Report," April 24, available online at <http://www.weightlossresources.co.uk/logout/news_features/cabbage_soup_diet.htm> (accessed May 2, 2006).

# Callas, Maria (1923–77)

Greek soprano known as *La Divina* to opera lovers the world over for her incredible vocal and stylistic range, Maria Callas was equally famous for her radical physical transformation. Deeply self-conscious about her "large build," Callas went on a strict diet in 1953, at the height of her career, losing a total of 68 pounds in nine months. Her metamorphosis was also part of a changing bodily aesthetic in the world of opera. More and more, thin was in.

Biographer Anne Edwards writes that Callas made the decision to lose weight after a conversation with director Luchino Visconti in which he told her she would make a "truer Traviata, who is after all dying of consumption" (2001: 115) if she lost weight. It was in the period following her weight loss that Callas met and fell in love with Greek shipping magnate Aristotle Onassis. She had become something of a style icon. Although she relished her weight loss and never regained any of it, some biographers suggest that the shock it caused to her system impacted her voice negatively. Michael Scott writes that "a voice reflects a physique" (1991: 111). Scott argues that her voice was most full-bodied when she was at her largest, eventually growing "thin and acidulous" as she slimmed down.

Just as the contemporary trend in Hollywood has been for starlets to slim down, the opera community continues to pressure its sopranos to do the same. More recently, dramatic soprano Deborah Voigt underwent gastric bypass in June 2004. Voigt was dismissed from a Covent Garden production of Strauss's *Ariadne auf Naxos*, because, Voigt claims, she had big hips, of which Covent Garden disapproved. This led her to follow in the path of Maria Callas in an attempt to slim enough to sing Strauss's *Salome* through bariatric surgery.

SLG/SHRUTHI VISSA

*See also* Bariatric Surgery; Celebrities

## References and Further Reading

Edwards, Anne (2001) *Maria Callas: An Intimate Biography*, New York: St. Martin's Press.

Huffington, Arianna (1981) *Maria Callas: The Woman Behind the Legend*, New York: Simon & Schuster.

Jinman, Richard (2006) "Diva Gives in to the Weight of Slender Expectations," *Sydney Morning Herald*, March 30.

Scott, Michael (1991) *Maria Meneghini Callas*, Boston, Mass.: Northeastern University Press.

# Calorie

A calorie is a scientific unit of measurement that describes the amount of energy contained in a substance. As a term, it has had a wide range of meanings. Coined in France in the 1830s, it was adopted into English in the 1870s. In 1870, Thomas Phipson translated a French science text, which noted that,

> The quantity of heat which is called a calorie is . . . the amount required to raise 1 kilogramme of water 1° centigrade . . . In England the . . . calorie is sometimes stated to be the quantity required to raise 1 lb. of water from 60° to 61° Fahr., the equivalent of which in work is 722 foot-pounds.
>
> (Phipson 1870: 43)

As late as LuLu Hunt Peters' *Dieting and Health, With Key to the Calories* (1918), the word was unfamiliar enough to the general public that a pronunciation guide was given ("pronounced Kal′-o-ri").

In terms of dieting, the word "calorie" also refers to the energy contained in food. These two measures are not exactly the same measurement. A calorie of food is actually 1,000 calories or 1 kilocalorie in terms of the way science measures energy. In contemporary culture, calories are used to describe how much energy a particular food contains. This measure can be used to compare one food to another, which has been particularly useful in dieting culture. In order to lose one pound of fat from the body, a dieter would need to consume 3,500 fewer calories in food than she actually burned from daily activities (Stipanuk 2000: 426). People have used this concept to design diets that allow people to lose weight and ultimately change the look of the body. Thus, a "calorie" has come to mean something dangerous to one's health and is the prime focus of dieting.

SLG/SUZANNE JUDD

**References and Further Reading**

Herbert, Victor and Subak-Sharpe, Genell J. (eds) (1995) *Total Nutrition: The Only Guide You'll Ever Need*, New York: St. Martin's Griffin.

Peters, Lulu Hunt (1918) *Diet and Health, with Key to the Calories*, Chicago, Ill.: Reilly and Lee.

Phipson, Thomas L., trans. (1870). Amédée Guillemin. *The Sun*, London: R. Bentley.

Stipanuk, M.H. (2000) *Biochemical and Physiological Aspects of Human Nutrition*, Philadelphia, Pa.: Saunders.

# Cannon, William Bradford, MD (1871–1945)

Cannon graduated from Harvard College in 1896, where he had studied with the psychologist William James and the physiologist Charles B. Davenport (with whom he had published a paper as an undergraduate). He took his MD at Harvard and worked there from 1896 in the laboratory of Henry Pickering Bowditch (1840–1911). Bowditch had recently introduced modern physiological research, developed by the German physiologist and psychologist Wilhelm Wundt, into the U.S.A. In 1902, Cannon became an assistant professor of physiology, and in 1906 he succeeded Bowditch as the George Higginson Professor of Physiology, a position he would hold until 1942.

Under Bowditch, Cannon began to investigate swallowing and stomach motility using the newly discovered X-ray technique. Wilhelm Röntgen had discovered "X-rays" on December 9, 1896; not a year later, Cannon was tracing the passage of a pearl button through the digestive system of a dog using them. Moving to human subjects, he found that he was able to correlate feelings of satiety to physiological responses. In 1911, he coauthored a study with Arthur Lawrence Washburn, which showed that stomach contractions were tied to hunger. Every morning, Washburn, then a medical student, swallowed a length of rubber tubing, to which was tied a condom, and recorded when he felt hungry, as he went about his usual activities. The condom was filled with air, and the tubing attached to a pressure gauge. The pressure gauge recorded the contractions, and Cannon found Washburn's subjective hunger pangs correlated to his stomach contractions. This study would be the most influential study about appetite for fifty years. It was later discovered that there was no causal relationship between these things. They were both caused by a drop in blood glucose levels. Cannon also published one of the earliest dieting articles in the very first issue of the *American Journal of Physiology* in 1898, recounting his research on swallowing and stomach motility.

Cannon's published books include *Bodily Changes in Pain, Hunger, Fear, and Rage* (1915) and *The Wisdom of the Body* (1939). During World War I, he published widely on shock among soldiers and documented the ways in which systems changed in response to shock. He argued strongly for the theory of homeostasis, which explained the self-correction of bodily systems, including hunger and digestion.

SLG

**References and Further Reading**

Cannon, W.B. (1898) "The Movements of the Stomach Studied by Means of the Röntgen Rays," *American Journal of Physiology* 1 (3): 359–82.

—— (1929) *Bodily Changes in Pain, Hunger, Fear, and Rage*, New York and London: D. Appleton & Co.

—— (1939) *The Wisdom of the Body*, New York: W.W. Norton & Company.

Cannon, W.B. and Lieb, C.W. (1911) "The Receptive Relaxation of the Stomach," *American Journal of Physiology* 29 (2): 267–73.

Cannon, W.B. and Moser, A. (1898) "The Movements of the Food in the Esophagus," *Journal of Physiology* 1 (4): 435 –44.

Cannon, W.B. and Washburn, A.L. (1912) "An Explanation of Hunger," *American Journal of Physiology* 29 (5): 441–54.

Cross, Stephen J. and Albury, William R. (1987) "Walter B. Cannon, L.J. Henderson, and the Organic Analogy," *Osiris* 3: 165–92.

# Carpenter, Karen (1950–83)

Member of the brother-sister duo "The Carpenters," Karen Carpenter achieved an iconic status in twentieth-century North American popular culture. Not only was she a Grammy- and Academy Award-winning recording artist, she also embodied a grim message regarding celebrity and the pursuit of thinness. In 1967, Karen Carpenter and her brother Richard Carpenter signed with RCA records, and by 1971, they embarked on their first world tour. The new pressure to maintain a certain public image as a thin celebrity forced Carpenter to reexamine her physical appearance. She believed that although she had talent, she needed to embrace a more feminine image, which at the time was thin and waif-like.

As a child, Carpenter was not overly thin; in fact, her own brother recalled her as a "chubby teenager." As her career threw her further into the spotlight, she began to become obsessed with her weight. She lost 20 pounds after a doctor placed her on a water diet. Not satisfied with the initial weight loss, she used laxatives, thyroid medication, and purging the little food that she ate. The rapid loss of weight weakened Carpenter and eventually led to her collapsing on stage in 1975. She was only twenty-five years old and at the time was down to 80 lbs.

Though the media had already begun to comment that Carpenter looked too thin, her collapse solidified her illness in the public's mind. She took some time off from performing and regained some of the weight that she had lost. However, the years of medications and malnourish-ment had weakened her heart. In 1983, at the age of thirty-three, she died of heart failure. This was both alarming and eye-opening for the public who thought that since she had gained weight, she was healthy again. Her dieting, highly visible weight loss, and dramatic death in 1983 drew anorexia nervosa into popular discourse and shaped the ways in which eating disorders continue to be represented and understood.

Carpenter's death was a major catalyst for the constitution of eating disorders as a public health issue (Brumberg 1988; Young 2006). Rapidly following her death, media coverage boomed and other celebrities "came out" about their eating disorders. This moment marked the dawn of support groups and specialized clinics for eating disorders (Young 2006). With public knowledge and acceptance of the disease anorexia nervosa came funding for treatment and research into the causes of the disease. Carpenter's death came at a time when the after-school special on television could be used to deliver messages to teenagers of the perils of public health issues like smoking, drinking, drug use, and anorexia. Her story was made into a made-for-television movie, entitled *The Karen Carpenter Story* by Joseph Sargent in 1989 with Cynthia Gibb as Karen. The popularity of the film heightened public interest in her story and dramatically increased sales of her albums.

SLG/ANGELA WILLEY

*See also* Anorexia; Celebrities; Cheyne; Developing World; Hornby; Metabolism; Smoking

**References and Further Reading**
Brumberg, Joan Jacobs (1988) *Fasting Girls: The Emergence of Anorexia Nervosa as a Modern Disease*, Cambridge, Mass.: Harvard University Press.
Desjardins, Mary (2004) "The Incredible Shrinking Star:

Todd Haynes and the Case History of Karen Carpenter," *Camera Obscura* 19 (3): 22–55.
Sargent, Joseph (dir.) (1989) *The Karen Carpenter Story*. Central Broadcasting Station (broadcast January 1).
Young, Adena (2006) "Battling Anorexia: The story of Karen Carpenter." Available online at <http://atdpweb.soe.berkeley.edu/quest/Mind&Body/Carpenter.html> (accessed May 9, 2006).

# Celebrities

In American culture today, celebrities are often revered as icons of beauty. A celebrity should be understood as someone who is famous during his or her own lifetime, often famous for being famous. Most contemporary celebrities achieve their fame through acting, singing, modeling careers, or being a wealthy socialite. Moreover, celebrities' bodies have, for over a century, set the tone for the nation in terms of what is in vogue. Celebrities, by definition, are in the public eye and, therefore, can act as spokespeople for various diets and body images, often in relation to their own appearance. While many celebrities advocate svelte bodies, others champion "curvy" bodies as being healthy, natural, and beautiful. Most often, a celebrity uses his or her own body as a billboard of sorts to communicate to the public their personal ideals of beauty.

## Celebrity diets

Because celebrities so often set the standards of beauty around the world, their respective diets are viewed as vehicles to attain such standards. Often individuals who admire a particular celebrity's body will follow the diet they are reported to follow in the hope of achieving a similar figure. Due to the power of their marketing influence, celebrities have served as spokespeople for diets, raising both their own earnings, as well as the earnings of the particular diets. As pop culture's boundaries are spreading to further global limits, the influence of celebrity power is spreading as well, which, in effect, spreads diet culture.

For example, when Kirstie Alley (1951–) first became famous on the television show *Cheers* as the svelte and beautiful Rebecca Howe, no one would have guessed that years later she would balloon to over 200 pounds and become the source of tabloid criticism for weight gain. After Alley's initial weight gain, she hoped to capitalize on it through a comedic television show called *Fat Actress*, in which the main character is loosely based on herself. Alley contacted Jenny Craig and in January 2005, she signed on not only to be their spokeswoman, but also to lose weight in the limelight. Alley gradually and healthfully lost weight through the Jenny Craig plan, successfully promoting the diet as one that works. In Alley's second appearance on *Oprah*, after she had lost 33 pounds on Jenny Craig's diet, she said, "Jenny Craig has been a godsend . . . I needed a game . . . this has been so much fun because they have 8,000 things you can order to eat, and you get your own consultant!"

Another example of celebrity weight loss is Jennifer Aniston (1969–). On the television show *Friends*, Aniston's body transformed from one commonly described as voluptuous to stick-thin right before America's eyes. As the change became ever more apparent to Aniston's fans and the *Friends* viewing audience, questions arose as to how this happened. Both Aniston and her publicist responded that Aniston had started on the Zone Diet, which is based on a food ratio of 40 percent carbohydrates, 30 percent protein, and 30 percent fat (Jegtig 2006). Aniston's changing body has no doubt served as an advertisement for the Zone Diet because Aniston, like most other celebrities, serves as a role model for her fan base. Not only has Aniston popularized the Zone Diet, but she has also popularized the "stick thin" image that has become desired not only by celebrities but by many "average" women as well.

Hollywood culture is also very interested of late in the innovative and obscure diets of celebrities, and Gwyneth Paltrow provides an excellent example. Aside from her pregnancy, there has not been a moment since Gwyneth Paltrow (1975–) hit the Hollywood celebrity scene that she has not been incredibly slender. Paltrow, who is viewed as a fashion icon by many, has publicly spoken about following a strict macrobiotic diet plan in order to keep her figure in tip-top shape (Field 2006). The macrobiotic plan is a diet based on the Chinese cosmological principles of yin and yang and consists primarily of whole grains.

Renee Zellweger (1969–) is another celebrity famous for her weight fluctuations. She is an American actress who won the Oscar in 2004 in the Best Supporting Actress category for her performance in the film *Cold Mountain*. The native Texan is perhaps best known for her recurring role as Bridget Jones, a British everywoman who is self-admittedly "a little bit fat," in *Bridget Jones' Diary* (2001) and its sequel *Bridget Jones: The Edge of Reason* (2004). The first film was based on Helen Fielding's novel. Bridget Jones is a self-deprecating character who is ironic and insecure. She has very little self-confidence and constantly worries about her appearance, specifically her weight. Although Zellweger's performances in the films themselves were worthy of acclaim— she received an Academy Award nomination for the first one—it was the hype surrounding her change in appearance to personify her character that gained the most publicity. The actress gained an excess of 20 pounds in order to look like the "average-sized" Jones. Zellweger claims to have lost the weight via portion control and frequent visits to the gym. Interestingly, she returned to an even more svelte size than her pre-Bridget size four. In the next film she shot, *Chicago* (2002), after the first Bridget Jones movie, she was practically emaciated. Caryn James of the New York Times comments on the absurdity of our culture that Zellweger had to gain weight to be the size of an "average person." James further argues that in regard to Zellweger and her weight, "of course she's not average; she a movie star paid millions to pack it on or lose it" (James 2004).

## Surgery

Gastrointestinal surgery is considered a last resort for those who are severely obese after diet and exercise regimes have failed. According to the U.S. Department of Health and Human Services, gastrointestinal surgery alters the digestive process of the stomach, thereby limiting caloric intake (Connor 2002). In the view of many, celebrities are responsible for the recent popularity of the surgery. Randy Jackson (1956–) and Al Roker, for example, are two celebrities who have publicized their success with gastric-bypass surgery. They, along with shrinking stars, have popularized both general familiarity with the surgery and the procedure itself. In essence, the "no-longer-larger-than-life" (Contreras et al. 2002: 58) act as walking billboards for the operation. In 2003, Jackson, a judge on *American Idol*, underwent the surgery and lost over 100 pounds, and Roker weighed 325 pounds before he underwent gastric-bypass surgery. Roker, in an interview with *U.S.A. Today*, noted that it is just as difficult to overcome an addiction to food as an addiction to alcohol or drugs. Roker cleverly explained that, "you can stop drinking, you can stop sticking a needle in your arm, [but] you cannot not eat" (Johnson 2004). Therefore, it is impossible to avoid the source of addiction completely.

## Eating disorders

Due to the demand for tremendous beauty among celebrities, severe extremes are often sought in order to attain specific beauty standards. Among various celebrities, the pressures to maintain a low weight in Hollywood have led to the occurrence of eating disorders. The scrutiny of weight in Hollywood among celebrities has no doubt transferred onto pop-culture followers. At the same time, celebrities who have publicly spoken about their personal battles with eating disorders have often helped those out of the limelight who suffer.

While many models claim their waif-like bodies are natural and a result of a fast metabolism, current plus-size model Kate Dillon was never part of that crew. As a child, Dillon was always overweight, with the nickname, "Overweight Kate." This all changed starting at age twelve, when Dillon watched a television movie, ironically called, *Kate's Secret*, which, for Dillon, glamorized anorexia (NOVA online). From that point on, until age nineteen, Kate continuously struggled with anorexia. Speaking on behalf of National Eating Disorders Awareness Week at the University of Michigan in 2002, Dillon explained how she felt during her battle with anorexia (when she was a high-fashion model, rather than a plus-size model). Dillon explained that during this time, she was overwhelmed by the images and expectations that she felt media and society held. Dillon also spoke about her reality check, which happened when *Harper's Bazaar* magazine praised her after a fashion show for which she had starved herself for weeks. After consulting a nutritionist, and eventually recovering from anorexia, Dillon was no longer desired as a "skinny" model, but instead as a plus-size model. Dillon has served as a role model to many young girls who are currently battling eating disorders and to those who are recovering and struggling to accept their new bodies and lives.

But eating disorders don't just affect female models and celebrities; men can fall victim to Hollywood pressures to be thin as well. In 1998, the Hollywood bad boy Billy Bob Thornton (1955–) shocked the public when he talked openly for the first time about his battle with anorexia (Ryan 1998). Not only is it unusual for a celebrity to admit to having an eating disorder, but the occurrences of a male celebrity admitting to or having an eating disorder are even more exceptional. Thornton first told *The Los Angeles Daily News*, "Frankly, for a while there, I think had a little mental problem . . . I got anorexic; of course I denied it to my girlfriend [then Laura Dern] and everyone else who said I had an eating disorder." Thornton trimmed down 59 pounds, from 197 to 138, during his battle with anorexia. Thornton public admittance of an eating disorder popularized the notion and reality that men can and do have eating disorders.

Mary-Kate Olsen (1986–) is another member of the "young Hollywood" elite. She is an actress and an entrepreneur along with her twin sister Ashley. The pair made their television debut in infancy on the sitcom *Full House*. As a result of the twins' clothing line, home videos, and other commercial items, they are reportedly worth $150 million each. Due to overall thinness, the public began to question an eating disorder in Mary-Kate. Her publicist made a statement in June 2004 admitting that the actress did indeed have an eating disorder, though declined to comment on which one specifically. Tabloids worldwide cite anorexia as the source of Mary-Kate Olsen's rapid weight loss; however, she has never admitted to this (Thomas 2004).

## Obesity

As in the rest of the world, there exists a double standard in Hollywood regarding beauty ideals. At the turn of the nineteenth century, Lillian Russell, who weighed over 200 pounds, was the reigning sex symbol. However, today a woman of that size is considered unattractive and obese. These categories are not mutually exclusive or inclusive for that matter. Today, men in Hollywood who are by the common standard considered obese are still regarded as sexy. Men like John Goodman (1952–), John Candy (1950–94), and other large male celebrities have been able to maintain roles—as love interests no less—despite their weight. For instance, in the 1990s, *People Magazine* rated Goodman as one of the "sexiest men alive" (Sharma 1996). Writer Dana Gioia observed, "Funny is okay, but what does it say about our culture that at a time when the average American has never been heavier the only part an overweight actor can play is a clown?" (Gioia 1999).

## Rebels against body image

Both Queen Latifah and Kate Winslet have been outspoken in their desires to pursue "natural bodies." While Queen Latifah (1970–) is currently thought of as a strong woman—who is proud of and comfortable with her body size and shape—she has not always been that way. In 1999, in an interview with *Ebony* magazine, Queen Latifah admits that it took her years to accept her body image. The article quoted her saying,

> People look at me now and think, "Wow, there's a full-sized woman who has it together." Puh-lease! It took me years to get to the point where I love my body . . . I hated my breasts. I hated my butt. I even hated the way I walked . . . And although society tells me I'm too big, what I try to keep in my head are the words from Maya Angelou [in her poem "Phenomenal Woman"].

In May 2004, Queen Latifah was featured on the cover of *Glamour* magazine, which typically displays thin actresses. In the interview with her, *Glamour* focused largely on body image. Queen Latifah expressed that she felt satisfied she had been able to portray a different image to young girls who are struggling with their "natural" body types. She has come to represent pro-natural stance on body types, leading a healthy and happy life on her own terms.

Kate Winslet (1975–) is another actress who has often been quoted with championing statements such as, "Obviously I have my fat days and days where I go, 'Oh my God, I've got such floppy boobs and my bum's too big.' But at the same time I would never try to really physically change how I'm built to get more work or different work" (in an interview with U.K. *Elle* in December 2005). She is recognized by the public as beautiful actress, with a "normal" body, a body that can be attained by a "normal" person. In 2003, Winslet fought back against *GQ Magazine*, which digitally altered her body on their cover, presenting her as skinnier and taller. In response to the cover, Winslet stated,

> I don't want people to think I was a hypocrite and had suddenly gone and lost 14 kilos which is something I would never do, and more importantly don't want to look like that. They made my legs look quite a bit thinner. They also made me look about six feet tall, which I'm not, I'm 5′ 6″, and you know I have got muscly legs, me and my sisters and my mum are quite proud of our muscly, strong legs and hips and all the rest of it.

Winslet, like Queen Latifah, serves as a role model to young girls in search of body acceptance.

SLG/Jessica Elyse Rissman and Laura K. Goldstein

*See also* Anorexia; Bariatric Surgery; Craig; Men; Russell; Zone Diet

## References and Further Reading

Alley, Kirstie "Kirstie's Blog," *Jenny Craig, Inc*, available online at <http://www.jennycraig.com/kirstie/012505.asp> (accessed April 26, 2006).

Alley, Kirstie and Winfrey, Oprah "Kirstie Drops the Pounds," *Oprah.com*, available online at <http://www.oprah.com/tows/slide/200505/20050516/slide_20050516_106.jhtml> (accessed April 26, 2006).

Connor, Tracy (2002) "Staple of Celebrity Diets: Stars Put Fat-Fighting Surgery in the Spotlight," *New York Daily News*, November 17, p. 32.

Contreras, Joseph, Noonan, David, and Carmichael, Mary (2002) "The Diet of Last Resort," *Newsweek*, June 10.

Dillon, Kate "Dying to Be Thin: Ask the Experts," *Nova Online*, available online at <http://www.pbs.org/wgbh/nova/thin/ask_d_001215.html> (accessed April 26, 2006).

Field, Melissa "Diets A-Z: Celebrity Diet Secrets." Available online at <http://www.ivillage.co.uk/dietandfitness/wtmngment/diets/articles/0,235_657401,00.html#gwyneth> (accessed April 26, 2006).

Finnigan, Kate (2006) "A New Woman," *Elle* (U.K. edition), January.

Gioia, Dana (1999) "Warner Brothers' Fat Men," *Dana Gioia Online*, available online at <http://www.danagioia.net/essays/efatmen.htm> (accessed April 29, 2006.

Hensley, Dennis (2004) "Long Live the Queen," *Glamour*, May.

James, Caryn (2004) "Gaunt to Gargantuan and Back: The Atkins Method of Acting," *New York Times*, October, p. E1.

Jegtig, Shereen "Jennifer Aniston and the Zone," *About.com Nutrition*, available online at <http://nutrition.about.com/od/celebritydietsandfitness/p/jennifer_anisto.htm> (accessed April 26, 2006).

Johnson, Peter (2004) "The Skinny on Roker's Weight Loss," *U.S.A. Today*, available online at <http://www.usatoday.com/life/columnist/mediamix/2002-11-03-media-mix_x.htm> (April 26, 2006).

Norment, Lynn (1999) "Queen Latifah Has a New TV Show, a New Movie, and New Sass," *Ebony*, November, p. 3.

Raymond, Clare (2005) "How I Got Rid of Fat Jack," *Daily Mirror*, U.K., August 17.

Ryan, Joal (1998) "Billy Bob: I 'Got Anorexic.' " *E! Online News*, available online at <http://www.eonline.com/News/Items/0,1,4047,00.html> (accessed April 26, 2006).

Sharma, Vijai P. (1996) "Be Kind to Overweight People," *Mind Publications*, available online at <http://www.mindpub.com/art227.htm> (April 29, 2006).

Thomas, Karen (2004) "Celebs Haunted by Anorexia," *U.S.A. Today*, available online at <http://www.usatoday.com/life/people/2004-06-22-anorexia-rumors_x.htm> (accessed April 26, 2006).

U.S. Department of Health and Human Services (2004) "Gastrointestinal Surgery for Severe Obesity," *National Institutes of Health Publication*, No. 04–4006, available online at <http://win.niddk.nih.gov/

publications/gastric.htm#howdoes> (accessed April 26, 2006).

Winfrey, Oprah (2004) "Incredible Transformations," *The Oprah Winfrey Show* (broadcast January 12).

# Cheyne, George (1672–1743)

English physician and diet therapist, personal physician and friend to Samuel Richardson, and the author of *An Essay on Health and Long Life* (1724). George Cheyne's autobiography is appended not to his book on longevity but also notably to his 1733 handbook, *The English Malady, or, a Treatise of nervous diseases of all kinds, as Spleen, Vapours, Lowness of Spirits, Hypochondrical, and Hysterical Distempers* (1733). Life experience becomes the basis for his claim to the authenticity of his understanding of how to cure the obese body. But it is also vital to realize that the portrayal of Cheyne's body evoked in his autobiography is the caricature of the fat man, such as Trulliber in Henry Fielding's parody of the novel of female sensibility, *Joseph Andrews* (1742):

> he was indeed one of the largest Men you should see, and could have acted the Part of Sir John Falstaff without stuffing. Add to this, that the Rotundity of his Belly was considerably increased by the shortness of his Stature, his Shadow ascending very near as far as in height when he lay on his back, as when he stood on his legs.
>
> (Fielding 1987: 127)

In this depiction, the fat man is a comic character, a figure larger than life who can exist only on the stage or in the comic novel. Cheyne was described by Alexander Pope in 1739 in a letter to their mutual friend Lord Lyttelton as "a Perfect Falstaff" (Macmichael 1828: 56–7).

Cheyne, born in Scotland in 1673, studied medicine in Edinburgh and established himself in London by the beginning of the eighteenth century as one of the most successful (and interesting) figures on the medical scene (Guerrini 2000). Wracked with self-doubt after a number of his books were either ignored or attacked, he had a massive breakdown at the age of forty-two. The cause of the ailments is clear in Cheyne's account. While he came from healthy parents, one side of his family was corpulent. He himself was not as a child, because he lived the life of the mind "in great Temperance" (Cheyne 1733: 325). His predisposition to fat, he states, was triggered when he moved to London, where he fell into the company of "Rottle-Companions, the younger Gentry, and Free-Livers" (Cheyne 1733: 325). The sole purpose of this companionship was to eat and drink. Taken up by them, Cheyne "grew daily in Bulk," and, after a few years, he grew "excessively fat, short-breathed, Lethargic and Listless" (Cheyne 1733: 326). He then began to suffer from a series of illnesses, each of which more difficult than the last to cure. Fits followed fever. As he became more and more ill, his friends abandoned him, "leaving me to pass the melancholy Moments with my own Apprehensions and Remorse" (Cheyne 1733: 326). Such friendship, founded on "sensual pleasures and mere Jollity," were false, as they were not rooted in "Virtue and in Conformity to the Divine Order" (Cheyne 1733: 328).

Forced to retire to the country, Cheyne began to diet, stripping his daily food down to the barest, and he "melted away like a Snow-ball in Summer." He became an adept of the growing craze for vegetarianism, ascribing his new health to a diet of milk, fruit, roots, and seeds. In many ways, he was the first celebrity "diet doc." But Cheyne also claims this was easier for him as he had been led astray rather than having given himself into the vices of London society. He was able to cure himself because he remained an outsider to the "Vices and Infidelity" that were the modern, urban world. In this, Cheyne sees society as the cause for his ailments, and the countryside and the acknowledgment of "natural Religion" (Cheyne 1733: 331) as the cure. Cheyne's image of the country as the refuge from a life of dissipation and the place where the obese, ill body could be reconstituted as a healthy, male body is a reflection on the newly emerging belief that the ideal state of nature is the only place where healthy, thin, and beautiful bodies exist.

Cheyne's cure was not limited to the countryside, but he also attempted to be cured by waters at Bath and at Bristol (Cheyne 1733: 334). He dieted, and he regularly vomited and purged—and he lost weight. And yet, he continued to have illness after illness. He finally went onto a "milk diet" suggested by one of his physicians who had used it himself. No alcohol in any form, no meats, only milk, and the physician claimed that he could play six hours of cricket without tiring. Cheyne reduced his meat and alcohol intake, adding vegetables, seeds, bread, "mealy roots, and fruit" (Cheyne 1733: 337). And the weight continued to come off. He became "Lank, Fleet and Nimble" (Cheyne 1733: 338). Riding 10 to 15 miles a day, he felt he was fit, even though he continued to purge and vomit. He suddenly felt that he could add some meat, chicken, and a few stronger liquors. He also stopped exercising and soon became very ill again. He then returned to his diet for twenty years and continued "sober, moderate and plain" (Cheyne 1733: 342). And yet, over time, he fell into the habit of adding more and more foods, alcohol, meat, nuts; his weight returned and he again became "enormous": "I was ready to faint away, for want to Breath, and my Face turn'd Black." Upon trying to walk up a flight of stairs, he was "seiz'd with a Convulsive Asthma" (Cheyne 1733: 342). His body was covered in ulcers, and he began to suffer from gout. The pain forced him back on his milk diet. He suffered from "Sickness, Reaching, Lowness, Watchfullness, Eructation, and Melancholy" (Cheyne 1733: 346). His mental state was as bad as his physical one.

Yet, all along he continued to practice as a physician: "I attended indeed (in a manner) the Business of my profession, and took Air and Exercise regularly in the Daytime; but in such a wretched, dying Condition as was evident to all that saw me" (Cheyne 1733: 348). He was persuaded to return to London at the end of 1725 where he then met with his medical friends who were not the dandies that had abandoned him. He tried to return to the earlier diet, but was suddenly aware that the flexibility of youth had diminished and that he had to be ever more watchful and vigilant in his present state (Cheyne 1733: 350). This meant no meat, little alcohol, and a modicum of medicinal port. While a healthy diet, it is only one that one comes to in extremity: "no one will ever be brought to such a Regimen as mine is now, without having been first extremely Miserable; and I think Com-

mon Life, with temperance, is best for the Generality, else it would not be Common" (Cheyne 1733: 353). What he ate is familiar to us from Cornaro: "the Simplicity of the Alimentary Gospel." He avoided "onions and garlick" (Cheyne 1733: 355). Still, he continued to suffer from flatulence and eruction—belching—for a time. But he became fit, able to "be abroad in all Weathers, Seasons or Times of the Year, day or Night, without much Dread or Hazard of Cold" (Cheyne 1733: 358). More importantly, when he had a carriage accident and was knocked unconscious, he was able to recover, according to him, because of the new state of his health (361). Dieting preserves life in all cases and makes one a better and more moral human being. Cheyne's powerful view that only vegetarianism furthers the sensitive nature of man became part of the image of the vegetarian. Jean-Jacques Rousseau was to argue, using a Cheynian view, that the English were "cruel and ferocious" because of the "roast beef" (Guerrini 1999: 38 and Stuart 2006: 234).

SLG

*See also* Cornaro; Vegetarianism

## References and Further Reading

Cheyne, George (1724) *An Essay on Health and Long Life*, London: George Strahan.

Cheyne, George (1733) *The English Malady, or, a Treatise of Nervous Diseases of All Kinds, as Spleen, Vapours, Lowness of Spirits, Hypochondrical, and Hysterical Distempers*, London: G. Strahan.

Fielding, Henry (1987) *Joseph Andrews*, ed. H. Goldberg, New York: Norton.

Guerrini, Anita (1999) "A Diet for a Sensitive Soul: Vegetarianism in Eighteenth-Century Britain," *Eighteenth-Century Life* 23 (2): 34–42.

—— (2002) *Obesity and Depression in the Enlightenment: The Life and Times of George Cheyne*, Norman, Okla.: University of Oklahoma Press.

Macmichael, William (1828) *The Golden-Headed Cane*, London: John Murray.

Stuart, Tristram (2006) *The Bloodless Revolution: Radical Vegetarianism and the Discovery of India*, New York: HarperCollins.

# Children

Children seem to be in a precarious position in the contemporary global dieting culture. Threatened with rising rates of obesity and related diseases (Wilfley and Saelens 2002), young people, from toddlers to teens, must wrestle with body image in a culture that worships slenderness. Much is being done in schools and homes to reduce obesity numbers in children (Goldfield and Epstein 1995: 573–7); however, the preoccupation with preventing overweight may distract parents and doctors from the equally important problems of body-image disturbance and dieting behaviors in children and adolescents.

While dieting and disordered eating are generally thought to emerge during adolescence, studies show the onset of dieting behaviors can be found in preadolescent children (Truby and Paxton 2002). A study in 2000 of body dissatisfaction amongst third- to sixth-grade children using interviews and questionnaires found that 50 percent of them wanted to lose weight (Schur et al. 2000: 74).

In addition, interviews with eight-year-old girls have revealed a concern about weight gain and a desire to be thin, while similar interviews with five-year-old boys revealed that they were aware of body size and desired a muscular body type (Grogan 1999: 119–20; Harris 1997: 15). Finally, studies reveal that even second-grade boys and girls report preoccupation with food and dieting (Cherene et al. 1999). Taken together, the results from these body-image satisfaction studies show that, without a doubt, awareness of (gendered) expectations for body size develops early and frequently results in dissatisfaction.

Children do not, however, only internalize adult body standards. They also develop a fairly sophisticated awareness of the imperative to diet and methods of losing weight prior to adolescence. Schur et al. (2000) found that, out of sixty-two elementary school students surveyed, 16 percent reported having attempted to lose weight. Perhaps even more surprisingly, the study indicated that 42 percent of boys surveyed had attempted to either lose or gain weight through dieting methods. Clearly, onset of dieting and eating disordered behavior may precede adolescence and affect young children.

In the study by Schur et al., children who dieted in order to lose or gain weight expressed diverse motivations, including being teased, feeling pressure from family, feeling embarrassed about their weight, and having a desire to look "better," improve sports abilities, and "be healthier" (Schur et al. 2000). However, popular culture, specifically diet commercials and diet-related teen magazines, have also been implicated in dieting and eating disordered behavior in adolescents. In the Schur study, 55 percent of children reported learning about dieting from the media, and several children actually cited specific commercials for weight-loss products, like Jenny Craig and Slim Fast. A 2003 study also found that "girls who read magazine articles about dieting and weight loss are more likely to engage in weight control behaviors" (Field 2003: 906).

Adult-like body dissatisfaction and dieting behaviors can be measured in children as young as five to seven, and the methods that children use to diet may also resemble adult dieting practices. Schur et al. also found that, while children do not generally conceive of dieting in terms of caloric restriction, they did define dieting as "eating less" and exercising more, and some even mentioned the use of diet pills as a method of weight loss (Schur et al. 2000).

The early onset of dieting in school-age children has various consequences, including unanticipated weight gain and the development of eating disorders. A 2003 study published in the classic journal of childhood medicine *Pediatrics* demonstrated that dieting in childhood may be predictive of weight gain during three years of follow-up. Reasons for potential weight gain were cited as changes in metabolic rate and dietary attrition (Field 2003).

While weight gain in children is certainly a concern in the context of a growing obesity epidemic, perhaps of more concern is the possible link between the early onset of dieting and the development of eating disorders in children and adolescents. A 1987 study of bulimia and binge-eating behavior in school-age populations found that, of 126 school children surveyed, 53 percent reported engaging in some form of binge behavior. While not directly linked to dieting behaviors, the prevalence of binge-eating was found to be closely associated with "unwanted thoughts about food" (Lakin and McClellan 1987). The "predominance of young people at risk for bulimic behavior" was also found to be high in a 1999 study of unhealthy eating behaviors in adolescents (Martín 1999). Studies have also shown that rates of anorexia amongst preadolescent girls have been increasing every decade since the 1950s (Inoko 2005; Emans 2000; American Academy of Pediatrics 2003). These studies and others demonstrate that even young children in a dieting culture are susceptible to eating disorders, such as anorexia, bulimia, and binge-eating disorder.

Children have become one of the main focuses of diet culture, yet they are often the main targets of "junk-food" marketing. Foods such as Kraft's Macaroni and Cheese, Dunkaroos, Gushers, Fruit by the Foot, and Chex Mix have little if any nutritional benefits, yet are nevertheless marketed to children, who need proper nutrients in order to grow. Because "junk-food" marketing has made these specific foods so exciting and appealing to children, there is no wonder that children are one of the groups who are subjected to the diet culture.

Pressures of the dieting culture have extended and heightened for children in recent years as obesity has come to be seen as a growing problem for children. One of the main concerns about obesity in children is that obese children are at substantial risk for remaining obese throughout their lives (Kolata 1986). At the National Institute of Child Health and Human Development, participants advocated that physicians should "intervene," and attempt to control this problem among their patients. In the past, it has been argued that fat children outgrow their obesity, but due to the rising rate of obesity in children and adults, this idea has recently been countered. Leonard Epstein of the Western Psychiatric Institute and Clinic in Pittsburgh notes that 40 percent of children who are obese at age seven become obese adults (Goldfield and Epstein 1995: 577), and 70 percent of obese adolescents become obese adults. There have been various hypotheses as to why the childhood obesity rate has been rising. William Dietz of the New England Medical Center Hospitals in Boston feels that, "Children eat more while they are watching TV and they eat more of the foods advertised on TV. The message that TV conveys is that you will be thin no matter what you eat. Nearly everyone on television is thin" (Dietz 2002). This message is obviously false. In addition to the marketing effects of television, it also causes inactivity among children, as they give up outside activity for inside sitting.

Obesity among children is by no means random. Fat parents tend to have fat children, not only because they set an example of poor eating habits to their children but also because of genetic predisposition. Focusing more on the behavioral aspect of obesity, more research has been

suggesting that children are also strongly influenced by their parents' attitudes to being overweight and their approaches to dieting (McAllister 2006). Many health authorities recommend that parents, teachers, and other influential adults set a pattern and example for healthy eating habits during childhood. With increasing independence, older children eat more meals out of the home, therefore reducing the effect of the household on the child. In order to positively affect health and nutrition of children, nutritional education should be targeted toward mothers with young children and toward school-age children who make their own eating choices (Variyam et al. 1999).

The obesity problem among children is being examined outside of the U.S.A. In the U.K., in particular in Hull, which is the country's most obese city, a slimming club has started for children. The club, Slimming World, invites children from eleven and up to attend weekly classes which will help them lose weight. Director Clare White stated, "It's not about dieting, it's about healthy eating and education" (Bingham 2005). Schoolchildren in Hull are given one piece of free fruit each day to help promote a healthy diet and to contend obesity.

Schools around the world are making changes in their lunch programs and vending machines in the hope of promoting healthier eating habits among their student body. While this movement within schools is quite recent, there has been speculation for years that healthy diet leads to better performance in school. A study of the diet and health of schoolchildren in South Carolina over fifty years ago showed those with better diets to be superior in health, in posture, and in scholastic progress (Everitt 1952). While posture is no longer a main concern in the twenty-first century, health and scholastic progress certainly are.

For this reason, celebrity chef Jamie Oliver began something of a revolution in various London schools in 2004. Oliver had taken on the challenge of going into schools and swapping the usual unhealthy foods with healthful, and tasty foods. His ideas, struggles, and successes have created another successful television show for Oliver. Oliver's campaign, Feed Me Better, was launched on the Internet. Within weeks of the television airings and site creation, people all over England were sharing Oliver's disgust with the lack of quality and nutrition in the food being served at schools for lunch and dinner. The revolution Oliver started became the talk of the nation. Unlike earlier Europeanwide attempts to change the politics of school lunches, Oliver's approach paid off, as British Prime Minister, Tony Blair, announced that the Government would take immediate action over school meals by upping the per pupil cost from 37 pence (70 cents) to 50 pence (95 cents) (Young 2003).

An analogous approach to reform the eating habits of children was undertaken by Arthur Agatson, the creator of the "South Beach Diet," a version of the low-carbohydrate diet, in 2004. Using the Osceola County (Florida) school district as his "laboratory," he created HOPS (Healthier Options for Public School Children). Working on the assumption that a change in diet would impact the short- and long-term health of the child, Agatson created gardens to show children how food was grown and to encourage them to eat "fresh." They included nutritional information in other classes, such as math or social sciences, so that it became a general topic of conversation. Most importantly, HOPS provided the cost difference between the school district's food budget and the increased budget for healthier foods. Thus, white bread was replaced by whole-grain bread; "Tater tots" by sweet-potato fries. While the program was successful in changing the eating patterns of most children, there seems to be little evidence that such changes actually reduce "obesity," which was the public health rationale for such undertaking (Belkin 2006).

Children's nutrition has become a concern all over the world. While it is important not to place weight pressures on children, because they can lead to several psychological and emotional problems, it is just as important at the same time for healthful eating to be part of a child's daily routine. In order to change the obesity and weight-related health problems, changes need to be made among children. Overweight children today may well lead to overweight adults tomorrow.

SLG/C. Melissa Anderson/Laura K. Goldstein

*See also* Advertising; Anorexia; Binge-eating; Craig; Epidemic; Genetics; Media; Men

## References and Further Reading

American Academy of Pediatrics (2003) "Identifying and Treating Eating Disorders," *Pediatrics* 111 (1): 204–11.

Belkin, Lise (2006) "The School-Lunch Test," *New York Times Magazine* August 20: 30–5; 48; 52–5.

Bingham, L. (2005) "Never Too Young to Start Slimming," *Hull Daily Mail* December 30, p. 4.

Cherene, Kelly, Ricciardelli, Lina A. and Clarke, John D.

(1999) "Problem Eating Attitudes and Behaviors in Young Children," *International Journal of Eating Disorders* 25 (3): 281–6.

Dietz, William (2002) "An Interview with William Dietz." Available online at <http://www.esi-topics.com/obesity/interviews/DrWilliamDietz.html> (accessed June 1, 2007).

Emans, S.J. (2000) "Eating Disorders in Adolescent Girls," *Pediatrics International* 42 (1): 1–7.

Everitt, Viola (1952) "Food Habits and Well-Being of School Children," *The Elementary School Journal* 52 (6): 344–50.

Field, Alison E. (2003) "Relation between Dieting and Weight Change among Preadolescents and Adolescents," *Pediatrics* 112 (4): 900–6.

Goldfield, Gary S., and Epstein, Leonard H. (1995) "Management of Obesity in Children," in Kelly D. Brownell and Christopher G. Fairburn (eds), *Eating Disorders and Obesity: A Comprehensive Handbook*, New York: Guilford Press, pp. 573–7.

Grogan, Sarah (1999) *Body Image: Understanding Body Dissatisfaction in Men, Women, and Children*, London: Routledge.

Harris, Tracy A. (1997) *Eating and Dieting Attitudes of Elementary School Children*, Fayetteville, Ark.: University of Arkansas.

Inoko, Kayo (2005) "Effect of Medical Treatments on Psychiatric Symptoms in Children with Anorexia Nervosa," *Pediatrics International* 47 (3): 326–8.

Kolata, Gina (1986) "Obese Children: A Growing Problem," *Science* 232 (4746): 20–1.

Lakin, Jean A., and McClellan, Eleanor (1987) "Binge Eating and Bulimic Behaviors in a School-Age Population," *Journal of Community Health Nursing* 4 (3): 153–64.

McAllister, Rallie (2006) "Mom's Diet Impacts Kids: We Innocently Deliver a Running Commentary About Our Weight, Our Waistlines and Our Lack of Willpower," *The Buffalo News*, April 3: C3.

Martín, Amelia Rodríguez (1999) "Unhealthy Eating Behavior in Adolescents," *European Journal of Epidemiology* 15 (7): 643–8.

Oliver, Jamie (2005) "How It Happened. Feed Me Better." Available online at <http://www.jamieoliver.com/schooldinners> (accessed March 22, 2007).

Schur, Ellen A., Sanders, Mary and Steiner, Hans (2000) "Body Dissatisfaction and Dieting in Young

Children," *International Journal of Eating Disorders* 27 (1): 74–82.

Truby, Helen, and Paxton, Susan J. (2002) "Development of The Children's Body Image Scale," *British Journal of Clinical Psychology* 41 (2): 185–203.

Variyam, Jayachandran, Blaylock, N. James, Lin, Biing-Hwan, Ralston, Katherine and Smallwood, David (1999) "Mother's Nutrition Knowledge and Children's Dietary Intakes," *American Journal of*

*Agricultural Economics* 81 (2): 373–84.

Wilfley, Denise E. and Saelens, Brian E. (2002) "Epidemiology and Causes of Obesity in Children," in Christopher G. Fairburn and Kelly D. Brownell (eds), *Eating Disorders and Obesity: A Comprehensive Handbook*, 2nd edn, New York: Guilford Press, pp. 429–32.

Young, Ian (2003) *Eating at School: Making Healthy Choices*, Strasbourg: Council of Europe Publishing.

# China in the early twentieth century

In early twentieth-century China, there was a popular fascination with diet, perhaps as a result of the images of "famine" that marked Western and Chinese views of the pathological body in the nineteenth century (Edgerton 2002; Mallory 1926). Indeed, when you systematically read the standard "Western" medical journal published in China, the *China Medical Journal*, from the beginning of the twentieth century to the Japanese invasion of China, the central medical discourse concerning "diet" and the body is that of famine and starvation. In a 1912 article in the *China Medical Journal*, the physicians of the Chinese Medical Missionary Association are concerned that the food made available in their hospitals has sufficient protein and fat, to the extent that they advocate "crossing foreign and native cows," or the introduction of canned milk to improve the local diet. That diet seems to be regionally differentiated. One physician notes that the "rich have rice, vegetables, and meats. The poor have rice, vegetables, and substitutes for meat." It is only "when floods overtake the people year in and year out that so many are driven to our doors for charity" (Stone 1912: 299). It is the distribution of foods that seem to be at the heart of famine from the standpoint of the physicians. In this rather contemporary view, it is the poor distribution network that causes famine (Read 1921). Amartya Sen's 1981 *Poverty and Famines: An Essay on Entitlement and Deprivation* argues that famine occurs not from a lack of food, but from inequalities built into mechanisms for distributing food (Sen 1981). But there is

also some suspicion that the indigenous foods may not be "suitable" enough to maintain a healthy diet (Embrey and Wang 1921). Though the soybean is proposed over and over again as an adequate substitute for other forms of protein in the form of local foods such as "Toh fu" (Adolph and Kiang 1920; Adolph 1923), when the concern is starvation, the sense is that "Western" cures, such as a rich, milk-based diet are most appropriate. The physicians see the child as most at risk from the effects of famine. They are at risk both in terms of their mortality and morbidity as well as their social status. The selling of children is seen as a major result of the famine culture of China (Dow 1922). "Cannot the famine relief associations . . . take this matter into consideration and put an end to it," writes one irate physician (Sargent 1920). In all of the myriad concerns about the pathological effects of the "Oriental" diet, not a single word is spent on the dangers or effects of obesity.

Yet, the concern with obesity appears in Chinese popular magazines, where it is already seen as a response to the past and contemporary, allopathic medicine view of China as a famine culture (Beahan 1975; Nivard 1986). This is not to say that there has not been a constant and intense concern with the "immoderate body" in the medical and dietetic literature of traditional Chinese medicine. In the sixteenth century, Li Shizhen (1518–93) wrote in his *Bencai gangmu* (*Systematic Materia Medica*) that the consumption of fresh crabs was healthy "in small quantities," but "gluttons will consume a dozen or more at a sitting together with various kinds of meat and other foods. They eat and drink twice as much as they need . . . then blame [their upset stomachs on] the crabs. But why blame the crabs?" (Lo and Barrett 2005: 417). The culture of excess in the world of traditional Chinese medicine became a hallmark of the degenerate Chinese body in need of regeneration by the early twentieth century.

Immediately before the revolution that overthrew the Qing dynasty on October 10, 1911, the word "reform" was everywhere, and a new fantasy of the body had begun to emerge in China. Obesity came to be viewed as one of the signs of the degenerate Chinese body, a body clearly in need of reform. Following the model of "regeneration" that captured most of the ideologies of the day (from Zionism to Marxism to social Darwinism to colonialism), obesity defined the ability of the society to reform the individual. In one of the most widely read columns "Ziyoutan" (Unfettered Talk) in the renowned newspaper *Shenbao*, the author Wang Dungen explored the reform of the body. He was a well-known writer who was a key figure in the "Mandarin Ducks and Butterflies School," attacked by the May Fourth progressive writers in the late 1910s and early 1920s, and in 1914 created the comic journal *Saturday*. In this comic essay, "Reforming the Human Body," Wang Dungen envisions a grotesque ideal of the "new" body. He imagines a body with newly configured mouth, tongue, ear, eyes, nose, skin, eyebrows, hair, teeth, neck, shoulders, arm, hands, fingers, and feet. He sees it as having hundreds of mouths so that a person can eat more and still be able to talk (Wang Dungen 1911). This is an ironic response to the starved body, which desires a reform that can consume more. "Western" models of regeneration, such as structured physical exercise, become the means of reforming the too fat body. Such an approach was advocated by the leader of the New Cultural Movement, Chen Duxiu, and in 1917 Mao Zedong published a full-scale manual of physical activity to reform the body (Mao Zedong 1992).

By 1913, the classical Chinese medical literature on obesity was beginning to be summarized for an intellectual readership in China. The essay "On Obesity," by Shuhui and Weiseng, was written in classical Chinese for a leading women's magazine. Such magazines arose to shape and be shaped by the images of the so-called New Woman (*xin nuxing*) and Westernized Modern Girl (*modeng nulang*) who came into prominence in the first decade of the twentieth century in China as well as in the West. They were defined in many ways, and to no little extent by their "thin" body form. The essay presents the argument that obesity is an illness that women must not take lightly (Shuhui and Weiseng 1913). The authors refer to male figures and texts from ancient China, such as a man named "Zilong" who lived in the warring-state period. Zilong felt he was too fat, so he took *Phragmites communis Trirn* (a traditional medicine) to lose weight. The authors use this example to prove that obesity is an illness treatable by medical intervention even in the premodern period. One source they mention is *Hanshu* (*The History of the Former Han Dynasty*) written by the historian Bangu. They argue that according to Hanshu, too much body fat is the cause of obesity. But there are two kinds of obesity: one is obesity with too many blood cells and the other not enough blood cells. The causes the former are (1) not eating appropriately; (2) not having a balanced life style; and (3) not enough sex. Not eating appropriately means that one eats too many foods such as flour, sugar, and alcohol that contain water. Obesity of the second type is caused by external injury, overworking, stress, or sometimes after giving birth.

As with the Western literature of the late nineteenth century, there are stages of obesity. For the authors, obesity has three phases. Initially, when the person looks acceptably plump, this indicates prosperity and others admire him; then he looks overtly obese and funny; and finally, he is in danger and others take pity on him. This final stage of obesity presents with symptoms including sweating, fatigue, backache, heart disease, sexual incompetence, etc. The "cure" for obesity is a balanced eating and lifestyle: Avoid eating things that contain too much fat; don't sleep more than eight hours; take a warm bath two or three times a week; walk two or three hours everyday; and be persistent. In terms of medication, one should take either traditional medication such as wodu or, better yet, thyroid tablets. The later are the classical pharmaceutical intervention which certainly can reduce weight by making the individual hyperthyroidic, increasing basal metabolism. This will lead to weight loss but can lead to a wide range of other pathological symptoms, such as Grave's disease, with its physiological and psychological symptoms.

The modern creeps into this world of classical Chinese view on the obese with the suggestion of treating it as an endocrinological deficiency, one of the most up-to-date views in early twentieth-century medicine. The obese body is the antithesis of the beautiful and healthy body. And this is a special problem for contemporary women.

In an essay "Keep the Body Slim," published in a women's magazine in 1922, the author, Daizuo, stresses that people with obesity are not beautiful, especially women: "A person who is too fat looks very ugly. Women especially can't be fat. If a woman gains too much weight and became fatty, where can one find her beauty?" (Daizuo 1922). In addition, obesity is an important medical problem. Obesity is seen as the result of faulty metabolism, the result of hormone imbalance. Yet, obesity is not a random occurrence, as some people are more at risk: Specifically, people who eat rich and abundant food, people who are not physically active, people with a family inheritance of obesity and alcoholics.

Obesity is dangerous as it leads to heart disease. People with obesity have shortness of breath and rapid heartbeats even after walking a few steps. They are more likely to have stroke. People with obesity have urinary and kidney problems. Dieting is, again, the solution. One should not overeat; one should avoid foods that contain too much fat; and one should eat less meat. Other suggestions the essay gives for weight loss are physical exercises, the use of laxatives, and electric steam therapy to reduce body fat, which, according to the essay, is very popular abroad. Electrotherapy was a standard late-nineteenth-century Western treatment for the "failure or perversion of nutrition," including diabetes (Hedley 1921: 209–20).

It is clearly women who are the target of the growing anti-obesity anxiety of Republican China. In one essay, the author, Zhou Zhenyu, states that he is a doctor who often has female patients who need help to lose weight (Zhenyu 1926). Zhou Zhenyu comments

> when I was a doctor in Beiping, I often had women patients come asking for the method of losing weight. I would tell them the method, some of them went home and practiced following my suggestions, others would come visit again and want medication. The effects differ because the causes of their obesity vary.
>
> (Zhenyu 1926)

"The cause and danger of female obesity" is seen either in overindulgence and the absence of exercise or imbalance of hormones. This is the classic argument about obesity that dominated the late-nineteenth-century discussion of the causes of obesity. By 1924, the editors of the *Journal of the American Medical Association* published an editorial entitled "What Causes Obesity?" In it they argue, following a powerful antipsychological strand in obesity research that began in the late nineteenth century, for its etiology in malfunctions of normal metabolic processes. Seeing obesity as a "scientific problem," they write, will free the "fat woman" from the stigma that she "has the remedy in her own hands—or rather between her own teeth" (Anon. "What Causes Obesity?"). That new object of scientific interest is the fat woman, who had been charged with carrying "that extra weight about with her unless she so wills" (Anon. "What Causes Obesity?"). Women, not "men" or "people" are at risk from obesity, a far cry from the evocation of Falstaff as the exemplary sufferer from obesity in the mid-nineteenth century. According to the anonymous Chinese physician in 1922, although fat people usually eat less than thin people, they do not burn enough calories. There are still large amounts of fat accumulated and stored in their body. While the obese do not eat much every meal, they snack often. Women specifically can suffer from hypothyroidism, hypopituitarism, or a loss of estrogen. Pregnant women are especially at risk. One woman, after giving birth, had to get up and eat every night. She quickly gained weight and became obese.

The danger of female obesity is the collapse of one's health and thus one's ability to bear children. This remains the classic definition of women's health. Obese women have compromised immune systems, are likely to catch cold and coughs, which lead to tuberculosis. They have heart disease. There is danger to their nervous systems. The obese are usually slow and lazy, but often they laugh and seem happy. Obese women have problems conceiving, have problems when having sex, and are likely to have miscarriages.

By 1941, as the war raged and famine haunted China, a public discourse on obesity remained part of the popular register of the changes of Chinese attitudes toward the body. They come to be labeled as a "tragedy at the dinner table" (Qihui 1941). The essay with this title seems to be a free adaptation of a number of foreign medical and popular articles, especially American ones. It presents the harm of overeating and its pathological consequences. The author identifies middle-aged people as being most at risk, because they seem to be more easily taken by the desire for fine eating. The essay defines pathology by quoting a saying attributed to an American congressman: "fifty, fifty, fifty," which means if a 50-year-old person is 50 pounds overweight, his life span will be reduced 50 percent. The author also quotes statistics by an American doctor that out of 2,000 cases of sudden death, 90 percent of people died of heart disease. "Most of them eat too much, are overweight, which causes heart disease." While other foreign cases of overeating are mentioned, such as the ancient Romans, the American Thanksgiving is picked out as a moment of public gluttony:

> Around Thanksgiving time, there are often a few cases of death caused by overeating in the mortuary. People in charge of postmortem examinations are often busy rushing to luxurious banquets to do their work. It's also quite dangerous to eat too much after fasting. One should definitely divide all the nice dishes into several meals, and never eat everything up at once. It is nice to be able to enjoy a full table of luxurious food, but one should remember not to gamble with one's own life. Otherwise, tragedy would take place in the holiday season, and one would sadly fall into the bosom of the death.
>
> (Qihui 1941)

The result of such gluttony is death, through sudden death, chronic heart disease or diabetes. A litany of diseases is the result of obesity: High blood pressure, lung disease, cancer, even suicide and accidental death. For, according to the author, people with obesity often have psychological problems and are very slow in reacting to what is going on—thus, they are susceptible to accidents. The overweight should consult qualified doctors to decide his or her individual diet. Yet, the "cure" proposed in the essay of 1941 is to pay minute attention to what and how much one eats. The formula does not have much to do with any specific type of food; rather, as one gets older, one should eat less. When one gets very old, one should only eat light and simple food, returning to the diet proscribed to infants. Being a child is being in the state of health.

SLG

*See also* Electrotherapy; Genetics; Metabolism

## References and Further Reading

Anon. (1912) "Preliminary Report of Committee on Infant and Invalid Diet." *China Medical Journal* 26: 133–44.

Anon. (1924) "What Causes Obesity?" *Journal of the American Medical Association* 82: September 27: 1003.

Anon. (1924) "Relation of Oriental Diet to Disease," *China Medical Journal* 38: 834–6.

Adolph, William H. (1923) "Diet Studies in Shantung," *China Medical Journal* 37: 1013–19.

Adolph, W.H. and Kiang, P.C. (1920) "The Nutritive Value of Soy Bean Products," *China Medical Journal* 34: 268–75.

Beahan, Charlotte L. (1975) "Feminism and Nationalism in the Chinese Women's Press: 1902–11," *Modern China* 1: 379–416.

Daizuo (1922) "Keep the Body Slim," *Jiating Zizhi [Family Magazine]* 3: 1–4.

Dow, Jean I. (1922) "Maternity Famine Relief," *China Medical Journal* 36: 59–67.

Dungen, Wang (1911) "Reforming the Human Body," *Shenbao Ziyoutan* 3.

Edgerton, Kathryn Jean (2002) "The Semiotics of Starvation in Late-Qing China," dissertation, Indiana University.

Embrey, Hartley and Wang, Tsou Ch'ing (1921) "Analysis of Some Chinese Foods," *China Medical Journal* 35: 247–57.

Hedley, W.S. (1921) *Therapeutic Electricity and Practical Muscle Testing*, Philadelphia, Pa.: P. Blakiston's Son & Co.

Lo, Vivienne and Barrett, Penelope (2005) "Cooking Up Fine Remedies," *Medical History* 49: 395–422.

Mallory, Walter H. (1926) *China: Land of Famine*, New York: American Geographical Society.

Nivard, Jacqueline (1986) "L'Évolution de la presse féminine Chinoises de 1898 à 1949," *Études Chinoises* 5 (1–2): 157–84.

Qihui (1941) "Tragedy at the Dinner Table," *Liangyou* 167 (June).

Read, B.E. (1921) "Some Factors Controlling the Food Supply in China," *China Medical Journal* 25: 1–7.

Sargent (1920) "The Trade in Chinese Children," *China Medical Journal* 34: 695.

Sen, Amartya (1981) *Poverty and Famines: An Essay on Entitlement and Deprivation*, Oxford: Clarendon Press.

Shuhui and Weiseng (1913) "On Obesity," *Funu Shibao* 10: 26–8.

Stone, Mary (1912) "Hospital Dietary in China," *China Medical Journal* 26: 298–301.

Zedong, Mao (1992) "A Study of Physical Education," in

Stuart R. Schram (ed.), *Mao's Road to Power: Revolutionary Writings 1912–1949*, 5 vols, Armonk, NY: M.E. Sharpe, Vol. I, pp. 113–27.

Zhenyu, Zhou (1926) "The Cause and Danger of Female Obesity," *Xin Nuxing*: 42–5.

# China Today

The fear of obesity has reappeared in China during the past decade in an age that remembers another moment of famine against which it defines itself. Mao Zedong's famine from 1958 to 1961, which resulted from the collectivization of the peasants killed millions in China and evoked the horrors of the famines of the 1940s during the war against the Japanese, the civil war, and the policies of the nationalist government (Becker 1996). For adults in today's China, "famine" evokes their own experiences under Mao and the tales of starvation during the war by their parents and grandparents.

What is fascinating is how recent studies of obesity in China have come to reverse the claim that such food-borne diseases invade from the primitive "Orient." These Chinese-based studies are often rooted in the view that obesity and its attendant symptoms are the result of the recent pathological "Occidentalization" of China and the Chinese. This obsession with the "contamination from the West" has come to be part of the imagined etiology of obesity in contemporary medicine in China (People's Republic of China, PRC) as well as in Western (U.S./U.K.) medicine dealing with the diaspora Chinese.

The obesity epidemic seems to be the next great fear of Chinese public health officers following smoking. Chronic diseases now account for an estimated 80 percent of deaths and 70 percent of disability-adjusted life-years lost in China. Cardiovascular diseases and cancer are the leading causes of both death and the burden of disease, and exposure to risk factors is high: More than 300 million men smoke cigarettes, and 160 million adults are hypertensive, most of whom are not being treated. Children in the twenty-first century are at risk of being in a poor state of health. The transition from smoking to obesity as the most important threat to public health clearly parallels the argument in Western sources, such as the World Health Organization, that had identified obesity as the next great danger—having "eliminated" smoking as a public health hazard (Reid 2006).

For China, with an exploding number of people now smoking, but where tobacco remains a major source of state revenue, obesity is the new danger. The fat child not the Marlboro Man is the source of anxiety (Chen and Dietz 2002). Indeed, smoking is popularly seen as a "positive" reflection of the process of modernization, while obesity has come to represent the corruption imported from the West. The official journal of "preventive medicine," *Zhonghua Yu Fang Yi Xue Za Zhi*, acknowledged in 2005 that

> the prevalence of overweight and obesity among people living in rural areas was lower than that of their urban counterparts, while the increment of overweight and obesity prevalence among rural people was greater than that of their urban counterparts. It was estimated that another 70 million overweight and 30 million obese Chinese people emerged in China from 1992 to 2002. The prevalence of overweight and obesity of Chinese people was increased rapidly in the past decade, which had affected 260 million Chinese people. It would continue to increase in the near future if effective intervention measures have not been taken.
>
> (Ma et al. 2005)

Chinese medical and epidemiological studies argue that "obesity has become a global epidemic" though there seems to be little knowledge of the state of affairs in China (meaning the PRC). Looking at "a group of 2776 randomly selected adults (20–94 years of age) living in the Huayang Community in Shanghai, China," a 2002 study argued that while "the prevalence of obesity [using Western standards] was lower in China than in the West," the "overall fat mass-related metabolic disorders were also common" (Jia at al. 2002). The Chinese, unlike the Japanese over the past fifty years, seem to be growing "fat" without developing greater height or frame size. Rather than the positive aspects of a change in diet being measured, only the pathological results of overweight preoccupy the medical scientists. The diseases of "modernity," such as diabetes, are often the proof of a decaying, decadent population, just as it was in the nineteenth century in studies of diabetes, then labeled the "Jewish" disease. Today, the argument is that diabetes is more than twice as frequent in the Chinese (urban) overweight population, even though this population was of a lower weight than the equivalent Western population. The visible pathology of obesity was immediately translated into the invisible disease of diabetes. But what is the cause?

Westernization and "economic success" in the new China or among diaspora Chinese is seen as the ultimate cause of the disease. "Americanization" is the cause of obesity rather than, as in the early twentieth century, the place from where "cure" may come. Tsung O. Cheng of George Washington University's medical school has made the claim concerning even the recent work on obesity in China that "the proportion of obesity among children under the age of 15 increased from 15% in 1982 to 27% today" because of "fast food and physical inactivity." "All of the children in China recognize the image of Ronald McDonald, even though they may not be able to read English" (Cheng 2004). Zumin Shi of the Jiangsu Provincial Center for Disease Control and Prevention looks at the expansion of obesity-related illnesses such as anemia among adolescents in the new China and correlates this to parental attention and "overnutrition" (Shi et al. 2005). J.X. Jiang at the National Center for Women's and Children's Health examines a similar problem in terms of family structure for etiology and intervention (Jiang et al. 2005). Bin Xie, a social worker who is based in California, looks at data from Wuhan to correlate mental state (depression) and obesity among the newly successful that now lack an adequate social network. The claim is that "the findings of this study may contribute to our understanding of the influences of psychological correlates in pediatric overweight in the Eastern cultural environment" (Xie et al. 2005: 1137). All imagine that obesity is a reflex of the altered status of individual, family, and society to the most recent changes in the economic system.

What happens when we leave (for a moment) China and move with the Chinese Diaspora to that land of McDonald's, America? Jyu-Lin Chen and Christine Kennedy examine correlative material in an analysis of overweight Chinese-American children:

a more democratic parenting style contributes to a higher BMI in Chinese-American children. First, several studies have shown that an authoritarian parenting style in Chinese families may not necessarily reflect the strict parenting that was measured in Western society. Conversely, parents' involvement, care, supervision, and encouragement of academic achievement, all of which typically have been identified as components of an "authoritarian" parenting style in Western society, are, in fact, a reflection of caring and loving parenting in the Chinese culture.

(Chen and Kennedy 2005: 111)

American-type success breaks down the "parental control and warmth" that constitutes Chinese child-raising and leads to fat Chinese children who are a pathological sign of that success: "a democratic parenting style, and poor family communication contribute to higher BMI in Chinese-American children" (Chen and Kennedy 2005: 115). All obesity comes from the West. Chinese families, understood as a traditional society (certainly not in terms of the cultural revolution), simply don't produce fat kids. Only American children raised "Chinese" (not "Asian-American") children are at risk, unless, of course, you live in Shanghai.

There are, of course, large numbers of "Asian Americans" who fall below the poverty line. They are seen to be at risk for the obesity associated in contemporary medical argument with poverty. In this way, too, they mimic "typical" American dietary patterns. In one study, "Asian American ethnic groups," defined as the Chinese, Vietnamese, and Hmong in California, were the focus. In the study,

the concept of good health [in these communities] included having a harmonious family, balance, and mental and emotional stability. All groups also expressed the general belief that specific foods have hot or cold properties and are part of the Yin/Yang belief system common to Asian cultures. The lure of fast food, children's adoption of American eating habits, and long work hours were identified as barriers to a healthy, more traditional lifestyle.

(Harrison et al. 2005: 2962)

Yet the results here are virtually identical with those whose belief systems were very different: The classification of the "poor" as those at risk for the pathologies of obesity. Indeed, one recent study has argued that children in China stunted by malnutrition are at substantially greater risk from obesity as they mature (McCarthy 1997).

"America" serves as more than the place where obesity has its origin. In many Chinese studies, the model of a multiethnic America, with different rates of risk, becomes the model for understanding different groups' responses to obesity. What was once a monolithic risk to the "Chinese" becomes a more differentiated risk, where ethnic subgroups are seen as being at greater risk because of their implied genetic or cultural difference. Looking at "ethnic" populations in Xinjiang, a recent study documented that more "obese" Kazak people developed hypertension, whereas more "obese" Uygur people developed diabetes. Implicitly, the different "genetic" background was suggested as the cause using the American studies of African-American and Mexican-American obesity and the resultant increase in cases of Type II diabetes in these communities. (The People's Republic of China includes fifty-six national minorities, but the "majority" Han is itself a composite category.) But it is also clear that the Uygur subjects were from rural south Xinjiang and the Kazak subjects from suburban north Xinjiang (Yan et al. 2005). Thus, the "Han" become the unspoken parallel to the labels in American majority culture: epidemiologically rarely differentiated and labeled "white" or "Caucasian." This is just as constructed a "majority" category in opposition to the other minority and therefore "racial" ones, as is the Han (Dikötter 1992). The "rural versus urban" question of healthy versus unhealthy is here a muddy one as the studies reveal that for ethnic minorities, as in the U.S.A., ethnicity trumps geography.

There are numerous questions, which seem to go unanswered in these studies. Is "obesity" in "Asia" the same phenomenological category as in the "West"? Not only are there different histories of the "large" body and its meaning in "Asia," but are there different physiological measures which would be used for the definition of the obese body? I use the label "Asia" in this context rather than "Chinese," as, in 2002, the World Health Association called a meeting in Hong Kong to examine whether the obese body was to be defined differently among "Asians." This "led to the proposal that adult overweight could be specified in Asia when the body mass index exceeded 23.00 and that obesity should be specified when the BMI exceed 25.00" (James 2002). This is substantially (almost 10 points) lower than the American criteria, which should include that new category "Asian-Americans." It is clear that the Asian-American population is being measured by Western public health definitions of overweight and obesity. What are the boundaries of "Asia"? Do they now contain Taiwan, which sees itself in the context of the Pacific islands? Does it reach north into Mongolia and Siberia? To the Ainu? To the west to India? Or is it a composite that rests in an American fantasy of the "Asian"? Bodily changes among Japanese-Americans over three generations after immigration have been demonstrated. Yet, there seems to be no increase in obesity except over the past decade with the imposition of "Western" definitions of "obesity" (Tahara et al. 2003). Indeed, "Japanese Women Don't Get Old or Fat," the title of a recent book claiming that Japan has the lowest obesity rate in the developed world, the longest life expenditure and the lowest per-capita health care cost (Moriyama 2005). It postulates a "Japanese Paradox" (analogous to the "French paradox" and the claim of universal thinness in France): "How can the world's most food-obsessed nation have the lowest obesity rates in the industrialized world—and the best longevity on Earth?" The answer given is diet: "the Asian diet is probably the best on earth" (Moriyama 2005: 8). Yet, the take-out foods available are Western: "Italian, Chinese, French, and Indian, since food in Japan has been a global affair for many centuries" (Moriyama 2005: 25). No such claims are made about the low impact of Western foods on China. Indeed, a recent popular American study claims that the Chinese diet is the answer to Western obesity (Campbell and Campbell 2005: 69–110).

Westernization in both China and the Chinese diaspora may well play a role, but it is a secondary cause— the primary cause is the long-established one-child policy in China and the change in the status of urban children. This change is analogous to the attitudes of many first-generation immigrants in the American urban diaspora (not only the Chinese). There is a preoccupation with the diseases of obesity, specifically diabetes (Type II) found within this literature on China. In a paper from 2001, a study of adults in a population of northeastern China, specifically in Da Qing City, argued,

> increasing waist measurements predicted 10-fold increases in hypertension and a three-to-five times

increased risk of diabetes. Suitable waist cut-off points were 85cm for men and 80cm for women, with statistical analysis showing waist as the more dominant predictor of risk than age, waist-to-hip ratios or BMIs. Hence, small increases in BMI, and particularly in waist circumference, predict a substantial increase in the risk of diabetes . . . in Chinese adults.

(Li et al. 2002: 167)

What is being seen is the shift in body size because of the accessibility of different foods and the so-called "thrifty genotype" hypothesis that had been suggested in 1964. Simply stated, it has been observed that when mice are transferred from a harsh to a benign environment, they gain weight and are hyperglycemic. When one thus measured first-generation groups of immigrants to the U.S.A. in the late nineteenth century, there was a substantially higher rate of diabetes. The initial groups showed an extremely low index of obesity and the resultant diabetes. This index, however, skyrocketed after just a short time of living in their new environment. Thus, diabetes and obesity seem to be an index of a failure to adapt rapidly to changed surroundings (Schmidt-Nielsen et al. 1964). It is the rapidity of change that lies at the heart of the matter.

In China today, rural children are suffering from malnutrition. The Beijing-based Institute of Nutrition and Food Safety found that more than 29 percent of children under five years old in China's poorest regions were growing at a slower than normal rate. This is quite different to the cities where too rich a diet has increased the level of obesity. In China's larger, wealthier cities, milk, formula milk powder, yogurt, and many other types of food are available which would prevent childhood malnutrition. Yet, of course, the availability of such foods seems also to be viewed as causal for the new Chinese "obesity epidemic." According to Chinese public-health sources, severe obesity now affects some 16–20 percent of urban youngsters. (Malnutrition hits 30 percent.) But, of course, "urban" itself is a highly problematic category for it includes the rural diaspora, living marginal lives in the large cities as well as cities which have had little share in the new boom economy.

Now, in a China with a growing urban middle class, obesity seems to have been uncoupled from the official demand under Mao Zedong in 1979 that only one child per couple be allowed which radically reduced the average

three to four children per family in rural areas and two to three in urban areas. China, unlike most societies in transformation that have a reduction in birth rate as a reflex of increasing economic status, saw the reduction in the number of children per family prior to the development of the new economic modernization begun under Deng Xiaoping. More food and more television are today indeed a means of pampering these children, often called the "Little Emperors" (*xiao huangdi*)—but the number of children and their status are independent of economic change. These "Little Emperors" are "used to getting plenty of candy, lavish praise from grownups, and pretty much anything else [they] want" (Chandler 2004: 138). And what they want is food, at least as imagined from the perspective of a Western observer writing for a Western audience accustomed to critiques of the "Fast Food Nation" (Schlosser 2002). They are imagined being "weaned on cheeseburgers from McDonald's, pizza from Pizza Hut, and fried chicken from KFC," (Chandler 2004: 138). Their growing obesity has become not only a public-health problem but also a source for a new "weight-loss business."

At the Aimin Fat Reduction Hospital in Tianjin, a former military institution that launched China's first weight clinic in 1992, doctors treat 200 patients, most of them under 25, with a daily regimen of acupuncture, exercise, and healthy food. Fifteen-year-old Liang Chen reports proudly that he has lost 33 pounds in less than a month at Aimin. But he can't stop reminiscing wistfully about his regular visits to KFC. (Indeed, his favorite T-shirt is a souvenir from China's largest KFC store.) "I used to be able to eat an entire family-size bucket all by myself," he recalls. "Just one?" snorts his roommate, 14-year-old Li Xiang. "That's nothing. I used to be able to eat four buckets—sometimes five, if I didn't eat the corncobs and bread."

(Chandler 2004: 140)

Childhood obesity is not the only curse of the "Little Emperors," as anorexia nervosa seems also to be present. In 1993, researchers reported 200 cases of radical underweight among children from 1988 to 1990 brought to an eating disorders clinic in the Fujien area. The gender balance was remarkable from Western criteria for anorexia nervosa, as 112 cases were boys and only eighty-eight were girls. It was not the case that these were the product of a starvation culture but rather of "non-fat phobic anorexia" caused, according to the researchers by the single-child policy as the children were spoiled by their parents and developed unhealthy eating habits which contributed to their underweight (Cheng 2004).

Here the problem is not "Western" food but the absence of moderation, an absence fostered by the "Little Emperor" syndrome. The number of children is a result of the "Old" Communist system and maybe exacerbated by the availability of "Western" fast foods. There are studies that minimize the shifts of diet in regard to a "Westernization" of the Chinese diet. One such study argues that while in the U.S.A. snacks contribute "more than one-third of their daily calories and a higher proportion of snack calories from foods prepared away from home," in

> China . . . snacks provide only approximately 1% of energy. Fast food plays a much more dominant role in the American diet (approximately 20% of energy vs. 2% to 7% in the other countries), but as yet does not contribute substantially to children's diets in the other countries. Urban-rural differences were found to be important, but narrowing over time, for China . . . whereas they are widening for Russia.
>
> (Adair and Popkin 2005: 1281)

What has changed in contemporary China? Moderation is what has been sacrificed—not traditional foods. The status of the child may be linked to the new status of what the child eats, but childhood obesity is not the result of the availability of alternative, Western foods but the perceived special status of the child. No such parallel state existed in Japan, where the reduction in the birthrate was concomitant to the increase of economic status. In Japan, American fast food has been omnipresent since the 1960s. If there is an increase of childhood obesity (and the argument is that this is then reflected in adult obesity), then it has occurred only over the past decade. In the National Survey of Primary and Middle Schools in Japan, between 1970 and 1997, obesity in nine-year-old children increased threefold, but the focus has been on the past decade, a decade of economic retrenchment (<http://ific.org/foodinsight/2001/jf/globesityfi101.cfm>).

Today in China, no one would imagine tying childhood obesity to anything but perceived economic improvement in the "New Economy" as part of "Jiang Zemin's legacy." This, of course, mimics the Western *Super Size Me* rationale that sees all obesity as a result of the global "epidemic" of "junk food." The introduction of Westernized forms of "traditional" Chinese medicine, such as "electroacupuncture" for the treatment of overweight has melded traditional views of obesity and the newest research on human metabolism including serum total cholesterol, triglyceride, high-density lipoprotein cholesterol and low-density lipoprotein cholesterol (Cabioglu and Ergene 2005). What comes from the West can be cured now by that which (seems) indigenous to the East (but, of course, is not—just like obesity).

China, like America, is suffering from a new epidemic but one that documents its modernity—no model of Oriental, primitive infectious diseases here. Rather, a claim of the "invasion from the West," the negative aspects of the new economy which can be confronted through the importation of models of obesity from Western public health. Obesity and its treatment are both to be understood as part of a system of modernization with all of the pitfalls recognized and the "cure" in sight.

SLG

*See also* Developing World; Electrotherapy; Jews; Obesity Epidemic; Smoking

## References and Further Reading

Adair, L.S. and Popkin, B.M. (2005) "Are Child Eating Patterns Being Transformed Globally?" *Obesity Research* 13 (7): 1281–99.

Becker, Jasper (1996) *Hungry Ghosts: China's Secret Famine*, London: J. Murray.

Cabioglu, M.T. and Ergene, N. (2005) "Electroacupuncture Therapy for Weight Loss Reduces Serum Total Cholesterol, Triglycerides, and LDL Cholesterol Levels in Obese Women," *The American Journal of Chinese Medicine* 33 (4): 525–33.

Campbell, T. Colin and Campbell, Thomas M., II (2005) *The China Study: The Most Comprehensive Study of Nutrition Ever Conducted and the Startling Implications for Diet, Weight Loss and Long-Term Health*, Dallas, Tex.: Benbella Books.

Chandler, Clay (2004) "Little Emperors: China's Only Children—More Than 100 Million of Them—Make

Up the Largest Me Generation Ever. And Their Appetites Are Big," *Fortune* October 4, pp. 138–42.

Chen, Chunming and Dietz, William H. (eds) (2002) *Obesity in Childhood and Adolescence*, Philadelphia, Pa.: Lippincott Williams & Wilkins.

Chen, D.G., Cheng, X.F. and Wang, L.L. (1993) "Clinical Analysis of 200 Cases of Child Anorexia," *Chinese Mental Health Journal* 7: 5–6. (In Chinese.)

Chen, Jyu-Lin and Kennedy, Christine (2005) "Factors Associated with Obesity in Chinese-American Children," *Pediatric Nursing* 31 (2): 110–15.

Cheng, Tsung O. (2004) "Obesity in Chinese Children," *Journal of the Royal Society of Medicine* 97 (5): 254.

Dikötter, Frank (1992) *The Discourse of Race in Modern China*, Stanford, Calif.: Stanford University Press.

Harrison, G. G., Kagawa-Singer, M., Foerster, S.B., Lee, H., Pham Kim, L., Nguyen, T.U., Fernandez-Ami, A., Quinn V. and Bal, D.G. (2005) "Seizing the Moment: California's Opportunity to Prevent Nutrition-Related Health Disparities in Low-Income Asian American Population," *Cancer* 104 (suppl): 2962–8.

James, W.P.T. (2002) "Appropriate Asian Body Mass Indices," *Obesity Reviews* 3: 139.

Jia, W.P., Xiang, K., Chen, L., Xu, J. and Wu, Y. (2002) "Epidemiological Study on Obesity and Its Comorbidities in Urban Chinese Older Than 20 Years of Age in Shanghai, China," *Obesity Reviews* 3 (3): 157–65.

Jiang, J., Xia, X.X.L., Greiner, T., Lian, G.L., and Rosenqvist, U. (2005) "A Two Year Family Based Behaviour Treatment for Obese Children," *Archives of Disease in Childhood* 90 (12): 1235–8.

Li, G., Chen, X., Jang, Y., Wang, J., Xing, X., Yang, W. and Hu, Y. (2002) "Obesity, Coronary Heart Disease Risk Factors and Diabetes in Chinese: An Approach to the Criteria of Obesity in the Chinese Population," *Obesity Reviews* 3 (3): 167–72.

Ma, G.S., Li, Y.P., Wu, Y.F., Zhai, F.Y., Cui, Z.H., Hu, X.Q., Luan, D.C., Hu, Y.H. and Yang, X.G. (2005) "The Prevalence of Body Overweight and Obesity and Its Changes Among Chinese People During 1992 to 2002," *Journal of Preventive Medicine* 39 (5): 311–15.

—— (2005) "Malnutrition Hits 30 Percent of China's Poverty-Stricken Children," *Agence France Presse*. October 8.

McCarthy, Michael (1997) "Stunted Children Are at High Risk of Later Obesity," *Lancet* 349: 34.

Moriyama, Naomi (2005) *Japanese Women Don't Get Old or Fat: Secrets of My Mother's Tokyo Kitchen*, New York: Delacorte.

Reid, Roddey (2006) *Globalizing Tobacco Control: Anti-Smoking Campaigns in California, France and Japan*, Bloomington, Ind.: Indiana University Press.

Schlosser, Eric (2002) *Fast Food Nation: The Dark Side of the All-American Meal*, New York: Perennial.

Schmidt-Nielsen, K., Haines, H. and Hackel, D.B. (February 14, 1964) "Diabetes Mellitus in the Sand Rat Induced by Standard Laboratory Diets," *Science* 143: 689.

Shi, Zumin, Lien, Nanna, Kumar, Bernadette Nirmal, Dalen, Ingvild, and Holmboe-Ottesen, Gerd (2005) "The Sociodemographic Correlates of Nutritional Status of School Adolescents in Jiangsu Province," *Journal of Adolescent Health* 37 (4): 313–22.

Tahara, Y.K., Moji, S., Muraki, S., Honda, S., and Aoyagi, K. (2003) "Comparison of Body Size and Composition Between Young Adult Japanese-Americans and Japanese Nationals in the 1980s," *Annals of Human Biology* 30 (4): 392–401.

Xie, B., Chou, C.P., Spruijt-Metz, D., Liu, C., Xia, J., Gong, J., Johnson, Y., and Li, C.A. (2005) "Effects of Perceived Peer Isolation and Social Support Availability on the Relationship Between Body Mass Index and Depressive Symptoms," *International Journal of Obesity* 29: 1137–43.

Yan, W., Yang, X., Zheng, Y., Ge, D., Zhang, Y., Shan, Z., Simu, H., Sukerobai, M. and Wang, R. (2005) "The Metabolic Syndrome in Uygur and Kazak Populations," *Diabetes Care* 28: 2554–5.

# Chittenden, Russell Henry (1856–1943)

## Researcher and pioneer in area of daily protein requirements for humans

In 1880, Chittenden received his Ph.D., and in 1882 he started his career as the Professor of Physiological Chemistry in the Sheffield Scientific School of Yale University. Chittenden's initial research dealt with the chemical nature of proteins. In collaboration with the German physiologist Wilhelm Friedrich Kühne (1837–1900), the two studied the enzymatic splitting of proteins, which has contributed to the understanding of the complexity of protein molecules. His initial studies sparked his interest in nutritional science and further led to his most important research, that on the protein requirements of humans.

The early nineteenth-century belief was that people needed an extensive amount of protein (118 grams) in their daily diet. After Chittenden encountered Horace Fletcher who maintained a low-calorie and low-protein diet, Chittenden's interest was sparked. He began a widespread study of low-protein diets, in which his subjects were Yale athletes and army volunteers. His volunteers consumed 2,600 calories a day and 50 grams of protein. In 1905, Chittenden enthusiastically published his results in his *Physiological Economy in Nutrition*.

While Chittenden passionately believed in a lower protein diet, there were many skeptics. He defended his findings through a study on dogs, which are primarily carnivorous animals. Unfortunately, the diet did not prove to be healthy for the dogs, as many began to suffer from ill health. Even so, Chittenden maintained enthusiasm for a low-protein diet, and once again defended his position in *The Nutrition of Man*, a course of eight lectures delivered before a general public at the Lowell institute of Boston in the early part of 1907. While nutritionists did eventually disregard the initial high protein requirements (118 grams), they continued to doubt Chittenden's findings. Throughout his career, Chittenden continued to be involved in nutritional studies and discussions and was regarded as an expert in nutritional sciences.

In 1918, he represented the U.S.A. on an Inter-Allied Scientific Food Commission, which met to discuss the nutritional needs of the allied forces in World War I. He was not able in his lifetime to prove his theories on protein requirements, though his research was continued by others.

SLG

*See also* Fletcher; Ornish

## References and Further Reading

Anon. (1971) "Russell Henry Chittenden," *Dictionary of Scientific Biography*, New York: Charles Scribner's Sons, Vol. III, pp. 256–8.

Chittenden, Russell H. (1905) *Physiological Economy in Nutrition: with Special Reference to the Minimal Protein Requirement of the Healthy Man: An Experimental Study*, London: Heinemann.

—— (1907) *The Nutrition of Man*, London: Heinemann.

# Christianity

Health becomes one of the powerful metaphors in early Christianity, especially in terms of the relationship between the newly healthy body of the Christian and the sick body of the Jew (Avalos 1999). Jesus's cures are his most powerful miracles. Fasting, practiced among the Jews, becomes a means to salvation, as Paul writes in the epistles, "we gain nothing by eating, lose nothing by abstaining" (1 Cor. 8:8). With the establishment of the early Church (most readily seen in St. Augustine's *Confessions*), the submission to the temptation to overeat was written on the body in the form of fat. "Gula" is one of the seven deadly sins (Sawyer 1995). In many ways, it is the most difficult of the deadly sins to combat.

Augustine (354–430), the Bishop of Hippo in North Africa, struggled against lust and begged for chastity in his early youth: "But I wretched, most wretched, in the very commencement of my early youth, had begged chastity of Thee, and said, 'Give me chastity and continency, only not yet.'" (Augustine 1961: 235–7). When he turned sixteen, Augustine moved to Carthage, where, again, he was plagued by desire:

Where there seethed all around me a cauldron of lawless loves. I loved not yet, yet I loved to love, and out of a deep-seated want, I hated myself for wanting not. I sought what I might love, in love with loving, and I hated safety . . . To love then, and to be beloved, was sweet to me; but more, when I obtained to enjoy the person I loved. I defiled, therefore, the spring of friendship with the filth of concupiscence, and I beclouded its brightness with the hell of lustfulness.

(Augustine 1961: 235–7)

He writes that he struggles each day with the desire to eat and to drink even more than he does with sexual lust: "In the midst of these temptations I struggle daily against greed for food and drink. This is not an evil which I can decide once and for all to repudiate and never to embrace again, as I was able to do with fornication" (Augustine 1961: 235–7). For the seduction of food and what it signifies, the fat body, haunts Augustine's sense of himself. He sees food as both necessary for health and a force for healing, but only in strict limits:

I look upon food as a medicine. But the snare of concupiscence awaits me in the very process of passing from the discomfort of hunger to the contentment, which comes when satisfied. For the process itself is a pleasure and there is no other means of satisfying hunger except the one, which we are obliged to take . . . Health and enjoyment have not the same requirement.

(Augustine 1961: 235–7)

The desire for food is itself the Devil present in the body. He cites Paul in that "we gain nothing by eating, lose nothing by abstaining" (1 Cor. 8:8). This is a basic struggle to control desire and the very form of the body.

Augustine makes the ideal body the body divine, much as in the Platonic notion of beauty it is beyond the material.

In his *City of God*, Augustine links the carnal pleasures of the flesh to sins of the soul. They are the same. He condemns with equal verve the Epicurean philosophers who "live after the flesh, because they place man's highest good in bodily pleasure" and the Stoics who "who place the supreme good of men in the soul, live after the spirit" (Augustine 1957: II, 247). The Epicureans also claim that "pleasure is very largely a matter of physical health" and the Stoics that "only the wise are beautiful" (Augustine 1957: III, 37). Augustine quotes Paul over and over again on the need to control carnality and the fallen nature of the soul. There is a compelling case for understanding the Pauline letters themselves as sites of a thoroughly allegorical anthropology. Among the binary oppositions of Pauline allegory stand the analogous pairs, flesh–spirit, literal–figurative, signifier–signified, in which the first element is a mere pointing to the privileged, second element. And so, for Paul, the Torah is but pointing to its fulfillment in Christ (Boyarin 1994). The ideal body is to be found only in Heaven when he describes heavenly bodies as possessing "a wondrous ease of movement, a wondrous lightness" (Daley 1991: 144). Here the image of the perfectly light and slim body of the divine is in contrast to the mortal and sinful one.

The crucial early Christian text is again from Paul's letters in 1 Cor. 8:1: "knowledge puffs up, but love builds up." Fat, as a sign of gluttony, is a reflection of prideful nature of humans. It is often linked to *acedia*, sloth, the deadly sin which is part of the tradition of the representation of madness in the West. The puffed-up body is also the spirit that is so unwilling to act as to be a sign of moral decay and mental instability. For Augustine, it is his body, in which all desires seem confused and interchangeable. It is the body most at risk from inaction and desire.

Here it is St. Thomas Aquinas (1225–74) who must rethink these limitations in Pauline terms when he preaches that "meditating upon all these things, let us not give our minds to delights, but to what is the end of delights. Here on earth it is excrement and obesity, hereafter it is fire and the worm" (Toal 1957: III, 315). If for Paul all humans are damned by their flesh, Aquinas needs to stress this once again, by seeing us trapped in our fallen bodies by our natural functions—eating and excreting. And yet it is St. Teresa who says, that the soul "finds everything cooked and eaten for it; it has only to enjoy its nourishment" (St. Teresa 1957: 90). This now being the pure food of the spirit, not of the flesh.

SLG

*See also* Jews

### References and Further Reading

Augustine (1961) *Confessions*, trans. R.S. Pine-Coffin, London: Penguin Books.

Augustine (1957–72) *The City of God*, 7 vols, Cambridge, Mass.: Harvard University Press.

Avalos, Hector (1999) *Health Care and the Rise of Christianity*, Peabody, Mass.: Hendrickson.

Boyarin, Daniel (1994) *A Radical Jew: Paul and the Politics of Identity*, Berkeley, Calif.: University of California Press.

Daley, Brian E. (1991) *The Hope of the Early Church: A Handbook of Patristic Eschatology*, Cambridge: Cambridge University Press.

St. Teresa of Avila (1957) *The Life of Saint Teresa of Avila by Herself*, Harmondsworth: Penguin.

Sawyer, Erin (1995) "Celibate Pleasures: Masculinity, Desire, and Asceticism in Augustine," *Journal of the History of Sexuality* 6 (1): 1–29.

Shaw, Teresa M. (1997) "Creation, Virginity and Diet in Fourth-Century Christianity: Basil of Aneyra's on the True Purity of Virginity," *Gender and History* 9 (3): 579–96.

Toal, W.F. (ed.) (1957–63) *The Sunday Sermons of the Great Fathers*, 4 vols, Chicago, Ill.: Regnery.

# Cornaro, Luigi (1463–1566)

Cornaro's autobiography is certainly the earliest and most influential text of dieting literature that still has a readership today. His elegantly written Italian text, *Discorsi della vita sobria*, translated as the *Discourses on a Sober Life*, the *Art of Living Long* and also the *Temperate Life*, first appeared in 1558. He began the book in 1550 when he was eighty-three and the final installment appeared when he was ninety-five.

Cornaro's books became instant bestsellers and remain in print today. As Joseph Addison and Richard Steele writing in 1711 note in *The Spectator* his texts "are written with such a spirit of cheerfulness, religion, and good sense, as are the natural concomitants of temperance and sobriety" (Addison and Steele 1711: 4). Nearly two hundred years later, the German philosopher Friedrich Nietzsche in the section on "four great errors" in his *Twilight of the Idols* (finished in 1888) doubted the efficacy of Cornaro's diet, having tried it (and many other interventions including electrotherapy) to cure his own ailments. He accused Cornaro of underestimating the fixity of predisposition to illness, believing that his long life was due to his diet rather than to his very nature:

Cornaro mistakes the effect for the cause. The worthy Italian thought his diet was the cause of his long life, whereas the precondition for a long life, the extraordinary slowness of his metabolism, was the cause of his slender diet. . . . A scholar in our time, with his rapid consumption of nervous energy, would simply destroy himself on Cornaro's diet. *Crede experto*—believe me, I've tried.

(Nietzsche 2003: 58)

This debate about inheritance, health, and weight loss continues to be waged and Cornaro's texts continue to be read as first-hand accounts of what works and what does not work to lose weight and thus prolong life.

Cornaro confesses to the reader that at middle age, he was dissipated by forty years of gluttony and overindulgence in sensual pleasures. He was at death's door. For him, gluttony was a killer, not merely a sin, for it "kills every year . . . as great a number as would perish during the time of a most dreadful pestilence, or by the sword or fire of many bloody wars" (Cornaro 1903: 41). In the depths of his illness, he turned to physicians. They advised him to be temperate. He thus cured his obese body through a strict limitation of his diet. While the cure is for him proof of the beneficence of God, it is equally proof that living longer allows one to develop those "splendid gifts of intellect and noble qualities of heart" (Cornaro 1903: 42). In a sense, the evidence for God's grace and the best use of his gifts comes at the end of life. It is a "natural death," at the time when one's vital powers have diminished and one dies well—peacefully and without struggle.

Cornaro's text is a handbook for a good life (and death). Its power lies in its autobiographical, indeed, confessional mode, which echoes Augustine. He observes, and carefully chronicles, his symptoms as a younger man from his perspective as an old, healthy, thin man. He was certainly ill with many of the diseases attributed to obesity in the Galenic tradition: "I had pains in the stomach, frequent pains in the side, symptoms of gout, and, still worse, a low fever that was almost continuous; but I suffered especially from disorder of the stomach, and from an unquenchable thirst" (Cornaro 1903: 43–4). But he also lost his ability to reject temptation, having become addicted to eating and drinking. He turned to the physicians whose advice was quite clear; they "declared there was but one remedy left for my ills—a remedy which would surely conquer them, provided I would make up my mind to apply it and persevere in its use. That remedy was the temperate and orderly life" (Cornaro 1903: 44). This is what the physicians admonished and what the patient followed to success.

Sobriety after a life of indulgence is a cure for the physical effects of obesity, not obesity itself. Cornaro sees himself as typical of the men of his age. The riches of their lives have led to the brink of death as a result of what he identified as the three evil customs or sins widespread in sixteenth-century Italy: "adulation and ceremony . . . heresy and . . . intemperance" (Cornaro 1903: 40). Only through the good counsel of the doctors does he find a cure for all three. For gluttony is understood as the cause of the list of infirmities found in the fat man. The overindulgence of the man in his best years is the cause of his fat, and his fat is the sign of his sick body. There is a strong moral tradition that owes its form to Paul and the Christian abnegation of the body. The society in which he lives, however, does not understand this simple rule:

These false notions are due entirely to the force of habit, bred by men's senses and uncontrolled appetites. It is this craving to gratify the appetites which

has allured and inebriated men to such a degree that, abandoning the path of virtue, they have taken to following the one of vice—a road which leads them, though they see it not, to strange and fatal chronic infirmities through which they grow prematurely old. Before they reach the age of forty their health has been completely worn out—just the reverse of what the temperate life once did for them. For this, before it was banished by the deadly habit of intemperance, invariably kept all its followers strong and healthy, even to the age of fourscore and upward.
(Cornaro 1903: 41)

It is not knowledge of the world that cures, but simplicity and temperance. Cornaro bemoans the fact that

friends and associates, men endowed with splendid gifts of intellect and noble qualities of heart, who fall, in the prime of life, victims of this dread tyrant; men who, were they yet living, would be ornaments to the world, while their friendship and company would add to my enjoyment in the same proportion as I was caused sorrow by their loss.
(Cornaro 1903: 42)

He is now cured of his illnesses and fat by his strict regime. The world of simplicity may have its roots in the advice of physicians, but when Cornaro, at the age of seventy, was in a carriage accident and dislocated an arm and a leg, he rejected his physician's suggestion that he be bled. He was convinced that his now healthy body would heal itself and, according to his account, it did. As a result of his own diet, he believes to know his body so well, that he is aware of what it needs to evince a cure.

Moderation is now his model for men to regain again their manhood, a manhood defined by longevity. And Cornaro was long-lived. This indeed was the key to his claim on authenticity in writing his autobiographical text. After the beginning of the sixteenth century, this anxiety about premature death was heightened. Cornaro's rejection of excess in food parallels Augustine's anxiety that gluttony was even worse that sexual license, for one did not have to fornicate (to use Augustine's concept), but one did have to eat. But what is excessive in the intake of nourishment for one man may not be for another. One can eat anything one wants but in moderation.

I began to observe very diligently what kinds of food

agreed with me. I determined, in the first place, to experiment with those, which were most agreeable to my palate, in order that I might learn if they were suited to my stomach and constitution. The proverb, "whatever tastes good will nourish and strengthen," is generally regarded as embodying a truth, and is invoked, as a first principle, by those who are sensually inclined . . . In it I had hitherto firmly believed; but now I was resolved to test the matter, and find to what extent, if any, it was true. My experience, however, proved this saying to be false.

(Cornaro 1903: 46)

Since we must eat, as Augustine noted, we cannot suffer only to eat those things that give us pleasure, for that will only make us more gluttonous. Appetite is but a form of desire. Cornaro translates this into the discourse of health and illness. Eat for pleasure, and you will become ill. But it is also clear that the ability to eat exactly those things that he wants is linked with his idea that certain foods are simply healthy.

Those foods, such as meat and fish, clearly evoke the wealth that was part of the temptation of Cornaro's youth. A member of the powerful Cornaro family of Venice, he could earlier afford to be gluttonous and now he can afford to eat fish.

Of meats, I eat veal, kid, and mutton. I eat fowls of all kind; as well as partridges and birds like the thrush. I also partake of such salt-water fish as the goldney and the like; and, among the various fresh-water kinds, the pike and others. . . . Old persons, who, on account of poverty, cannot afford to indulge in all of these things, may maintain their lives with bread, bread soup, and eggs—foods that certainly cannot be wanting even to a poor man, unless he be one of the kind commonly known as good-for-nothing. Yet, even though the poor should eat nothing but bread, bread soup, and eggs, they must not take a greater quantity than can be easily digested; for they must, at all times, remember that he who is constantly faithful to the above-mentioned rules in regard to the quantity and quality of his food, cannot die except by simple dissolution and without illness.

(Cornaro 1903: 87–8)

Cornaro resolved to restrict his diet drastically. Initially,

it was reduced to a daily intake of twelve ounces of food and fourteen ounces of wine. Eventually, however, it was reduced to a single egg a day. However, he also understood the relationship between the outward manifestation of the body and its spirit. He resolved to control his temper and the "melancholy, hatred, and other passions of the soul, which all appear greatly to affect the body" (Cornaro 1903: 48). Assuming that he was in fact born in 1564 (contesting some accounts that claim his age at death was 103), Cornaro lived to be ninety-eight and, according to his autobiography, it is the accomplishments in old age that reveal the character of man. He muses on what it is to be old and healthy. This is defined by his ability to work and to concentrate on questions of private as well as public health:

My greatest enjoyment, in the course of my journeys going and returning, is the contemplation of the beauty of the country and of the places through which I travel. Some of these are in the plains; others on the hills, near rivers or fountains; and all are made still more beautiful by the presence of many charming dwellings surrounded by delightful gardens. Nor are these my diversions and pleasures rendered less sweet and less precious through the failing of sight or my hearing, or because any one of my senses is not perfect; for they are all—thank God!—most perfect. This is especially true of my sense of taste; for I now find more true relish in the simple food I eat, wheresoever I may chance to be, than I formerly found in the most delicate dishes at the time of my intemperate life . . . With the greatest delight and satisfaction, also, do I behold the success of an undertaking highly important to our State; namely, the fitting for cultivation of its waste tracts of country, numerous as they were. This improvement was commenced at my suggestion; yet I had scarcely ventured to hope that I should live to see it, knowing, as I do, that republics are slow to begin enterprises of great importance. Nevertheless, I have lived to see it. And I myself was present with the members of the committee appointed to superintend the work, for two whole months, at the season of the greatest heat of summer, in those swampy places; nor was I ever disturbed either by fatigue or by any hardship I was obliged to incur. So great is the power of the orderly life which accompanies me wheresoever I may go! Furthermore, I cherish a firm hope that I shall live to witness not only the beginning but also the completion, of another enterprise, the success of which is no less important to our Venice: namely, the protection of our estuary ... These are the true and important recreations, these comforts and pastimes, of my old age, which is much more to be prized than the old age or even the youth of other men; since it is free, by the grace of God, from all the perturbations of the soul and the infirmities of the body, and is not subject to any of those troubles which woefully torment so many young men and so many languid and utterly worn-out old men.

(Cornaro 1903: 69–70)

Cornaro's autobiography is at its heart a handbook of dietetics to reform the fat boy's body and turn him into a healthy and abstentious man who can in turn create a healthy world.

Building on Cornaro's work, modern science has begun to examine the role of calorie restriction in life expectancy and development of chronic disease (Gerstenblith 2006). Scientists have demonstrated that animals that are fed calorie-restricted diets have longer life expectancies than animals fed higher-calorie diets (Couzin 2005). Although at the time of publication of this book, some doctors and scientists are recommending low-calorie diets, there have not been any studies in humans to confirm the results. Additionally, some in the contemporary press have questioned this notion of calorie restriction that began with Cornaro. Although calorie restriction may increase life expectancy, some argue that indulging

in food is a part of leading a full life and would rather not choose a life of temperance (David 2004). Regardless, Cornaro was a pioneer in examining the role of diet and life expectancy in Western culture.

SLG

See also Christianity; Medical Use of Dieting

## References and Further Reading
Addison, Joseph and Richard Steele, *The Spectator* 195: Saturday, October 13, 1711, p. 4.
Benecke, Mark (2002) *The Dream of Eternal Life: Biomedicine, Aging, and Immortality*, trans. Rachel Rubenstein, New York: Columbia University Press.
Cornaro, Luigi (1903) *The Art of Living Long*, Milwaukee, Wisc.: William F. Butler.
Couzin, J. (2005) "How Much Can Human Life Span Be Extended?" *Science* 309 (5731): 83.
David, G. (2004) "Caloric Restriction. Extreme Makeover. Eating Like a Bird May Extend Your Life. But Is It Worth It?" *Fortune* 149 (8): 138.
Gerstenblith G. (2006) "Cardiovascular Aging: What We Can Learn from Caloric Restriction," *Journal of the American College of Cardiology* 47 (2): 403–4.
Gruman, Gerald J. (1966) *A History of Ideas About the Prolongation of Life: The Evolution of Prolongevity Hypotheses to 1800*, Philadelphia, Pa.: American Philosophical Society.
Nietzsche, Friedrich (2003) *Twilight of the Idols and The Anti-Christ*. trans. R.J. Hollindale, Harmondsworth: Penguin.

# Craig, Jenny (1932–) and Craig, Sid (1932–)

Founders of Jenny Craig, Inc., one of the world's largest weight-management companies. Jenny Craig's "official" account of her life stated that she wanted to share her philosophy of balancing nutrition, physical activity, and lifestyle, which helped her embark on a career that brought her international acclaim as a weight-loss expert and author, as well as gave her the ability to help millions of people live healthier lives. Jenny Craig had an

experience that many of her followers seemed to share. After giving birth to her second daughter, she looked in the mirror and decided that she did not like what she saw: She was 45 pounds overweight. In the mirror, she saw another image, which was that of her mother who died at the age of forty-nine from a stroke, possibly related to her overweight condition. Jenny had many reminders in the family that weight was the primary health problem.

Once Jenny got her weight under control, she started to work for fitness clubs, ultimately managing, owning, and selling one of her own. After divorcing her first husband and marrying Sid Craig in 1979, they quickly set up Jenny Craig, Inc. centers first in Australia and then in the U.S.A. Sidney Craig, a former dance instructor and child tap dancer, was in his senior year at Fresno State University majoring in business, financing his college education by teaching ballroom dancing in the evenings at an Arthur Murray dance studio. After graduation he acquired five Arthur Murray franchises, which he sold in 1970 to purchase Body Contour Inc. Figure Salons. Sid Craig's first opened a salon in New Orleans, and Genevieve "Jenny" Marie born Guidroz (then known by her married name of Bourcq) was the first person he hired in 1970. They were married in 1979, and Jenny helped Sid increase Body Contours, Inc. to nearly 200 centers, making it a company earning $35 million a year.

In 1982, Jenny and Sid Craig sold the Body Contour Company and moved to Australia to open the first Jenny Craig Weight Loss Center. Centers were opened in Melbourne, and then were expanded into the U.S.A. Currently, Jenny Craig remains very involved in the company she helped found in 1983. She still serves as Chairman of the Executive Committee. Although the company was sold in May 2002, it still bears her name since Jenny's personal weight-loss experience and her nutritional guidance philosophy provided the foundation on which the company was ultimately built. Today, Jenny Craig, Inc. is one of the largest weight-management service companies in the world. There are 652 company-owned and franchised centers in the U.S.A., Australia, New Zealand, Canada, Puerto Rico, and Guam.

SLG/RAKHI PATEL

## References and Further Reading

Erickson, Gregory K. (1994) "Excerpts from Women Entrepreneurs Only: 12 Women Entrepreneurs Tell the Stories of Their Success. How Jenny Craig Turned a Weight Problem into a Business Colossus," *Business Week Online* May 28.

Jenny Craig Inc., available online at <http://www.jennycraig.com/corporate/company/jcraig.asp> (accessed March 18, 2007).

# D

## Davis, Adelle (1904–74)

One of the early twentieth-century diet authorities who had a professional background in nutrition. Trained in dietetics and nutrition at the University of California at Berkeley, she received her M.S. degree in biochemistry from the University of Southern California in 1938. Her work piggybacked on that of Gayelord Hauser in that she was an early advocate of nutritional supplements as well as "natural" foods in specific combinations. In 1935, Stationers' Hall of London, England published her *Optimum Health*, and in 1939 her second book, *You Can Stay Well*. In 1942, the Macmillan Company published the most assertive of Davis's works of the period, *Vitality through Planned Nutrition*.

Davis's celebrity as a diet guide in the U.S.A. began with the release of the first in her series of "Let's" titles, *Let's Cook it Right* (1947). This series would eventually include four titles, all of which became international bestsellers. In *Let's Have Healthy Children* (1951) she argued for serious attention to prenatal diet. But, as with many of her serious suggestions, she overstated the case, claiming that "every woman, by her choice of foods during pregnancy, largely determines the type of baby she will produce" (Davis 1951: 5). If a woman had a poor diet, the results would be catastrophic: heart defects, clubbed feet, tumors, premature birth, to list a few (Davis 1951: 6). But a good diet assured an easy labor and a "happy mother" (Davis 1951: 9). Davis was also part of the cult of cow's milk as the ideal food, advocating that infants regularly drink milk from a bottle as its "absence creates illness" (Davis 1951: 183).

In *Let's Have Healthy Children*, she recommended the use of potassium chloride for colic, which caused the death of an infant. As a result of the lawsuit that followed, the book was withdrawn and reedited before being republished. In 1954, she published her *Let's Eat Right to Keep Fit*, and finally, in 1965, her final book, *Let's Get Well*. Davis argues there against the notion that "obesity is chiefly of psychosomatic origin," so popularly advocated by Hilde Bruch (Davis 1965: 65). Rather, she argues, "too few nutrients are supplied in our diets to burn fat readily" (Davis 1965: 65) and we can eliminate fat by making these available. She presents dietary "cures" for arthritis, diabetes, gout, high blood pressure, and disorders of the nervous system.

Davis' popularity remained so high that at the 1969 White House Conference on Food and Nutrition, she was identified as the most damaging source of false nutrition information in the nation. She has been called "one of this century's masters of the anecdote presented as factual evidence" (Mowbray 1992: 192). Yet her views on questions such as the drinking of unpasteurized milk, are still cited as authorities (Planck 2006). We should remember that she wrote in *Let's Get Well*: "I have yet to know of a single adult to develop cancer who has habitually drunk a quart of milk daily" (Davis 1965: 266). Indeed, "most cancer could probably be prevented if the nutritional knowledge now available were applied" (Davis 1965: 274). Such claims came over time to be seen as excessive.

SLG

*See also* Bruch, Hauser

**References and Further Reading**
Davis, Adelle (1935) *Optimum Health*, Los Angeles: California Graphic Press.

—— (1939) *You Can Stay Well*, Los Angeles: California Graphic Press.

—— (1947) *Let's Cook It Right: Good Health Comes from Good Cooking*, New York: Harcourt Brace.

—— (1951) *Let's Have Healthy Children*, New York: Harcourt, Brace & World.

—— (1965) *Let's Get Well*, New York: Harcourt, Brace & World.

Mowbray, Scott (1992) *The Food Fight*, New York: Random House.

Planck, Nina (2006) *Real Food: What to Eat and Why*, New York: Bloomsbury Publishing.

# Detoxification

Popular detoxification (detox) diets work under the assumption that people regularly and normally take in toxins from their environment. We worry about asbestos in insulation, lead in paint, and dioxins in tampons. The goal of detox dieting is to improve one's health by removing these accumulated toxins from the body, as they are the cause of ill health. The main idea is that by regulating food and water intake, and sometimes taking certain herbs and supplements, toxins are removed from the body, and it returns to its normal, healthy state. Religions and moral philosophies have detoxification diets as well. The focus in those diets is on moral reform, but the means of regulating food intake remains the same. Exponents of alternative medicine, such as Frank Ervolino, a doctor of naturopathic medicine, asserts that detoxing can "prevent disease" and lessen the effects of "autoimmune diseases, such as arthritis . . . and chronic fatigue syndrome" (Ervolino 2005: 32). There are many people who claim that detox diets work wonders, but there is also a strong voice against detox dieting.

The effects of toxins in the body are as numerous as they are hazardous. Americans are anxious about toxins, a theme inherent in alternative medical circles. This is summarized in the claim of Michael T. Murray, a naturopathic physician, that the environment is becoming increasingly toxic (2003: 9). It may also be that we are becoming more aware of that fact. There is much about our normal environment that is a potential hazard to our health: Radiation from cell phones, old color television sets, old smoke detectors, x-ray machines, and power lines are a small sampling. There is also the radiation from the sun, of course, and with holes in the ozone layer it is important to be extra mindful about protecting the skin from unnecessary exposure, which can lead to skin cancer, unattractive wrinkles, and "old age spots."

Even though radiation can be a hazard to one's health, chemicals in our food are a much more frequent reason given for detoxing. The U.S. Environmental Protection Agency (EPA), and the U.S. Food and Drug Administration (FDA) have focused research on the toxins in animals and animal products. Animals eat food which has been exposed to pesticides and pollutants, and when we eat those animals, we take in the toxins too. Oceanic animals, like salmon and shark, have dangerously high levels of mercury in their meat as a result of polluted runoff that seeps into aquatic vegetation, travels up the food chain, and results in mercury poisoning in humans. Sometimes what we eat is not even food at all. Gloria Gilbère raises the issue that plastic residue, from products like Saran™ Wrap and Styrofoam™ coffee cups, may be found in human fat (2004: 34).

Thus, detox diets take on a mammoth challenge by attempting to eliminate all toxins that we ingest. Fast foods as well as foods that have been processed or refined are avoided in the diets. They focus instead on replacing them with nonprocessed foods, which are intended to get our digestive system working efficiently again. With detoxes, there persists a notion that our intestines need cleaning. It is largely in them that the toxins manifest themselves, dirtying them and creating a source of ill health. According to Ervolino, the symptoms from a diet of overprocessed, refined, and fast foods are "low energy, pain (joint, headache or others), anxiety, irritability, heartburn or other digestive issues" (Ervolino 2005: 32), but other symptoms commonly attributed to excess toxins are extra fat, bloating, and shorter life.

A detox diet should include everything that a human body needs to live (Murray 2003: 9), even though it is followed for a definite period. The typical detox is almost exclusively "vegan," and some allow for eggs or small amounts of meat. Organic fruits, vegetables, and legumes are claimed to contain no chemical additives and are thus viewed as healthier because they do not. The essential proteins and fats lacking in a mostly fruit and vegetable diet come from seeds, nuts, unhydrogenated oils, and certain vegetables. Depending on the diet, various nutrients are prescribed to help the liver, kidneys, and other detoxifying organs, or to make up for vitamins and minerals not included in the diet. But it is not enough to consume just organic, vegan products. Many "organic" products contain "natural" toxins. Would "organic tobacco" be better for us than processed tobacco? Detox diets limit or exclude these from daily use. Detox diets include high-fiber foods (Murray 2003: 9), such as raw fruits, steamed vegetables, and crushed flax seed and soy nuts, to scrub and flush out the intestines, which can accumulate high levels of bacteria. Drinking plenty of water is also important to flush out the intestines as well as the rest of the body. Such views echo earlier medical claims from the Stoics to Upton Sinclair that the "effluence" of our waste products signals the corruption of the body, rather than being "natural" products of human metabolism.

Like other diets, detoxes have various requirements, mainly controlling food intake. They restrict which foods can be eaten and require certain foods to be eaten at certain times. Most require one to take in fewer calories than one is used to. The overall goal of these complex eating habits is to alter the body and improve physical and mental well-being. One advocate, Lynn Wallis, having tried a detox, remarks on the numerous physical changes due to the diet. She reports benefits to her hair and skin, that "(her) urine was completely colourless which is a very healthy sign," and she lost at least "a half inch of 'bloat' all over (her) body" (Wallis 2004: 23). And, the holy grail of dieting: she lost 8 pounds (Wallis 2004: 22), she claims. If the detoxer feels better, then the detox has worked. Wallis, like other detoxers, claims that the detox diet made her feel "fantastic" (Wallis 2004: 22). After all, a major part of being healthy is feeling healthy. She uses flowery language to emphasize her improved state of being. Wallis's "eyes were sparkling and clear" and her energy was "boundless" (Wallis 2004: 23).

The notion that the body needs to remove toxins is a good one. However, detox dieting is not straightforward. Certainly, it is healthier to include wholegrains in one's diet in place of processed grain, and there are plenty of toxins that one needs to watch out for when going through life: lead, mercury, and asbestos have already been mentioned, but there is no such thing as white-bread poisoning from Wonder® Bread. The toxins removed during a detox are not identified. Bernard Dixon makes this claim as well and adds, " 'detoxification' is a term legitimately applied only (to) . . . situations such as drug addiction and paraquat poisoning" (2005: 261). For millions of years, all life forms have been subject to toxins and, as a result, the human body has an array of organs to deal with detoxifying. The liver, the kidney, the tonsils . . . the entire digestive system has ways of dealing with the toxins it encounters. When organs cannot handle toxins, there are certain medical diets that can help in the detoxing process. Sometimes, even when organs can handle toxins themselves, there are medical ways of assisting the body. For instance, drug withdrawal is painful, and doctors medicate patients to ensure a successful and more pleasant detox to prevent the patient from reverting to his or her addiction.

Beyond considering whether or not it is legitimate to call these popular diets "detoxification," they are still not necessarily good. There are unpleasant aspects to them, such as headaches, which are caused by the fewer calories. Also, one can increase the level of toxins in one's blood by going on a detox diet. When ingesting fewer calories than one is used to, the body will use stored fat, which has toxins in it, as energy. On top of being potentially unhealthy, detoxing requires one to put excessive time into food preparation. Detox diets are typically for a set period of time and act as vacations from an unhealthy life, but this is not as effective as consistently pushing oneself toward becoming healthier.

However, there are other aspects of some detox diets that go beyond food restriction, such as exercise and even positive thinking; these play into a more complete view of good health. Detox diets are complex and have positive and negative impacts on different individuals' health. They are one aspect of what it means to lead a healthy life.

SLG/Benjamin D. Archer

*See also* Alternative Medicine; Kellogg; Religion and Dieting

## References

Dixon, B. (2005) "Detox, a Mass Delusion," *The Lancet Infectious Diseases* 5 (5): 261.

Ervolino, F. (2005) "Should You Cleanse?" *Better Nutrition* 10: 32.

Gilbère, G. (2004) "Understanding Pollution, in Your Body, That Is," *Total Health* 263: 34–5.

Murray, M.T. (2003) "Environmental Stress Factors on Your Health," *Total Health* 253: 9–10.

Wallis, L. (2004) "Detox Your Way to Health," *Nursing Standard* 17: 22–3.

# Developing World

In the developing world, undernourishment in the form of famine has historically been a bigger public health concern than overnourishment. There are serious health consequences when a person does not have enough food to eat or does not have sufficient variety in the diet. Malnourishment can lead to lack of energy, early death, and social disorder. Specific conditions of undernourishment can also exist when there is not enough of a specific type of nutrient such as protein or a particular vitamin. The case of pellagra, a disease caused by niacin (vitamin B3) deficiency, is a prime historical example. Endemic in the American South after the Civil War, it was argued by contemporaries that it was an "infectious disease of the poor." In 1918 at least 10,000 deaths were attributed to pellagra. Indeed, it was a disease of the poor as they ate the "three M's": meat (pork fatback); molasses; and meal (cornmeal). Its cure, as Joseph Goldberger discovered in the 1920s, was either to change one's diet by adding "real" meat, fresh vegetables, and milk or to augment it with a small amount of "brewer's yeast." The social impact had been catastrophic, as pellagra had as its symptoms mental illness as well as a wide range of physical debility, often ending in death (Kraut 2003). Although traditionally such types of malnutrition are associated with the developing world, especially with areas suffering from famine, overnourishment in the form of obesity has also become a problem. Indeed, where in the early twentieth century, pellagra was seen as a problem of the "New South," today obesity is most common in precisely those areas long haunted by undernourishment (Lopez et al. 2006). Pellagra continues to be a problem in developing countries where there is significant malnutrition or where niacin-deficient foods such as corn and rice are the primary sources of nutrition. Yet, there too, overnutrition may result in the diseases associated with obesity.

The complex nature of malnutrition in the developing world means that dieting interventions need to be developed for the specific state of nutrition in the population being targeted. Famines are not due to lack of food worldwide. They arise as a result of civil unrest affecting specific people. Amartya Sen's 1981 *Poverty and Famines: An Essay on Entitlement and Deprivation* argued that famine occurs not from a lack of food, but from inequalities built into mechanisms for distributing food. War and violence often prevent global relief agencies from delivering food to the people who are in need. Agencies such as the World Health Organization must negotiate with the local governments to allow food shipments to people. The main goal for this type of intervention is just to get people fed.

Sometimes, dietary interventions are needed because a particular population is deficient in a specific nutrient such as protein, vitamin A, or iron. In these cases, even though enough food is available to maintain caloric requirements, interventions are still necessary, as was the case with pellagra. Seasonal variations in the food supply can lead to deficiencies in protein. The results are classic images of emaciation, which have become the icons of famine. Two types of physical images of starvation exist, often appearing together. Marasmus, which is caused by the lack of energy due to insufficient food, presents with a "little old man" appearance in children, with obvious signs of emaciation: Radical thinness, prominent appearance of the ribs and spine, often accompanied by an alert but irritable behavior. Kwashiorkor, caused by the development of inefficient pathways through the protein deficiency disease often found in famine areas, provides further variations on the classic images of stunted children with its signs and symptoms of edema, with protruding stomachs that can be taken for plumpness on first glance; skin lesions; thick, easily bruised skin; thin, dry hair; lethargy and apathetic behavior (Eddleston et al. 2005: 594–5). They are the result of their not being able to meet the daily protein requirements for growth. Lack of protein leads to a weakened immune system and a greater chance of death from infection (Kleinman 2003). Often in areas of famine, therapeutic milk products, such as F75 and HEM (high energy milk), are employed. Interventions to target famine will then often consist of making further protein sources such as beans, meat, or eggs available.

Micronutrient (such as iron, folate, iodine, or vitamin C) deficiencies can lead to a variety of health outcomes such as mental retardation, maternal death in childbirth, and growth retardation. When micronutrients are the main source of deficiency, interventions often focus on supplementation of diet or fortification of foods. Fortification involves putting micronutrients such as iron, iodine, or folate in foods, like flour or salt, commonly consumed by the people. Most micronutrient deficiencies are reversible conditions and can be fixed with proper supplementation.

Overnutrition, a condition common to the developed world, is now affecting the developing world. Overnutrition often manifests itself in the form of obesity. As the developing world moves from rural to urban, from farming communities to manufacturing communities, individuals undergo a "nutrition transition." The nutrition transition occurs when a society moves away farming and the raising of livestock as the main source for their own food. Moderately developed countries have about 30 percent of their population engaged in farm work; affluent societies have only about 5 percent. Instead, food is often obtained secondarily, from markets, and, given the global expansion of food production and distribution, even supermarkets. Rather than obtaining food from the source, as much as 75 percent of the food is often processed and packaged, leaving it devoid of vitamins and minerals (James 2002). In addition to the change in access to the food supply, the nutrition transition is usually accompanied by a more sedentary lifestyle as people pursue work in offices or hi-tech manufacturing facilities.

People in countries undergoing nutrition transition are experiencing the same problems with obesity that has been seen in the U.S.A. In Latin America and the Caribbean as of 1995, there were still 6 million children under the age of five with low weight for their ages, yet the general tendency is now toward obesity: "In peri-urban areas it is normal to find a family in which the father has high blood pressure, may be fat or not, is short, and has a problematic history of malnutrition; the mother is anemic, probably obese, and short; and the child suffer frequent infections and show stunting" (Peña and Bacallao 2000: 3). The obesity rates in women there have increased more rapidly than in men. In Guatemala in 1995, 26.2 percent of women were overweight; 8 percent were obese (Peña and Bacallao 2000). The Food and Agriculture Organization of the United Nations (FAO) estimates that the burden of obesity in the developing world is becoming greater than the burden of not having enough food (see <http://www.fao.org>). Interventions to target these people are very different to those targeting people who do not have adequate food. Culturally specific interventions focus on teaching people about the importance of daily physical activity as well as moderate and diverse food intake. People in such populations very rarely have the wide variety of dieting choices available to the developed world. Therefore, the message is usually one of limiting food intake while maintaining energy requirements.

The movement of peoples also impacts on weight and disease. An example is the "Hispanic Paradox." Highly acculturated Mexicans have a marked higher rate of obesity in the U.S.A. than their Mexican cousins. Thus, Mexican-born men and women in the U.S.A. had the smallest waist circumference. Mexicans who were American-born speakers of English had intermediate waist circumference, but U.S.-born Spanish speakers had the largest waist circumference. Gender plays a role, as men were always larger than women (Sundquist and Winkelby 2000).

Thus, in such cultures, the very manifestation of eating disorders in addition to obesity reflects local concern. In China, for example, while anorexia nervosa is present in all of its "Western" appearance, patients attribute food refusal to "stomach bloating, loss of appetite, no hunger" and other rationales not concerned with body image (Lee et al. 1998). For these patients, "medical" symptoms such as "stomach bloating" are socially much more acceptable as a means for bodily self-control than anxiety about weight gain.

SLG/SUZANNE JUDD

*See also* China in the Twentieth Century; Emaciated Body Images in the Media

## References and Further Reading

Allen, L.H. (2006) "New Approaches for Designing and Evaluating Food Fortification Programs," *Journal of Nutrition* 136 (4): 1055–8.

Crawford, E. Margaret (1981) "Indian Meal and Pellagra in Nineteenth-Century Ireland," in J.M. Goldstrom and L.A. Clarkson (eds), *Irish Population, Economy, and Society: Essays in Honour of the late K.H Connell*, Oxford: Clarendon Press, pp. 113–33.

Drewnowski, Adam and Popkin, Barry M. (1997) "The Nutrition Transition: New Trends in the Global Diet," *Nutrition Reviews* 55 (2): 31–43.

Eddleston, Michael, Davidson, Robert, Wilkinson, Robert, and Pierini, Stephen (2005) *Oxford Handbook of Tropical Medicine*, Oxford: Oxford University Press.

Food and Agriculture Organization (FAO) (2001) "The Developing World's New Burden: Obesity." Available online at <http://www.fao.org/FOCUS/E/obesity/obes1.htm> (accessed March 18, 2007).

James, W. Philip T. (2002) "A World View of the Obesity Problem," in Christopher G. Fairburn and Kelly D. Brownell (eds), *Eating Disorders and Obesity: A Comprehensive Handbook*, 2nd edn, New York: Guilford Press, pp. 411–16.

Kleinman, Ronald E. (2003) *Pediatric Nutrition Handbook*, 5th edn, Elk Grove Village, Ill.: American Academy of Pediatrics.

Kraut, Alan M. (2003) *Goldberger's War: The Life and Work of a Public Health Crusader*, New York: Hill & Wang.

Lee, Sing, and Katzman, Melanie A. (2002) "Cross-Cultural Perspective on Eating Disorders," in Christopher G. Fairburn and Kelly D. Brownell (eds), *Eating Disorders and Obesity: A Comprehensive Handbook*, 2nd edn, New York: Guilford Press, pp. 260–4.

Lee, Sing, Lee, A., and Leung, T. (1998) "Cross-Cultural Validity of the Eating Disorder Inventory: A Study of Chinese Patients with Eating Disorder in Hong Kong," *International Journal of Eating Disorders* 23 (2): 177–88.

Lopez, A.D., Mathers, C.D., and Ezzati, M. (2006) *Global Burden of Disease and Risk Factors*, New York: Oxford University Press.

Peña, Manuel and Bacallao, Jorge (2000) "Obesity Among the Poor: An Emerging Problem in Latin America," in *Obesity and Poverty: A New Public Health Challenge*, Washington, DC: Pan American Health Orgainzation, pp. 3–10.

Popkin, Barry M. (2003) "The Nutrition Transition in the Developing World," *Development Policy Review* 21 (5–6): 581–97.

Sen, Amartya (1981) *Poverty and Famines: An Essay on Entitlement and Deprivation*, Oxford: Clarendon Press.

Sundquist J. and Winkelby, M. (2000) "Country of Birth, Acculturation Status and Abdominal Obesity in a National Sample of Mexican-American Women and Men," *International Journal of Epidemiology* 29 (3): 470–7.

Wahlqvist, M.L. (2005) "The New Nutrition Science: Sustainability and Development," *Public Health Nutrition* 8 (6a): 766–72.

# Diana, Princess of Wales (1961–97)

Diana Frances Mountbatten-Windsor, née Spencer, British philanthropist and ex-wife of Charles, Prince of Wales. She was an outspoken figure in the area of popular dieting culture. Lady Diana Spencer married Charles in 1981, at the age of nineteen. From the beginning, their marriage was under extraordinary pressures being in the media spotlight. The young Diana suffered the pressures of celebrity more than her spouse, as she was not from a court background and had to adapt to life constantly in the spotlight on her own.

She was a member of the upper-class, club scene, called by the media the Sloane Rangers (as they congregated about Sloane Square). They were characterized by their "sportiness" and "anti-intellectualism." There was a great emphasis on slimness for the women, who stressed physical rather than intellectual virtues. Later, Diana announced that she had suffered from bulimia nervosa as a means of explaining her psychological vulnerability during her marriage. She also confessed that she had a number of other stress-induced psychiatric conditions, including potential borderline personality disorder, postpartum depression, and self-mutilation. It is speculated that her abnormal eating patterns began around the time of her marriage, continued through the birth of her two children (William in 1982 and Henry in 1984), and until she sought treatment in the late 1980s. The late 1980s also marked the point when Diana began to gain acceptance by the people on her own terms for her charity work, most prominently with AIDS and landmine organizations. Here, the announcement about her psychological difficulties was part of a campaign to "humanize" her as she negotiated with the Court about her status. By speaking in public about eating disorders, she was able to place herself among the growing number of celebrities who were able to admit "failure," which was less and less seen as stigmatizing.

In 1992, Andrew Morton's confessional book *Diana, Her True Story*, in which she explicitly spoke to him about her bulimia, was released. In 1993, she spoke on the importance of destigmatizing eating disorders to an international congress. She also talked on television in a famous 1995 BBC interview with Martin Bashir about the problem. She had become a "poster-girl" for beating eating disorders. This position allowed her a moral superiority but was also a means of identification with an increasing number of young women self-aware of their position in the dieting culture. In 1997, Diana died in a high-speed car chase trying to escape paparazzi, together with international playboy Dodi Al Fayed, the son of the owner of Harrod's department store in London.

The *Oxford Dictionary of National Biography* situates Diana's impact on the perception of bulimia with the following:

> Where the life and death of Diana had perhaps their greatest impact was on the acceptability of public displays of emotion … Her adoption of the language of psychotherapy, her patronage of the culture of alternative therapies and lifestyle gurus, her confessional approach, all reflected and amplified the move of parts of British society away from the traditional culture of stiff upper lips and repressed emotion.
>
> (Reynolds 2004)

There is, however, controversy over her true impact. Laura Currin's recent study in the *British Journal of Psychiatry* showed that from 1988 until 2000, as the (self-reported) rate of anorexia remained roughly the same, the rate of bulimia went up drastically, which implies to some that more people were seeking help, perhaps because of the destigmatizing effect of the Princess of Wales's public stance on the issue. The rate declined after 1997, suggesting to some that people once again were unwilling to come forward.

SLG/Katherine Mancuso

## References and Further Reading

Currin, L., Schmidt, U. Treasure, J., and Jick, H. (2005) "Time Trends in Eating Disorders," *British Journal of Psychiatry* 186: 132–5.

Diana, Princess of Wales "Speech on eating disorders." Available online at <http://www.settelen.com/diana_eating_disorders.htm> (accessed May 11, 2006).

Morton, Andrew (1992) *Diana, Her True Story*, New York: Simon & Schuster.

Reynolds, K.D. (2004) "Diana, Princess of Wales

(1961–97)," in *Oxford Dictionary of National Biography*, Oxford: Oxford University Press. <http:// www.oxforddnb.com.proxy.library.emory.edu/view/ article/68348> (accessed June 1, 2007)

# Disability

Obesity is now considered a disability, though for a long period of time it was not. In 1973, Carolyn Soughers brought the first (but unsuccessful) size-discrimination lawsuit. She had been denied employment with a county civil-service agency on account of her size. It was only in 1993 that the federal Equal Employment Opportunity Commission ruled that "severely obese" people could claim protection under federal statutes barring discrimination against the disabled. A "friend of the court" brief based on this ruling was filed in the case of *Cook* v. *Rhode Island* (0 F.3d 17 [1st Cir 1993]), a suit brought by a Rhode Island woman, Bonnie Cook, who accused her state of illegally denying her a job on the basis of "perceived disability" because of her size. In this case, the Equal Opportunity Commission filed an amicus brief stating that "voluntary morbid obesity" is covered under the Americans with Disabilities Act. As obesity became a disability, by 2000, San Francisco, Calif., Washington, DC, Santa Cruz, Calif., and the state of Michigan had passed ordinances that added height and weight to the same antidiscrimination codes in addition to race, religion, sex, gender, sexual orientation, disability, and place of birth.

The Americans with Disability Act (1990) stated that impairment was a state that substantially limited major life activities. (Analogous definitions are used in the Canadian Charter of Rights and Freedoms [1994], the British Disability Discrimination Act [1995] and the Swedish Act Concerning Support and Services for Persons with Certain Functional Impairments [1993].) And obesity certainly does limit such activities. The obese, as we shall see,

continually encounter various forms of discrimination, including outright intentional exclusion, the discriminatory effects of architectural, transportation, and communication barriers, overprotective rules and policies, failure to make modifications to existing facilities and practices, exclusionary

qualification standards and criteria, segregation, and relegation to lesser services, programs, activities, benefits, jobs, or other opportunities.

*(Americans with Disability Act* 1990)

Under the regulations promulgated to enforce this act "morbid obesity," defined as body weight more than 100 percent over the norm, is "clearly an impairment" (*Equal Employment Opportunity Commission Compliance Manual* § 902.2 [c] [5]). This rather arbitrary line means that to be covered by the "Americans with Disabilities Act," the individual cannot just be too overweight for a specific occupation. In one case, the court held that the male "plaintiff cannot demonstrate that he was regarded as disabled on the basis of a specific job of his choosing" (*Clemons* v. *Big Ten Conference*, [1997] WL 89227 [N.D. Ill. 1997]). What that means is that the question of defining obesity as a disability still remains fluid.

One can add that not only is "fat" debated under the question of disability, but also that "too thin" is drawn into question. In 2000, a student, Keri Krissik, sued Stonehill College, a private Catholic college in Easton, Massachusetts "for refusing to let her register on the grounds of her anorexia," in violation of the Americans with Disabilities Act. At the time she was 5 feet and 6 inches and weighed 97 pounds, and had suffered a heart attack the preceding spring. The judge of the U.S. District Court, Rya Zobel, dismissed her suit saying that Krissik failed to show she would be irreparably harmed by not being allowed to attend the college. The judge did not, however, rule on whether Krissik could properly be classified as disabled (Roeber 2000).

The definition of a disability seems to be rather specific, even if the Supreme Court has been recently altering and limiting it. The World Health Organization (WHO), in its 1980 *International Classification of Impairments, Disabilities, and Handicaps*, makes a seemingly clear distinction between impairment, disability, and handicap.

Impairment is an abnormality of structure or function at the organ level, while disability is the functional consequence of such impairment. A handicap is the social consequences of impairment and its resultant disability. Thus cognitive or hearing impairments may lead to communication problems, which in turn result in isolation or dependency. Such a functional approach (and this approach was long the norm in American common and legal usage) seems to be beyond any ideological bias. This changes very little in the most recent shift to the idea that disability is to be redefined on a scale of "human variation" that postulates the difficulties of the disabled as the result of the inflexibility of social institutions rather than their own impairment.

When, however, we substitute "obesity" for "cognitive impairment" in the functional model, there is suddenly an evident and real set of implied ethical differences in thinking about what a disability can be. What is obesity? While there is a set of contemporary medical definitions of obesity, it is also clear that the definition of those who are obese changes from culture to culture over time. Obesity is more than the body-mass index (wt/ht$^2$), because even this changes meaning over time. Today in the U.S.A. and the U.K., people with a body-mass index between 25 and 30 kg/m$^2$ are categorized as overweight, and those with a body-mass index above 30 kg/m$^2$ are labeled as obese. Yet, when the National Health and Nutrition Survey in 1999 recorded a 55 percent increase in obesity over three decades in the U.S.A., they retrospectively used the body mass index of 30 to compute this figure. What is fat and what is obese (their two categories) shifts over time.

Let us apply the rather straightforward WHO standards of disability to the world of the obese. Is obesity the end product of impairment or is it impairment itself? If it must begin with impairment, what "organ" is "impaired"? Is it the body itself? Is it the digestive system? Is it the circulatory system? Or is it the mind, meaning, therefore, the obese suffer from that most stigmatizing of illnesses, mental illness? Is obesity a mental illness which is the result of an addictive personality (where food is the addiction)? Is addiction a sign of the lack of will? Is it physical dependency, as in heroin addiction? Is "addiction" a genetically preprogrammed "error" in the human body, which expresses itself in psychological desire for food or the mere inability to not know when one is no longer hungry?

Is the impairment of obesity like lung cancer in that it is the result of the voluntary consumption of a dangerous substance such as fat or carbohydrates? Certainly, WHO believes this. Having struggled against tobacco consumption, it is intent on launching a campaign against the rising levels of obesity by persuading manufacturers of processed foods to limit the amounts of added sugar. Is such food "addictive" like nicotine, or is it merely an interchangeable sign in society for those things we all desire but most of us can limit? Surely it is not possible to go without food as one could go without cigarettes. Is the obese person mentally or physically disabled? On the other hand, can you be obese and mentally stable? Is obesity a disease of "civilization" caused by too fat or too rich or too well-processed food? Is its "cure" a return to "real" food or the rejection of food in general? Has it become the new "epidemic" to be chartered by epidemiologists and combated by public health organizations? If it is an epidemic, is it contagious or ubiquitous? Are diet and exercise the sole cures for the myriad definitions of obesity? Is the social consequence of obesity isolation or a central place in the society? Where on the scale of "human variation" are you placed in a world completely shaped by and for those who are not fat? Is obesity exogenous or is it endogenous? Are you in the end treated like a social pariah or Santa Claus?

SLG

*See also* Celebrities; Fast Food; Obesity Epidemic; Smoking

## References and Further Reading

*Americans with Disability Act* (1990). Available online at <http://www.dol.gov/esa/regs/statutes/ofccp/ada.htm> (accessed June 1, 2007)

Garland-Thompson, Rosemarie (2001) *Extraordinary Bodies: Figuring Physical Disability in American Culture and Literature*, New York: Columbia University Press.

Longmore, Paul K. and Umansky, Lauri (2001) *The New Disability History: American Perspectives*, New York: New York University Press.

Mitchell, David T. and Snyder, Sharon L. (1997) *The Body and Physical Difference: Discourses of Disability*, Ann Arbor, Mich.: University of Michigan Press.

O'Brien, Ruth (2001) *Crippled Justice: The History of*

*Modern Disability Policy in the Workplace*, Chicago, Ill.: University of Chicago Press.
Roeber, Jessica (2000) "Anorexic Sues to Live on Campus," *The Boston Globe* December 21: B6.

World Health Organization (2001) *International Classification of Functioning, Disability and Health*, Geneva: World Health Organization.

# Dublin, Louis (1882–1969)

## Statistician and epidemiologist with the Metropolitan Life Company (MetLife)

Dublin was interested in the use of statistics to quantify the occurrence of diseases, thinking that knowing risk would help to increase people's life expectancy by changing their actions. In 1942, he examined the association between mortality and weight among the 4 million people insured by MetLife. He classified people based on height, weight, and body frame (small, medium, or large). At that time, the people insured by MetLife who maintained the average weight for twenty-five-year-olds tended to have greater longevity than those who were outside this weight range. Based on these findings, Dublin determined that people who maintained weight in an ideal range would live longer and be at lower risk for MetLife to insure. He published tables containing ideal weights for individuals based on their height and body frame.

Originally intended to separate people into favorable and unfavorable risk categories for the writing of life insurance, the MetLife tables became so popular among American physicians in the 1950s that they were renamed "desirable weight" tables in 1959. These tables enabled physicians to individualize a person's ideal weight based on that person's individual body height. People who were above the desirable weight for height were labeled unhealthy and were instructed to go on a diet to lose weight. Knowing one's desirable weight led to the increased popularity of weighing oneself at home to determine success when dieting. People now had a weight goal based on a "science" that provided them with an absolute barometer for dieting success and promised health and longevity. These tables ceased in 1983, and, thereafter, governmental or supra-governmental tables (such as those by the World Health Organization) have been used to measure the mortality and morbidity of people defined as excessively fat or excessively thin.

SLG/SUZANNE JUDD

*See also* Cornaro; Scales and Public Weighing

## References and Further Reading
Dublin, Louis I. (1966) *After Eighty Years: The Impact of Life Insurance on the Public Health*, Gainesville, Fla.: University of Florida Press.
Jarrett, R.J. (1986) "Is There an Ideal Body Weight?" *British Medical Journal* 293 (6545): 493–5.
McClellan, Patsy (2005) "Louis Israel Dublin, a Statistics and Social Welfare Titan," *Amstat News. Special Edition*. Available online at <http://www.amstat.org/about/statisticians/bios/dublinlouis.pdf> (accessed June 1, 2007).

# E

## Eating Competitions

On your marks . . . Get set . . . Eat! With thousands of fans screaming and ESPN cameras covering it all, off they go. A group of twenty or so adults, ranging from the small, fit, and trim to the big and tall football lineman, commence to gorge down, as fast as they can, about two dozen or so hot dogs piled high in front of each from Nathan's Deli. Buns and all! Is this an event at your local county fair? No, it's Nathan's Fourth of July Hot Dog Eating Contest in New York, with competitors from across the world, who have practiced all year long to down almost fifty hot dogs—not simply in one sitting, but in just twelve short minutes! Eaters' profiles can vary in age, weight, or gender. For example, Sonya Thomas, who holds the second-place rank of top eaters on the circuit worldwide, is a thirty-seven-year old, and 105-pound woman. In contrast, Joey Chestnut, who holds the third place rank, is a twenty-two-year-old male weighing 230 pounds.

In the past, informal eating competitions were about who could eat a certain amount of food in the shortest time, but it evolved into a formal competition to determine who could eat the biggest quantity of a certain food in a given amount of time. According to the International Federation of Competitive Eating (IFOCE), the situation of "30 hungry Neanderthals in a cave" fighting over a rabbit is a form of competitive eating that existed in the earlier days. It was not until the twentieth century that food-eating competitions became organized by and popularized at state and county fairs. The first documented hot-dog-eating contest was held in 1916 at Coney Island and has continued annually since, except in 1941 and 1971. In the early 1970s, the New York City publicist Max Rosey resuscitated the event to sell Nathan's Hot Dogs at their stand at Coney Island, then in a rapid state of decline. After Rosey's death in 1990, George and Rich Shea took over the Nathan's account and made the hot-dog-eating contest into a quasi-sport. In 1997, they created the IFOCE, based in New York City, to further their agenda of turning what had been a parody of sport into a competitive sport. The IFOCE's motto "In Voro Veritas," "In Gorging Truth," reflects the underlying parody of eating as a sporting event. With the support of sports writers such as Gersh Kuntzman of the *New York Post*, what had begun as a tongue-in-cheek joke quickly became a truly competitive sport. Today more than 6,000 professional eaters are registered with the IFOCE, with the best known having become celebrities. Ironically, at the moment when obesity became the world's newest "epidemic," binge-eating became a sport.

Organized competitive eating has become popular in a number of nations, including the U.S.A., Canada, Germany, Thailand, England, Ireland, the Ukraine, Russia, and Scotland. The most prestigious international event in competitive eating is Nathan's Fourth of July Hot Dog Eating Contest, which claims to be the Super Bowl or Olympics of competitive eating. A group of twenty skilled individuals annually compete at Nathan's flagship restaurant in Coney Island, where the world hot-dog-eating championship began. This twelve-minute contest is watched by fans, supporters, and media. The world record for this contest is held by Japanese, five-time champion, 132-pound Takeru Kobayashi (1978–), who ate 53 ½ of Nathan's Famous Hot Dogs and Buns in twelve minutes on July 4, 2004. Kobayashi also holds the world records for cow brains (17.7 pounds in fifteen minutes), hamburgers (sixty-nine Krystal Square Burgers in eight minutes), and rice balls (20 pounds of rice balls in thirty minutes).

Sports broadcasters on the popular cable network ESPN cover these events and identify the competitions as a sport and competitors as "athletes." The IFOCE spokesperson, Nancy Goldstein, defends the IFOCE referring to eating competitions as a sport because their athletes train to compete and acquire necessary skills for the craft. "Like any sport, the athletes train to compete . . . It is believed that [with] some of the heavier competitors, the extra weight doesn't allow their stomach to expand as much," she said. "Some of the skills needed are capacity to hold the large amount of food, and jaw strength is very important . . . having skill and great speed is very necessary as well."

Since safety is an important issue in any sport, the IFOCE has developed a set of rules. These rules include an age minimum of eighteen years. Also, authorized competitions may only take place in a controlled environment with fitting rules and appropriate medical assistance present. The IFOCE does not advise any in-home training or self-training of any kind and recommends only participating in sanctioned events.

As in any sport, there are conflicts regarding dangers and risks. Since competitive eaters eat and train at extreme levels, eating competitions may be a source of potential problems, seeing that it is not the healthiest thing to do. Overextending the stomach with this amount of food could damage the stomach lining. Depending on the competition, participants may consume anywhere from 4,000 to 12,500 calories in one sitting. The United States Department of Agriculture (USDA) recommends 2,300 calories a day for an average male. Some competitors do not completely digest all the food they eat; instead they vomit, which the IFOCE calls a "Roman incident." The IFOCE disqualifies any competitors who vomit before the time period has expired. This behavior is a form of binge-eating now understood as a sport.

Joseph Regan, MD and bariatric surgeon in Milwaukee went on record to say that by promoting competitive eating, a bad example is being set because it encourages binge-eating as a form of entertainment and sport. Regan and other doctors find it ironic that in an age where people are obsessing about weight and when obesity has emerged as one of the country's most significant health problems, media outlets, such as ESPN and MTV are reporting and glorifying these eating-competition events, recognizing binge-eating as a sport by referring to the competitors as "athletes."

Many people believe that a large body size is advantageous in this sport. However, George Shea, the Chairman of IFOCE contradicts this common notion, arguing that fat actually restricts the stomach from expanding to its greatest capacity. This theory is supported by the fact that today, three of the top competitive eaters in the world weigh less than 150 pounds.

SLG/Rakhi Patel

*See also* Binge-eating; Sports

## References and Further Reading

Alexander, William (2005) "Pig Out," September 1, available online at <http://www.enigmaonline.com/gbase/Expedite/Content?oid=oid%3A1520> (accessed March 18, 2007).

Anon. (July 2002) "A Man Who Can Stomach New York," *The Economist* 364: 29.

Caple, Jim (2006) "Competitive Eating a Man-Eat-Dog World," ESPN, available online at <http://www.espn.go.com/Page2/s/caple/020703.html> (accessed January 29, 2006).

Grabianowski, Ed (2006) "How Competitive Eating Works." Available online at <http://people.howstuffworks.com/competitive-eating.htm> (accessed April 6, 2006).

International Federation of Competitive Eating, available online at <http://www.ifoce.com> (accessed January 29, 2006).

Neary, Lynn (2005) "Interview with George Shea, Chairman of the IFOCE. Talk of the Nation," NPR Online, July 4, available online at <http://www.npr.org/templates/story.php?storyId=4730508> (accessed January 29, 2006).

# Electrotherapy

In the 1790s, based on the work of Luigi Galvani (1737–98), scientists began to study "animal magnetism." Galvani identified the movement of the muscles in a frog when it came in contact with two metals (brass and iron) (Pera 1992). The galvanic (direct) currents produced were seen as a "natural" phenomenon inherent to the very composition of the body. With the discovery by Alessandro Volta (1745–1827) in 1816 of the "voltaic pile" (battery), induced currents could be mastered in ways that static electricity never was. Volta showed that what was assumed to be a "natural" product of the body was in fact the result of the generation of a direct current of electricity through contact with metal. Joseph Carpue (1764–1846), one of the first modern cosmetic surgeons, used electricity as a medical treatment for somatic diseases (Carpue 1803). In 1827, Carlo Matteucci (1811–68) developed the theory of "counter-currents" for the treatment of muscular paralysis (Matteucci 1844: 266).

In 1831, Michael Faraday (1791–1867) discovered electromagnetic induction (the faradic coil), offering an enhanced electrotherapy through its alternating electric current. The German neurologist Paul Du Bois Reymond (1831–89) in 1849 formulated the law of electrical muscle stimulation and first employed the faradic coil for muscle stimulation. The French physiologist Guillaume Benjamin Amand Duchenne (1806–75) continued to investigate those points on the exterior of the body, triggering deep muscular reactions when stimulated with "localized faradization" (Duchenne 1855). This discovery led to a wide-ranging therapeutics of the body through the identification of trigger points where induced currents could stimulate the muscle tissue. In Germany, Robert Remak (1815–65) challenged Duchenne's use of "faradic" currents and advocated the use of Volta's battery, which produced direct current. Remak made extravagant claims for the therapeutic efficacy of electricity, which caused a cascade of anatomical and therapeutic studies of his "mystical points" of the body.

The "electrical treatment of obesity" was one of the applications of electrotherapy that treated almost every pathology diagnosed through the early twentieth century, understanding them all as having "somatic" rather than "psychological" causes. By the middle of the nineteenth century, "obesity" had become a common medical diagnosis based on the popularity of William Banting's

pamphlet. It was understood as a somatic disorder. The American electrotherapist George Miller Beard (1839–83) as early as 1869 treated a wide range of neurological illnesses, including the "American Disease," neurasthenia, with electrotherapy. All of these were understood as somatic diseases of the nervous system. One of Beard's most important disciples was S. Weir Mitchell. Mitchell, who strongly advocated diet as the primary treatment for "nervous" ailments, treated severely underweight patients (but not obese ones) with electricity "for the purpose of exercising muscles in persons at rest" (Mitchell 1877: 62). His case of Mrs. R showed rapid improvement, "gaining thirteen pounds on a weight of ninety-eight pounds . . ." (Mitchell 1877: 64). Mitchell followed the application of electrotherapy, being quite aware of the discomfort caused by such treatments, in the light of the anatomical views of the effect of electricity on the muscular system. For him, it was a physiological intervention, which enabled very thin (and therefore unhealthy) patients to gain weight. Little or no attention was paid to the psychological impact of such therapies.

By the beginning of the twentieth century, the radiologist Jean-Alban Bergonié (1857–1925) advocated the employment of electricity to create a general sense of stimulation of the body to improve overall health. There had been the use of static electricity to treat "neurasthenic patients with obesity" prior to that (Tousey 1915: 68). For Bergonié, electrification of the muscles was understood to be a surrogate for exercise. The treatment for obesity was in general the rapid contraction of the muscles of the body to maximize muscle strengthening while minimizing "one cannot say pain, for there is no pain with this treatment—sensation" (Humphris 1921: 209).

In the electrification of the muscles treatment, the patient was seated in a "semi-reclining chair" with fixed electrodes and was outfitted with a set of moveable, very large electrodes on the thigh, calf, abdomen, and arms. All were covered with damp towels to enhance conduction. The patient was covered with sacks of sand weighing up to 200 pounds. Treatments lasted from forty minutes to sixty minutes. According to the advocates of this approach, patients lost weight and gained "general well-being." In one case cited, a patient lost 1.5 inches around his neck, as well as 3 inches from his waist in three weeks. The fact that he only lost 7 pounds suggested he had gained muscle mass. While it was recommended that fruit, vegetables, and salad be consumed, diet was seen as a minor aspect of the overall treatment (Humphris 1921: 217). In addition, electrotherapy was often used to treat what was seen as the pathological results of obesity, the "failure or perversion of nutrition," including diabetes (Hedley 1900: 206–10). Alternative forms of therapy, such as "hydro-electric baths," were also employed, with the patient seated in a warm water bath while electricity was applied through the water for half an hour (Tousey 1915: 665).

Some physicians also advocated "cephalic electrization" which was "found to produce a loss of weight" as well as treat neurasthenia. The electrodes were placed at the nape of the neck and on the forehead; current was gradually applied for at least fifteen minutes. The result was both a "clearness of thought and ability to work" as well as a loss of weight (Tousey 1915: 418 and 507).

There was a powerful edge to the claims of electrotherapy. If obesity was primarily a process that could be reversed by a form of passive exercise, then its harmful side effects could be ameliorated. Many physicians of the time came to doubt the very premise of electrotherapy. Sigmund Freud (1856–1939) recalled that he "felt absolutely helpless after the disappointing results [of electrotherapy . . . T]he successes of electrical treatment in nervous patients are the results of suggestion" (Freud vol. 14: p. 9). Freud was among a growing number of physicians in the 1890s who found electrotherapy unsuccessful. Yet, its powerful associations with the newest technologies of mass electrification allowed electrotherapy to remain seductive until World War II.

The electrotherapy of obesity seems to have a similar placebo effect to that suspected by Freud in his patients. The patients undergoing electrotherapy for obesity may lose as much as 20 to 30 pounds but demanded a stricter regimen than the limitations imposed by the physician (Humphris 1921: 218). According to electrotherapists, patients are concerned with improvement in their general appearance and see the physical discomfort as vital to the perceived gain.

The "tingle" effect is the key to the psychological function of electrotherapy (Fishlock 1994). By the late nineteenth century, such shocks were associated with successful medical treatment for obesity. Electrotherapies for obesity have recently reappeared. Since 1995, a "Transcend Implantable Gastric Stimulator" (similar to a cardiac pacemaker) has been used to treat obesity in more than 700 patients. Implanted laparoscopically, the device provides ongoing electric shocks to the stomach. According to a study in France, the stimulator produced "satisfactory short-term weight loss . . . in a subset of patients" (D'Argent 2002). F.M. Ng of Monash University in Australia is exploring "the effect of subcutaneous electrotherapy in reduction of adipose tissue mass in cellulite" (Ng 2006). Electricity is still in the service of weight loss, without much consideration of its psychological implications.

SLG

*See also* Banting; Mitchell

## References and Further Reading

Carpue, J.C. (1803) *An Introduction to Electricity and Galvanism: with Cases, Shewing Their Effects in the Cure of Diseases: To Which Is Added, a Description of Mr. Cuthbertson's Plate Electrical Machine*, London: A. Phillips.

D'Argent, J. (2002) "Gastric Electrical Stimulation as Therapy of Morbid Obesity: Preliminary Results from the French Study," *Obesity Surgery* 12S (1): 21S–25S.

Duchenne, Guillaume Benjamin Amand (1855) *De L'Electrisation localisée*, Paris: J.B. Baillière et fils.

Fishlock, David (December 24, 1994) "The Tingle Factor," *New Scientist* 144: 58–9.

Freud, Sigmund (1955–74) *Standard Edition of the Complete Psychological Works of Sigmund Freud*, ed. and trans. J. Strachey, A. Freud, A. Strachey, and A. Tyson, twenty-four vols, London: Hogarth.

Hedley, W.S. (1900) *Therapeutic Electricity and Practical Muscle Testing*, Philadelphia, Pa.: P. Blakiston's Son & Co.

Humphris, Francis Howard (1921) *Electro-therapeutics for practitioners*, London: Henry Frowde and Hodder & Stoughton.

Matteucci, Carlo (1844) *Traité des phénomènes électro-physiologiques des animaux*, Paris: Fortin, Masson.

Mitchell, S. Weir (1877) *Fat and Blood and How to Make Them*, Philadelphia, Pa.: Lippincott.

Ng, F.M. (2006) "Intracellular signaling and cancer." Available online at <http://www.med.monash.edu.au/biochem/research/projects/obesity-diabetes.html> (accessed April 10, 2006).

Pera, Marcello (1992) *The Ambiguous Frog: The Galvani-Volta Controversy on Animal Electricity*, Princeton, NJ: Princeton University Press.

Tousey, Sinclair (1915) *Medical Electricity, Röntgen Rays and Radium with a Practical Chapter on Phototherapy*, Philadelphia, Pa.: W.B. Saunders.

# Elisabeth von Wittelsbach, Empress of Austria (1837–98)

Elisabeth Amelia Eugenia, Empress-Consort of Franz Joseph I, otherwise known as "Sisi," was one of the "beauty" celebrities of the nineteenth century. After her marriage to Franz Josef I, Emperor of the Austro-Hungarian Empire on April 24, 1854, she became "the reigning star of her age" (Sinclair 1998: 189). Like Diana, Princess of Wales, to whom she has been frequently compared, she became the symbol of celebrity beauty as the ultimate sign of tragedy (Daimler 1998: 241–52; Sinclair 1998: 200–4). Like Diana, Elisabeth stated often that her royal marriage had brought her in contact with the stifling nature of the court; and she later deeply regretted the marriage. As the mother of the thirty-one-year-old Crown Prince Rudolf of Hapsburg, whose suicide with his beloved Baroness Mary Vesta at Mayerling on January 30, 1889 shook the Empire, Elisabeth became a symbol of the tragic life of the beautiful. Indeed, after her death, she became the subject of a "Sisi-cult."

Sisi held herself up to extreme beauty standards, which included an 18-inch waist. Each day she was measured by her hairdresser Franziska Feifalik, who assured her that the waist, wrist, and ankle measurements of her 105-pound, five-foot and six-inch tall body fulfilled her and her world's ideal. Fasting was one of the penalties if she exceeded the measurements she thought ideal. Her perfect food was milk, to the extent that she actually travelled with her own milk cow, often living on a single glass a day for sustenance. Otherwise, she ate oranges, at the time expensive and difficult to obtain, or a glass of the newest "health" food, beef broth made from a powder.

Living in Imperial Vienna, Sisi had weight-loss instruments created for her personal living quarters in the Hofburg castle. She exercised every day and ordered a gym be made available to her when she traveled. Constantin Christomanos, who was the "Greek Reader" to the Empress, noted in a diary entry that the end result was an extremely thin body: "I just saw her in her gym. She cre-ated the impression of a being somewhere between a snake and a bird" (Christomanos 2005: 124).

Indeed, by the late 1890s, her physician Viktor Eisenmenger diagnosed her as having the tell tale breath of the anorexic, a diagnostic category only recently introduced by William Gull.

While her tiny waist and low weight contributed to her role as a nineteenth-century beauty icon, the measures she took to achieve her appearance were both physically demanding and unhealthy. The constant use of purgatives and laxatives as well as her restricted diet cost Sisi her health, leaving her with symptoms of sciatica and painful foot complaints. Sisi was so obsessed with attaining the highest levels of beauty, she refused to allow any photographs of her after she turned thirty, for it was said that she suffered from premature wrinkles. During the nineteenth century, thinness was not the standard of beauty, yet Sisi was nevertheless admired and loved by women and men around Europe for her dashing beauty and thinness. Like Diana, the circumstances of her separation from the Emperor after 1860, for "reasons of health," and her murder by the anarchist Luigi Lucheni on September 10, 1898 in Geneva made her the ideal beauty celebrity of her age.

SLG

*See also* Anorexia; Diana; Gull

## References and Further Reading
Christomanos, Constantin (2005) *Le Livre de l'impératrice Elisabeth*, Paris: L'Harmattan.
Daimler, Renate (1998) *Diana & Sisi: Zwei Frauen—Ein Schicksal*, Vienna: Deuticke.
Hamann, Brigette (1986) *The Reluctant Empress: A Biography of Empress Elisabeth of Austria*, New York: Knopf.

Schilke, Franz E. (1993) *Elisabeth und Ludwig II: Im Spiegel von Medizin und Kunst*, Munich: Verlag Medizin+Kunst.

Sinclair, Andrew (1998) *Death by Fame: A Life of Elisabeth, Empress of Austria*, London: Constable.

# Emaciated Body Images in the Media

The pop culture industry's idealization of stick-thin body types has received a large amount of attention in recent years, especially due to increasing evidence that American women are less satisfied with their bodies than ever before. Eating disorders are commonly discussed in the U.S.A., and body image is distorted to the point that 45 percent of healthy-weight women believe that they are overweight (and many of those report being "on a diet"). The literature attributes a large portion of this problem to the extremely large number of airbrushed images of stick-thin models bombarding the American population every day. Considering that average model is 5 foot 9 inches and 110–15 pounds and the average American woman is 5 foot 4 inches and 138 lbs, none of this is very surprising (Rowland).

The issue has reached a point where even some fashion magazines have begun to publish articles condemning unhealthy-looking models, some even going as far as to employ "plus-sized" models. Hilary Fashion, North America's most popular online women's magazine since 1995, is an example of this new trend. In a recent article entitled "Obsessed with Thin: Has the Media Gone Too Far?" the author puts magazine covers featuring stick-thin models side by side with quotes from models and actresses testifying that the pictures are not realistic.

The irony in this idealization of an emaciated body image is that only a few centuries ago in Western culture, and continuing today in some non-Western cultures, a starving body was associated with disease and poverty. In every human population besides the one of rare over-abundance in the contemporary Western world, to be fat was to flaunt one's wealth. The classic artistic representations of larger women by the seventeenth-century Flemish painter Peter Paul Rubens (1577–1640) ("the Rubenesque woman") offered a very different body image that was equally idealized. His highly charged *Rape of the Sabine Women* represented exaggerated and sexualized female figures reflecting middle-class aesthetic norms of the day. In contemporary American culture, however, highly caloric food is inexpensive, and time has become far more valuable. Today, unlike in the age of Rubens, it is no mark of status for a woman to be able to be seen as (or to see herself as) overweight; to be thin shows she has money to buy the more expensive, lower caloric foods, as well as the free time to prepare it. Furthermore, few people can appear fit and thin without exercise, which takes up more time, and many forms of exercise require the luxury of a trip to the gym. The end result is that in the Western world, upper-middle-class women tend to be significantly thinner than women of lower socioeconomic status. The irony is that the "peasant" pictures of Flemish artists of Ruben's age, such as Pieter Brueghel the Younger (1564–1638), do not reflect the exaggerated size of Ruben's idealized, erotic female figures. Thus, in his *The Peasant Wedding*, the festivities are presented without any reflection of exaggerated body types.

However, it is important to keep in mind that this phenomenon of a heavier lower class is confined to the modern Western world where food shortages are nonexistent. In much of the developing world, access to food is limited, leading to undernourished, thin people. However, overweight has also become a major problem in the developing world.

The greatest hypocrisy of all is that when Americans are bombarded with images of stick-thin models, they yearn to look like them, but foreign-aid agencies and news agencies use very similar pictures of people in developing countries for shock value. Fashion vs. Famine is a great contradiction in the world today, and one that has received surprisingly little attention.

SLG/Sarah Gardiner

*See also* Celebrities; Developing World; Hornby; Media

**References and Further Reading**

Andrist, Linda C. (2003) "Media Images, Body Dissatisfaction, and Disordered Eating in Adolescent Women," *Maternal and Child Health* 28: 119–23.

Rowland, Hilary "Obsessed With Thin: Has the Media Gone Too Far?" Hilary Fashion, available online at <http://www.hilary.com/fashion/bikini.html> (accessed May 10, 2006).

Seale, Clive (2003) "Health and Media: An Overview," *Sociology of Health & Illness* 25 (7): 513–31.

Spitzer, B.L., Henderson, K.A. and Zivian, M.T. (1999) "Gender Differences in Population Versus Media Body Sizes: A Comparison over Four Decades," *Sex Roles* 40 (7–8): 545–65.

Wells, Jonathan C.K. and Nicholls, Dasha (2001) "The Relationship Between Body Size and Body Composition in Women of Different Nutritional Status," *European Eating Disorders Review* 9 (6): 416–26.

Wilkinson, Richard G. (1994) "The Epidemiological Transition: from Material Scarcity to Social Disadvantage," *Daedalus* 123 (4): 61–78.

Wright, Terence (2002) "Moving Images: The Media Representation of Refugees," *Visual Studies* 17 (1): 53–66.

# Enlightenment Dietetics

What had been a religious obsession about moral corruption in Martin Luther's sixteenth-century understanding of obesity and the body came in the Enlightenment to be the stuff of the science of dietetics dealing with illness. The meaning of the fat body came to be the focus of science with all of the moral quality ascribed to secular questions of health and illness, rather than to the moral readings of gluttony and obesity.

By the seventeenth century, there was the first, modern creation of a specialized literature of "healthy" and "unhealthy" foods such as Johann Sigismund Elsholtz's (1623–88) *Diaeteticon* (1682). His tabulation of every possible food and drink that was (or could be) consumed for its healthy and unhealthy properties had become a standard for the classification of foods. Indeed, he quotes Galen to the effect that every physician should become knowledgeable in the art of cooking (Elsholtz 1984: xx2). Toward the end of his book, he advises on the appropriate diet for men—they should combine eating with work or exercise, such as fencing. He also ends his book with a warning, following Hippocrates, that the athletic body of the man can more easily age and become ill when he overeats (Elsholtz 1984: 345).

The moral questions remained, but slowly were loosed from the overt religious rhetoric of obesity. The French essayist Jean de La Bruyère (1645–96) presents us a series of portraits of men who are types, or "characters," in 1688. Among them is Clito who

had, throughout his life, been concerned with two things along: namely, dining at noon and supping at night; he seems born to digest; he has only one topic of conversation: he tells you what entrées were served at the last meal he was at, how many soups there were and what sort of soups.

(La Bruyère 1970: 208)

He is "the arbiter of good things." But sadly, La Bruyère notes, "he was giving a dinner party on the day he died. Wherever he may be, he is eating, and if he should come back to this world, it would be to eat" (La Bruyère 1970: 208). The deadly sin of "gula" (gluttony) has become gormandizing, but the result is the same—death.

By the Enlightenment, Christoph Wilhelm Hufeland (1762–1836) had captured in his extraordinarily popular *The Art of Prolonging Life* (in two volumes, 1796–7) the "good" and "moral" aspects of the physical nature of man (Hufeland 1797: I, 169). Fat is simply bad for Hufeland and the Enlightenment philosophers because most people eat much more than they need. "Immoderation" is one of the prime causes of early death (Hufeland 1797: II, 43). Invoking the golden mean, eating too much and eating too richly will kill you. "The first thing which, in regard to diet, can act as a shortener of life, is *immoderation*" (Hufeland 1797: II, 43). Too much food and food that is too "refined" are the cause of the shortening of life. Food that tastes too good makes one eat too much. Simple is better than complex: "Eggs, milk, butter and flour are each, used by itself, very easy of digestion; but when joined together, and formed into a fat, solid pudding, the produce will be extremely heavy and indigestible" (Hufeland 1797: II, 45–6). "People in a natural state . . . require few rules respecting their diet" (Hufeland 1797: II, 242). Balance in diet is vital: Vegetables and bread must be eaten with meat. Indeed, the avoidance of "flesh" and of wine is advocated (Hufeland 1797: II, 248). Healthy is simple; simple is long life.

"Idleness" is also a cause (Hufeland 1797: II, 64). Human beings have lost their natural ability to determine how much we need by childhood overindulgence. Natural man, notes Hufeland, in plowing the fields has purpose, exercise, and food appropriate to long life. "His son becomes a studious rake; and the proportion between countrymen and citizens seems daily to be diminished" (Hufeland 1797: II, 217). The fat child is now the father (and mother) of the fat adult. Indeed, Hufeland places at the very beginning of his list of things that will certainly cause early death—a "very warm, tender, and delicate education" in childhood in which children are stuffed "immoderately with food; and by coffee, chocolate, wine, spices, and such things" (Hufeland 1797: II, 9). Not sin but middle-class overindulgence begins to be seen as the force that creates fat boys. In the nineteenth century, the "science" of diet seems to replace the morals of diet. The hidden model remains the same: The normal, reasonable man is always contrasted with the fat boy and always to the fat boy's detriment. And the reward for the thin man is life, life extended (and if Augustine is to be believed, life eternal), while the fat person dies young and badly.

Immanuel Kant (1724–1804), in his essay on "Overcoming Unpleasant Sensations by Mere Reasoning" (1797), argued that dietetics could only become philosophy "when the mere power of reason in mankind, in overcoming sensations by a governing principle, determines their manner of living. On the other hand, when it endeavors to excite or avert these sensations, by external corporeal means, the art becomes merely empiric and mechanical" (Kant 1991: 371–93). This is his direct answer to Hufeland's empiricism. Hufeland had sent him his book on diet and longevity in the winter of 1796, and Kant recognized in it Hufeland's attempt to fulfill Kant's demand that the physical (and physiological) aspects of the human being be treated "morally." Kant's recognition that Hufeland's argument for prophylaxis is to avoid illness, rather than using specific foods for treatment in a philosophy of moral life. He relates this to the Stoic notion of "endurance and moderation" (Kant 1991: 375).

Kant's essay (as with many of these presentations concerning diet and longevity) is highly autobiographical. His discussion of diet is tangibly tied to his awareness of his own aging body (Kant 1991: 383). He compares himself to the men in their prime, and he defines aging specifically in gendered terms. He speaks of the increased amount of liquid that "aged men" seem to need to drink, which then disturbs their sleep. For Kant, the power of the rational mind to avoid illness rests in the control that the mind has not only over that which one ingests, but also the very control of breathing and the body. It is the will that controls the body. Part of this rationale is explained in the final footnote in which Kant speaks of the blindness in his one eye and his anxiety about the failing sight in the other. He distances this fear by asking whether the pathologies of vision are in his eye or in the processing of the data in his brain, and notes that he has not actually felt the loss of the blind eye. Unlike diet, which can be manipulated to control the health (and weight) of the body, the aging body seems to have its own rate of decline for which there is no control, even in rationality. Kant's essay, which begins with Hufeland's dietetics, ends with the aging, half-blind philosopher ruminating on the irresistible but fascinating decay of his own body.

The beginning of a "modern" (i.e., materialist) science of medicine saw the development of the view that human beings proceed along an arc of development and that there is a specific moment where the body is most at risk from obesity. In 1757, the Dutch physician Malcolm Flemyng (1700–64) argued for the inheritance of a tendency toward obesity in a presentation to the Royal Society of Physicians in London. His *A Discourse on the Nature, Causes, and Cures of Corpulency* (1757) argued for a physiological rather than a moral definition of obesity: Fat people are not inherently lazy or sinful. His cure is exercise early on as "persons inclined to corpulency seldom think on reducing their size till they grow very bulky and then they scarce can or will use exercise enough to be remarkable serviceable" (Flemyng 1757: 34). Thomas Jameson in 1811 felt that the period from the twenty-eighth to the fifty-eighth year was the height of male perfection (Jameson 1811). Kant would have agreed with this. And yet this is also the age of the most danger as "we … find corpulency steals imperceptibly on most men, between the ages of thirty and fifty-seven. In many instances the belly becomes prominent, and the person acquires a more upright gait" (quoted in Jameson 1811: 90). Yet this is not necessarily a bad thing as "a moderate degree of obesity is certainly a desirable state of body at all times, as it indicates a healthy condition of the assimilating powers" (quoted in Jameson 1811: 91). Obesity "also diminishes the irritability of the system, since fat people are remarked for good humour, and for bearing cold better than those who are lean, on account of the defensive coat of fat surrounding their nerves" (quoted in Jameson 1811: 91). But fat can become dangerous: "when the heart and great vessels are so oppressed with fat, as to render the pulse slow and feeble, and the respiration difficult, the cumbrous load becomes of more serious import to the health" (quoted in Jameson 1811: 92). The "prominent belly" is "considered as the first symptom of decay, particularly as it is generally observed to continue through a great part of old age" (quoted in Jameson 1811: 105). Here again the shadow of the Greek humors reappears to claim that the phlegmatic body and the aged body have the same, underlying pathology, that of obesity.

SLG

*See also* Greek Medicine and Dieting; Luther; Natural Man; Roman Medicine and Dieting

## References and Further Reading

Elsholtz, Johann Sigismund (1984) *Diaeteticon 1682*, Photo-reprint, Leipzig: Edition Leipzig.

Flemyng, Malcolm (1757) *A Discourse on the Nature, Causes, and Cures of Corpulency*, London: L. Davis and C. Reymers.

Hufeland, Christopher William (1796-7) *The Art of Prolonging Life*, 2 vols, London: J. Bell.

Jameson, Thomas (1811) *Essays on the Changes of the Human Body, at Its Different Ages*, London: Longman, Hurst, Bees, Orme & Brown.

Kant, Immanuel (1991) "Von der Macht des Gemüts, durch den blossen Vorsatz seiner krankhaften Gefühle Meister zu sein," in Wilhelm Weischedel (ed.), *Schriften zur Anthropologie, Geschichtsphilosophie, Politik und Pädagogik*, Vol. I, Frankfurt: Suhrkamp, pp. 371–93.

La Bruyère (1970) *Characters*, trans. Jean Stewart, Baltimore, Md.: Penguin.

# F

## Fashion

"If you attach no importance to weight problems, if not being able to wear new, trendy small-sized clothes does not cause you any regret, this book is not for you," states fashion designer Karl Lagerfeld (1933–). He gained fame or notoriety when he lost 80 pounds in one year. "I suddenly wanted to dress differently, to wear clothes designed by Hedi Slimane," he said. "But these fashions, modeled by very, very slim boys—and not men my age—required me to lose at least eighty pounds. It took me exactly thirteen months." He followed a diet created for him by Dr. Jean-Claude Houdret, which inevitably led to a book called *The Karl Lagerfeld Diet*. Thus, a fashion designer joined the countless numbers of people who invent and write books based on diets. However, some might argue that people in the fashion industry have always been influencing the world of dieting by perpetuating or creating bodily ideals.

In the late 1700s, Beau Brummell helped change British fashion by promoting a more natural look, reverting to the bodily ideal of the ancient Greeks (Hollander 1999: 137–8). Around 1815, tailors created standard measurements, based on standard proportions, in order to mass produce ready-to-wear clothing (Hollander 1999: 139–40). As a result, people could compare their bodies to the soldiers' bodies from which the norm was established. In the Victorian era, the Western world believed that women needed corsets in order to support their frame because their waists and spines were not strong enough. Tightly lacing their corsets also allowed women to attain the ideal body, which, from the 1820s, had a waist circumference of 18 inches and forced an upright posture. These corsets, despite inducing fainting, uterine and spinal disorders, muscle wasting, and crushed ribs, helped women achieve large hips and breasts. According to Germaine Greer's highly influential *The Female Eunuch* (1970) "Nineteenth-century belles even went to the extremity of having their lowest ribs removed so that they could lace their corsets tighter" (Greer 1970: 40). By the 1830s, padding was also used to enhance one's hips and breasts and was even used for one's arms and thighs (Banner 1983: 48, 60–1; see also Ogden 2003: 35). Meanwhile, New York couture toyed with the "willowy look, with a hint of frailty, as standards of appearance began to be more important for respectable women" (Stearns 1997: 7).

Then, from 1830 to 1870, the new ideal was a fuller figure, so clothing included puffed sleeves, heavier material, and strong colors (Lurie 1981: 64–9). Also at this time, Amelia Jenks Bloomer, with her Bloomer reform dress, attempted to change fashion with trousers and no corset for women. The damaging effects of corsets were also noted around this time (Thesander 1997: 98–9). From the 1870s, upper classes began trading in their corsets for a more natural, corsetless look with loose dresses that hid one's body size. In the 1880s, an electric corset was introduced to the market by "Dr. Scott," with an advertisement that claimed that it cured many diseases, including rheumatism, paralysis, liver and kidney troubles, and constipation. The corsets were declared to be "equalizing agents in all cases of extreme fatness or leanness, by imparting to the system the required amount of 'odic force' which Nature's law demands" (Rudofsky 1971: 107). That is, this magical corset claimed to be a body shaper in the both the mechanical and metabolic sense. But by the 1890s, the trend of going corsetless spread to the middle class and clothes became tighter, further encouraging thinness. In 1895, upper-class women still padded their clothing. In 1908, a French designer came out with corsetless dresses, although this sparked a controversy that lasted until the 1920s. One argument against corsetlessness was based on an aversion towards females and exercise. One author even wrote, "*What has the average girl to do with a gymnasium? Sweeping and scrubbing a floor and dusting out a room, is infinitely more beneficial and useful than going to a sanctified room to turn somersaults*" (Rudofsky 1971: 182). At the time, unless they exercised in a women-only facility, women wore corsets while exercising.

Gradually, a fuller figure was openly traded in for a thinner one. In 1912, the magazine *Journal des Dames et de Modes* vacillated in opinion by espousing both beliefs, that "fashion . . . only modifies very little the voluptuous silhouette of women of fashion" and that "thinness triumphs" (Steele 1985: 230). In the 1920s, the flapper look was firmly in vogue, so women desired a more natural, albeit asexual, shape, also known as the "modernist body." This streamlined figure may have been a reaction to the growing independence of women who earned the right to vote and were part of the workforce during World War I. The popularization of this shape can be seen in the changing display mannequins, from a natural, curved shape to a straight, boyish one. The consequence of this meant that sports and diet replaced corsets, although some women even used some sort of bodice to compress their bust. From 1925, legs became an indicator of one's fitness, so dresses became shorter and stocking production increased (Wollen 1993: 20–1; Thesander 1997: 107, 113, 118). After World War II, the corset returned to fashion. In the 1970s, a modern corselet, or combination of corset and brassiere, appeared, called the body stocking which fit one's natural shape. In the 1980s, fashion promoted fitness: Beauty meant youthful, slim, and active bodies; and dieting replaced corsetry (Thesander 1997: 201; Steele 1985: 241).

Since the early 1960s, fashion models have been thin. Photographers argued that thin bodies did not compete with the clothing, such that full interest could be devoted to the garments (Banner 1983: 287). In the 1960s, girls dieted for the extremely thin body of model Twiggy (Thesander 1997: 181). By this time, a transition occurred from corsets of wire and lace to rubber to no corsets at all. This so-called freedom actually meant that one needed more internal control of one's body, which resulted in expansion of the dieting industry (Ogden 2003: 106).

Clothing has continued to be used as a substitute for or supplement to a diet to achieve the illusion of one's desired body shape. For example, the Oprah episode titled "Look 10 Pounds Thinner—Instantly" advertised that viewers could "Look skinny! Look like you lost weight just by what you wear." One stylist suggests that plus-size women should wear capri pants because "it shows enough leg to look summery, and with a bit of a heel or wedge your legs will look longer so you will look leaner" (Bouchez 2005: 2). Similar fashion advice could be found in a *Men's Health* article called "Return of the Thin Man" (Dotson 1991: 45). Besides creating this illusion, Hillel Schwartz notes that this advice to "wear navy blue or black with vertical lines, slender jewelry, soft collars and noiseless materials. No large or glaring patterns, no jangling trim, no noisy taffeta or satin, no striking colors" served to do more than hide small flaws: "The clothing designed for the Stylish Stout was clothing designed to be inconspicuous, to fit in" (Schwartz 1986: 161).

In our current era of fashion, finding clothes that "fit" is of utmost importance. A new, state-of-the art invention that supports this trend is called "Intellifit." It is a see-through booth that uses radio waves to collect your body's measurements and suggest brands and sizes that best fit you (intellifit.com). In addition, many stores have added plus-sized clothing, and other stores have popped up that cater exclusively to this demographic in adults and children. Just as before, without corsets or, for men, without the slimming double-breasted suits, people are expected to maintain a thin look naturally through dieting.

Studies have not been able to clearly explain the relationship between fashion and dieting. While one study has shown a positive association between reading fashion magazines and having dieted or exercised in order to lose weight among U.S. preadolescent and adolescent girls (Field et al. 1999: 36), another study showed no such correlation between reading fashion magazines and dieting (Stice et al. 2001: 270). Despite the contradicting research, popular belief still holds that the fashion industry encourages dieting by promoting thinness. In 1953, *Vogue* editors wrote "Fashion is often reproached for this preoccupation with slimness—and, as a fashion magazine, we mind not at all sharing the accusation. For doctors agree that most women's desire to be slender is a vanity that can pay off in good health and a longer life" (Schwartz 1986: 334). The fashion industry has been criticized for the glorification of thin bodies and for size discrimination. In addition to fashion's influence on dieting, it is also true that the dieting industry has influenced fashion. With a greater emphasis on dieting, corsets are unnecessary, but fashions still attempt to be fitting and flattering, allowing the wearer to look thinner. Although fashion ideals came first, there is a definite association between fashion and dieting and a symbiotic relationship that has lasted for centuries.

SLG/DOROTHY CHYUNG

*See also* Hornby; Winfrey

## References and Further Reading

Banner, Lois W. (1983) *American Beauty*, New York: Alfred A. Knopf.

Bouchez, Colette (2005) "Plus-Size Panache: Spring Offers Fashions That Are Perfect for Every Body," *WebMD Weight Loss Clinic* April 22: 1–2. Available online at <http://www.webmd.com/content/Article/104/107585.htm?pagenumber=1> (accessed May 10, 2006).

Dotson, Edisol Wayne (1991) *Behold the Man: The Hype and Selling of Male Beauty in Media and Culture*, New York: The Haworth Press.

Field, Alison E., Cheung, Lilian, Wolf, Anne M., Herzog, David B., Gortmaker, Steven L., and Colditz, Graham A. (1999) "Exposure to the Mass Media and Weight Concerns Among Girls," *Pediatrics* 103 (3): e36.

Greer, Germaine. (1970) *The Female Eunuch*, London: MacGibben & Kee, Ltd.

Hollander, Anne (1999) "Suiting Everyone: Fashion and Democracy," in Arthur M. Melzer, Jerry Weinberger, and M. Richard Zinman (eds) *Democracy and the Arts*, Ithaca, NY: Cornell University Press, pp. 130–40.

Lagerfeld, Karl, Houdret, Jean-Claude, and Sischy,

Ingrid (2005) *The Karl Lagerfeld Diet*, New York: PowerHouse Books.

Lurie, Alison (1981) *The Language of Clothes*, New York: Henry Holt & Company, LLC.

Madacy Entertainment Group, Inc. (1998) *The Great Events of Our Century: Obsession: Health, Beauty, Fitness and Fashion—the Cult of Body Worship*, VHS.

Ogden, Jane (2003) *The Psychology of Eating: From Healthy to Disordered Behavior*, Malden, Mass.: Blackwell Publishing.

Rudofsky, Bernard (1971) *The Unfashionable Human Body*, Garden City, NY: Doubleday.

Schwartz, Hillel (1986) *Never Satisfied: A Cultural History of Diets, Fantasies, and Fat*, New York: The Free Press.

Stearns, Peter N. (1997) *Fat History: Bodies and Beauty in the Modern West*, New York: New York University Press.

Steele, Valerie (1985) *Fashion and Eroticism: Ideals of Feminine Beauty from the Victorian Era to the Jazz Age*, New York: Oxford University Press.

Stice, Eric, Diane Spangler, and Stewart, Agras W. (2001) "Exposure to Media-Portrayed Thin-Ideal Images Adversely Affects Vulnerable Girls: A Longitudinal Experiment," *Journal of Social and Clinical Psychology* 20 (3): 270–88.

Thesander, Marianne (1997) *The Feminine Ideal*, London: Reaktion Books.

Winfrey, Oprah (2005) "Look 10 Pounds Thinner—Instantly" *The Oprah Winfrey Show* (broadcast February 17). Details available online at <http://www.oprah.com/tows/pastshows/200502/tows_past_20050217.jhtml> (accessed June 24, 2007).

Wollen, Peter (1993) *Raiding the Icebox: Reflections on Twentieth-Century Culture*, Bloomington, IN: Indiana University Press.

# Fast Food

**W**ith the articulation of obesity as an epidemic came attempts to locate its origins. Fast food, as a rather obvious culprit, has emerged as the unscrupulous enemy of health (and thinness), especially for children. As a result, the industry has garnered all varieties of critical attention in recent years. In response to the outcry of scholars and activists, and, most directly, legal challenges, fast food has begun to reform its image.

A recent flurry of criticism addresses the linked ethical and nutritional failures of fast food and its increasingly global impact on eating habits and health. Eric Schlosser's critically acclaimed and widely taught *Fast Food Nation* (2001) paved the way for more recent and popular books like Greg Cristor's *Fat Land: How Americans Became the Fattest People in the World* (2004) and Morgan Spurlock's *Don't Eat this Book: Fast Food and the Supersizing of America* (2005). Perhaps most popularly damning the industry for its role in creating the obesity epidemic is Spurlock's 2003 Sundance award-winning documentary *Super Size Me*.

The film documents Spurlock's weight gain and ever-declining health as he embarks on a McDonald's-only diet in order to demonstrate the ill effects of fast food. He argues that encouraging overeating and frequent consumption of fast food is in fact the profit-hungry intent of McDonald's advertising, contrary to its legal defense, which suggested that consumers know that fast food is fattening and unhealthy and should be eaten in moderation. While many agree that lawsuits against the fast-food industry are outrageous, others have drawn parallels between anti-fast-food and anti-tobacco litigation, arguing that there must be corporate accountability for public health (Mello et al. 2003).

In the wake of bad PR, McDonald's and the rest of the fast-food industry have begun to clean up their image. Coca-Cola, PepsiCo, and Frito-Lay are among the big names that have in recent years sponsored campaigns to get kids more active and promote "healthy lifestyles." In addition, fast-food chains have introduced or vamped up the marketing of a variety of healthier alternatives. Most places are offering more salads and veggie burgers and are devoting more airtime to promoting them. McDonald's has been promoting its new white-meat chicken nuggets, while Wendy's has started including orange slices in its children's meals. Denny's and other fast-food diners have added vegetable and heart-smart sides to compete with their classic French fries.

Americans spend so much time eating away from home that a diet was even created for those who regularly consume fast food. Subway has cashed in on spokesperson Jared Fogle's extreme weight-loss success story, marketing itself as the fast-food alternative for adults and children (Buss 2004). After the success of the Subway diet and *Super Size Me*, most of the fast-food restaurants make healthy options very obvious on the menu. In addition, they publish information on the fat content of their foods so that the consumer can make an informed decision. The results of these changes in terms of childhood obesity remain to be seen. What is clear is that the diet industry is ever-expanding its reaches and is always big business, even for fast food.

SLG/Angela Willey

*See also* Children; Fogle; Food Choice; Obesity Epidemic; Spurlock

## References and Further Reading

Buss, Dale (2004) "Is the Food Industry the Problem or the Solution?" *The New York Times*, August 29: 3.5.

Critser, Greg (2004) *Fat Land: How Americans Became the Fattest People in the World*, New York: Houghton Mifflin Co.

Falit, Ben (2003) "Food Fighters Fall Flat: Plaintiffs Fail to Establish That McDonald's Should Be Liable for Obesity-Related Illnesses," *The Journal of Law, Medicine & Ethics* 31 (4): 725–51.

Mello, Michelle M., Rimm, Eric B. and Studdert, David M. (2003) "The Mclawsuit: The Fast-Food Industry and Legal Accountability for Obesity," *Health Affairs* 22 (6): 207–16.

Schlosser, Eric (2001) *Fast Food Nation: The Dark Side of the All American Meal*, New York: Harper Perennial.

Spurlock, Morgan (dir.) (2003) *Super Size Me*. Hart Sharp Video.

Spurlock, Morgan (2005) *Don't Eat This Book: Fast Food and the Supersizing of America*, New York: Penguin Adult.

# Fat Assessment in Adults

**W**eight assessment is a dynamic process by which the weight status of an individual or a group is evaluated. The process is considered dynamic because weight in terms of pounds may not be enough to predict health risks. However, this process enables a clinician or individual to identify risks and determine appropriate intervention. There are many measures used in weight assessment, all aiming to provide similar information.

Body Mass Index (BMI) is a number calculated from a person's weight and height, indicating presence of obesity and highly correlated with body fat and health risk. As BMI increases so does the risk of morbidity and mortality. BMI can be used to determine a "healthy weight" range for an individual or health risk, which is increased in persons with conditions such as diabetes, hypertension, or cardiovascular disease. BMI is a mathematical value calculated by weight in kilograms divided by height in meters squared ($kg/m^2$). The BMI value corresponds to a certain obesity class, applicable to both men and women:

| BMI | Obesity Class |
|---|---|
| 18.5 | Underweight |
| 18.5–24.9 | Normal weight |
| 25.0–29.9 | Overweight |
| 30–34.9 | Obesity (Grade I) |
| 35–39.9 | Obesity (Grade II) |
| 40 | Severe Obesity (Grade III) |

Even though BMI is considered a good estimate of body fat, it does misclassify elite athletes and bodybuilders as obese. Therefore, other measures have been created to better estimate body fat. Waist circumference (WC) is another measure that indicates an individual's relative risk for obesity related diseases. The indicator for obesity for males is a WC greater than 101.5 cm and for females a WC greater than 88.9 cm, and individuals with excess abdominal fat are at an increased risk for Type-2 diabetes, dyslipidemia, hypertension, and cardiovascular disease. WC is a specific measure of abdominal obesity, which is a stronger risk factor for many chronic diseases than other types of obesity. To determine WC, measure the circumference around the upper hipbone. The tape measure should be snug, but should not cause compressions on the skin. Measuring waist circumference is an inexpensive, convenient, and noninvasive method for estimating abdominal fat before and during weight-loss treatment.

Anthropometrics is a method used to establish whether BMI indicates muscle or fat. Common methods include measurements of wrist circumference and elbow breadth, which serve as criteria to determine body frame size. Frame size, useful in determining appropriate ranges of desirable body weight, is then calculated by dividing height by wrist circumference. Some people may find that they may have to lose more or less weight than they were originally led to believe since each person's bone structure and frame varies in size and density. Wrist circumference is measured at the bones of the wrist.

| | Small | Medium | Large (*cm*) |
|---|---|---|---|
| Men | <10.4 | 10.4–19.6 | >19.6 |
| Women | <10.9 | 10.9–19.9 | >19.9 |

When using elbow breadth measurement, the height corresponds with elbow breadth. The ranges fall in small frame (< range), medium frame (within range) and, large frame (> range):

Men

| Height | Elbow Breadth (cm) |
|---|---|
| 5'1"–5'2" | 6.35–7.30 |
| 5'3"–5'6" | 6.67–7.30 |
| 5'7"–5'10" | 6.98–7.62 |
| 5'11"–6'2" | 6.98–7.94 |
| 6'4" | 7.30–8.23 |

Women

| Height | Elbow Breadth (cm) |
|---|---|
| 4'9"–4'10" | 5.73–7.30 |
| 4'11"–5'2" | 5.73–7.30 |
| 5'3"–5'6" | 6.03–6.67 |
| 5'7"–5'10" | 6.03–6.67 |
| 5'11" | 6.35–6.98 |

In addition to the weight and length measures used to determine a person's weight, there are also ways to calculate body fat. Five common ways to calculate body fat are the bio-electric impedance, underwater weighing, bod pod, magnetic resonance imaging (MRI), and skin folds measures. Each of these measures has strengths and weaknesses in determining body fat. For example, MRI is considered the gold standard in terms of measuring abdominal obesity but costs thousands of times more than skin folds measures. And although either underwater weighing or the bod pod are considered the most accurate in terms of measuring total body fat, both are very invasive to the individual being tested. They involve taking off all one's clothes apart from a bathing suit or undergarments and then either submersing oneself in water (after exhaling all the air in the lungs) or lying in a confined space for anywhere from three to five minutes. Even though MRI, underwater weighing, and the "bod pod" are considered the gold standards for fat assessment, they are rarely used to measure fat because of cost and logistics. Therefore, even though skin folds and BMI (Body-Mass Index) are not nearly as accurate as the gold standards, they are far more commonly used.

Ever since Louis Dublin showed that weight is a strong risk factor for death, people have been trying to figure out if all weight is bad. In the later part of the twentieth century, it was believed that it was not weight alone that contributed to the increased risk but rather percentage of body fat. It is now believed that it is not just percentage of body fat but rather type and quantity of "bad" or abdominal fat that matters. As new ways of quantifying and qualifying fat become available, the definition will likely continue to evolve.

SLG/RAKHI PATEL

*See also* Brillat-Savarin; Dublin

### References and Further Reading
Anon. "Assessing Your Patient's Weight and Body Composition." Available online at <http://apps.medsch.ucla.edu/nutrition/weightassess.htm> (accessed May 1, 2006).
Anon. "BMI Calculator: Waist Circumference." Available online at <http://www.bmi-calculator.net/waist-to-hip-ratio-calculator/waist-circumference.php> (accessed May 1, 2006).
Anon. "Body Mass Index." Available online at <http://www.cdc.gov/nccdphp/dnpa/bmi/index.htm> (accessed May 1, 2006).
Anon. "Health calculators." Available online at <http://www.medindia.net/patients/calculators/framesize1.asp> (accessed May 1, 2006).
Anon. "Waist Circumference Measurement." Available online at <http://www.annecollins.com/lose_weight/waist-circumference.htm> (accessed May 1, 2006).

# Fat Camps

Over the past twenty years, American parents, educators, and health professionals have become increasingly concerned with the prevalence of overweight and obesity among children and adults in the U.S.A. and around the world. Results from the 2003–4 National Health and Nutrition Examination Survey (NHANES) indicate that an estimated 17 percent of children and adolescents aged two to nineteen are overweight (Johnston and Steele 2006: 1; National Center for Health Statistics 2003–4). The numbers for adults are even worse at an estimated 66 percent being overweight or obese. NHANES numbers also indicate that the problem of overweight in the U.S.A. is growing (Ogden et al. 2006).

With obesity numbers on the rise, popular and medical discourse on appropriate interventions and treatment methods for weight control are burgeoning. One increasingly popular treatment for overweight children and adults (who can afford it) is inpatient care at a residential weight-loss camp or facility, commonly known as "fat camps."

While there has certainly been an increase in the number of available camps, centers, clinics, and spas designed to treat overweight in recent years, residential health camps, themselves, are not a recent development. They have their historical roots in the spas, health resorts, and health farms of Europe and the U.S.A. It is likely that

European spa practices originally evolved from Roman baths, which grew out of southern Italian and Greek therapeutic bathing at volcanic springs (Delaine 1996: 236). In England, specifically, interest in hot water mineral spas as sites where health could be restored or promoted date to the sixteenth century (Hembry 1997: 1–2).

By the eighteenth and nineteenth centuries, European spas were popular destinations for members of the growing middle class who searched for disease cures and improved health (Hembry 1997: 2). At this time, newspapers and magazines advertised bathing in and drinking mineral water as a cure for such varied afflictions as scurvy, jaundice, indigestion, nervousness, and scrofula (Hembry 1997: Figure 5). Certainly, weight control and digestive difficulties were not the main focus of resort visitors; however, wealthy members of society did visit spas in search of a remedy for problems of overweight (Hembry 1997: 242). Corpulent individuals were encouraged to bath in and drink mineral water, which was bottled for sale and made available all across the country in the early 1800s (Hembry 1997: 242).

Health resorts were also popular destinations for middle-class leisure and recovery in Germany, France, and the U.S.A. In late-nineteenth and early twentieth-century America, doctors and lay enthusiasts developed health farms and institutions, which catered to patients suffering from infectious diseases and psychological ailments, as well as clients merely interested in "healthful living" (Jones 1967). Institutions, including the Agnes Memorial Sanatorium in Denver and the Battle Creek Sanatorium in Michigan among others, were especially popular destinations for patients seeking relief from tuberculosis (TB) (Jones 1967; Schwarz 1970). By the early twentieth century, the YMCA also established health farms in Denver, Dallas, Philadelphia, and other cities, where young men could recuperate from TB and other diseases; indeed, a nationwide series of "preventoria" were established so that urban children could strengthen their lungs in the healthful climate of rural American as a prophylaxis against TB (Anon., A Colorado Health Farm 1902; Anon., News and Notes 1903; Anon., Chicago Health Farm Proposed 1912).

These institutions emerged within the context of a growing medical and social concern about abnormalities in body weight, including the recognition of anorexia as a "wasting disease" apart from other conditions like TB and increasing cultural concern about overweight in children and adults (Brumberg 1988: 182–3 and 214–15).

While medical concerns about the health dangers of overweight can be dated to the early eighteenth century (Albala 2005), discourse about regulating body weight became more pronounced at the turn of the century (Sterns 1997: 27–32). Mothers, specifically, were encouraged to monitor the weight of their children against new standardized weight charts and to take measures to rectify weight problems (Brumberg 1988, 232–35). This context provided the impetus for medical professionals in the U.S.A. and Europe to develop dietary management routines for treating overweight and underweight patients (Brumberg 1988: 154–5; Sterns 1997: 38–47).

Treatments for abnormal body weight frequently included regimented eating and activity schedules designed to promote weight loss or weight gain depending on the patient's specific needs. For example, at Battle Creek, John Harvey Kellogg recommended excluding meat and dairy from one's diet and rigidly limiting caloric intake to one half the previous amount eaten. He espoused the virtues of eating only two meals a day and scheduled these meals at intervals of every six to seven hours. In addition, he prescribed increased activity and sweat baths to offset his dietary program (Schwarz 1970: 41–5). At the London Hospital and elsewhere, similarly regimented eating was used to treat underweight in anorexics. Patients were fed a diet of toast, vegetables, fish, and dairy at two-hour intervals, and their activity was severely restricted (Brumberg 1988: 154–6). This evidence suggests that in the late nineteenth and early twentieth centuries, individuals and families accepted inpatient residential programs as viable methods for treating abnormal body weight. William Howard Taft even spent time at "Professor" Izzy Winters's Health Farm in an attempt to reduce his impressive girth (Clark 1946; Hicks 1945).

By the 1950s, the practice of visiting health farms had combined with secular and religious summer-camp traditions begun in the late 1800s by Frederick W. Gull and others (American Camp Association 2006). As such, there were many summer camps for children that focused specifically on weight reduction (Sterns 1997: 82, 122). It is interesting that programs for children most inform our perceptions of residential weight-loss camps, despite the fact that the earliest residential treatment programs were designed for people of all ages. Even today, weight-loss camps are available for both adults and children, and new camps are emerging to treat entire families who are overweight. At all of these camps, counselors combine elements of structured activity, controlled diet, and behavior modification to force or facilitate dramatic weight loss over a short period of time (usually between four and eight weeks) (Brandt et al. 1980; Gately et al. 2005).

While summer weight-loss camps have evolved dramatically since their earliest incarnations, the prototypical "fat camps" of the 1950s probably most inform our contemporary conceptions of the environment, activities, and experiences of residential weight-loss programs for children. Specifically, weight-loss camps have been represented in popular media as miserable locations for pathetic social outcasts who need to reform their bodies to socially acceptable proportions. Some of the most recent and well-known parodies of the fat-camp experience appear in the popular television programs *The Simpsons* (2005) and *South Park* (2000), as well as in the 1995 film *Heavyweights* and the MTV documentary *Fat Camp* (2006). Yet, despite the frequently unsympathetic portrayal of fat camps in pop culture, these weight-reduction camps nevertheless have an important role to play in the efforts of children and their parents to treat obesity.

The role that residential diet camps have to play in the diet wars is evident in the increasing numbers and diversity of camps available. Between 2004 and 2005, there were about a dozen camps devoted strictly to weight loss, and four new camps opened in 2004 alone. Each summer, thousands of children and their parents put their hearts and dollars into this growing industry (Ellin 2005). However, the appeal of weight-loss camps is not confined solely to the Western world. In the context of increasing globalization and consumer culture, the appeal of these residential treatment programs is also evident in the emergence of camps in non-Western countries, such as China and Thailand (Jirapinyo et al. 1995). Camps in the U.S.A., Europe, and elsewhere are also receiving attention from major medical journals, such as the *International Journal of Obesity* and the *European Journal of Pediatrics*, and popular media outlets like the BBC, *The Oprah Winfrey Show*, *Dateline*, *The New York Times*, and the *LA Times*, among others (Ellin 2005; MSNBC 2006; Stein 2006).

Some of the most visible and talked-about sites in the U.S.A. and the U.K. include Camp Shane, which was established in 1968 and claims to be "the oldest weight-loss camp"; Camp La Jolla, a fitness-based camp in California; and Camp Wellspring, which is run by

Healthy Living Academies and has several locations across the U.S.A. and U.K. Typically, residential weight-loss programs or camps like these use physical activity, social support, and controlled diet within a cognitive behavioral framework to affect weight loss in children and adults (Braet et al. 2003). For example, Camp Wellspring, a typical weight-reduction camp, offers seven "state-of-the-science" weight-loss camps, including an adventure camp and a family weight-loss camp, in the U.S.A. and the U.K. (Wellspring Camps 2006).

Like all weight-reduction camps, this program promises campers permanent weight loss through changing eating habits and introducing daily activity, and, like most programs, it stipulates admissions requirements for its students. Children and young adults ages ten and older who want to attend Camp Wellspring "must be at least 20 pounds overweight and have been struggling with their weight for at least one year." However, the camp also admits younger clients ages five to nine to the Family Camp "if they are overweight." In addition to physical requirements of overweight, however, the camp also has "attitude requirements." Its promotional literature explains, "Campers must view Wellspring as an opportunity. Wellspring will not admit campers who are clearly opposed to attending, or who have a history of oppositional behavior or violence." This emphasis on the camper's own interest in treatment tacitly recognizes and addresses popular perceptions that children are forcibly committed to "fat camps" by their parents and presents Camp Wellspring, instead, as a place for overweight children who have made the choice to lose weight themselves (Wellspring Camps 2006).

Camp Wellspring's philosophy and program of treatment are also typical of the more recent weight-loss camps in the U.S.A. and U.K. and reflect new medical and scientific knowledge about dieting behavior and effectiveness. Their promotional material argues that "diets don't work" and, instead, introduces students to "foods that have the same flavor profile and feel as the foods that have contributed to weight gain, but that instead are very healthful." Nonetheless, eating at Wellspring, like at other camps, is controlled and restricted. The camp's promotional literature explains that "a typical day of controlled foods will include 1,200 calories, 10 g of fat, 50 g of protein, and 30 g of fiber." Wellspring's caloric goals are somewhat less than the typical weight-loss camp diet, which provides about 1,500 calories a day for overweight children (Ellin 2005); however, nutritional requirements vary widely from program to program (Gately et al. 2000: 1445–6). Like other programs Wellspring is committed to nutritional education and provides culinary training, as well as cognitive-behavioral sessions, which, it argues, will help children to monitor and moderate their eating habits after they leave the program, again, typical of most residential weight-loss camps (Brandt et al. 1980; Gately et al. 2000; Holt et al. 2004).

At all weight-loss camps, diet is combined with about three to four hours of exercise per day (Ellin 2005). More and more camps are moving toward a recreational sports model of exercise as opposed to the regimented intentional exercise of earlier programs (Holt et al. 2004: 222–3). For example, physical activity at Wellspring's general and adventure camps is provided through "fun" group sports, such as soccer and hiking. This newer model of physical activity reflects general physical-education findings that children are more likely to stick to an exercise routine when they enjoy it and represents a departure from earlier "boot camp" models for weight reduction.

Viewing the promotional literature alone suggests that a residential weight-loss camp just might be the answer for adults and children struggling with overweight and obesity. However, the cost of such programs is substantial. Most summer weight-loss camps cost about 7,500 dollars, which is approximately 1,500 dollars more than regular summer camps for children (Ellin 2005). Admittedly, a portion of these costs may be paid by major health-insurance providers; however, the out-of-pocket cost to families who choose this form of treatment is still substantial. Wellspring, for example, claims that the majority of PPO (Preferred Provider Organization, a common form of U.S. third-party health insurance) insured patients receive reimbursement of as much as 2,000 dollars (HMO [Health Maintenance Organization, a common form of U.S. third-party health insurance] patients are advised that they will not generally receive any reimbursement), but this covers only about a fourth of the total cost of the 8,650-dollar eight-week program (Wellspring Camps 2006). Clearly, the cost of attending a weight-loss camp like Wellspring is still prohibitive for many overweight families and individuals, especially those who are poor or uninsured (Johnston and Steele 2006: 4).

To many, treatment at a residential weight-loss camp may seem extreme. It is costly and requires that the patient be separated from his or her family and friends for a significant period of time. But to some families it may seem like the only choice, especially for obese children, who are generally not good candidates for surgical treatments or medication (Braet et al. 2004: 519). Researchers do agree that most residential weight-loss programs are effective in helping overweight/obese people lose weight in the short-term (Braet et al. 2003; Gately et al. 2000; Gately et al. 2005). However, the efficacy of these programs may be limited because many patients return to their previous eating and exercise behaviors upon leaving the controlled environment of the program (Snethen et al. 2006: 53–4). Factors, such as the duration of the program, the level of structure provided, weight at the time of entering the program, and the involvement/commitment of family members and the patient, contribute to the success or failure of individual participants in residential weight loss (Snethen et al. 2006: 53).

Studies of weight-loss camps also measure the psychological impact of these intervention programs on boys and girls because children "grow up in a climate of anti-fat attitudes and obesity stigmatisation" where they are "particularly vulnerable to body shape dissatisfaction, preoccupation with weight and shape, and low self-esteem" (Walker et al. 2003: 748). These studies show that "participation in a weight-loss camp improved rather than further impaired children's psychological state" (Walker et al. 2003: 752). Specifically, the patients' dissatisfaction with their body shapes also decreased, and self-esteem improved along with athletic competence and physical appearance esteem (Walker et al. 2003). In addition, patients may also have positive responses to peer and staff support and choice of activities at camp (Holt et al. 2004: 227–8).

However, studies have also shown that attending a weight-loss camp can have negative psychological effects on children. For example, residents experience homesickness and dietary concerns while at camp, which result in negative responses to the treatment program (Brandt et al. 1980; Holt et al. 2004). The little ethnographic work that has been done of children's weight-loss camps also suggests that these residential programs may contribute to campers' feelings that they are set apart from the rest of society because they are different or deviant (Millman 1980).

The treatment programs that we, today, call "fat camps" have a long history. From mineral baths to sanitariums and health farms, middle-class consumers have sought the controlled environments of residential retreats in their efforts to lose weight. While popular culture has constructed Fat Camp as a lonely place where the antisocial overeater can be rehabilitated, researchers tend to agree that "use of a structured fun-based skill learning program may provide an alternative method of exercise prescription to help children prolong the effects of . . . intervention" (Gately et al. 2000: 1445; Walker et al. 2003). In a time when childhood and adult obesity are on the rise and most obese children will continue to be overweight into adulthood, residential weight-loss camps are providing an evermore appealing, if costly, form of intervention and treatment.

SLG/C. Melissa Anderson

*See also* Anorexia; Cheyne; China Today; Globalization; Kellogg; Lindlahr; Obesity Epidemic; Socioeconomic Status; Taft

**References and Further Reading**
Albala, Ken (2005) "Weight Loss in the Age of Reason," in Christopher Forth and Ana Carden-Coyne (eds), *Cultures of the Abdomen: Diet, Digestion, and Fat in the Modern World*, New York: Palgrave Macmillan, pp. 169–84.
American Camp Association (2006) "The History of the Organized Camp Experience." Available online at <http://www.acacamps.org/media_center/about_aca/history.php> (accessed October 6, 2006).
Anon. (1902) "A Colorado Health Farm. Plans Made by the Young Men's Christian Association," *Philadelphia Inquirer*, June 15, p. 8.
Anon. (1903) "News and Notes," *Omaha World Herald*, August 12, p. 13.
Anon. (1912) "Chicago Health Farm Proposed," *Dallas Morning News*, July 7, p. 6.
Braet, Caroline, Tanghe, A., de Bode, P., Franckx, H. and Winckel, M.V. (2003) "Inpatient Treatment of Obese Children: Without Stringent Calorie Restriction," *European Journal of Pediatrics* 162 (6): 391–6.
Braet, Caroline, Tanghe, A., Decaluwé, V., Moens, E. and Rosseel, Y. (2004) "Inpatient Treatment for Children with Obesity: Weight Loss, Psychological Well-Being, and Eating Behavior," *Journal of Pediatric Psychology* 29 (7): 519–29.
Brandt, Gail, Maschhoff, Tom and Chandler, Nancy S.

(1980) "A Residential Camp Experience as an Approach to Adolescent Weight Management," *Adolescence* 15 (60): 807–22.
Brumberg, Joan Jacobs (1988) *Fasting Girls: The History of Anorexia Nervosa*, New York: Vintage Books.
Clark, Charles E. (1946) Untitled review, *Annals of the American Academy of Political and Social Science* 244 (March): 197.
Delaine, Janet (1996) "Baths," in Simon Hornblower and Anthony Spawforth (eds) *Oxford Classical Dictionary*, Oxford: Oxford University Press, pp. 235–6.
Ellin, Abby (2005) "For Overweight Children, Are 'Fat Camps' a Solution?" *New York Times*, June 28, F1.
Gately, Paul J., Cooke, C.B., Butterly, R.J., Mackreth, P. and Carroll S. (2000) "The Effects of a Children's Summer Camp Programme on Weight Loss, with a 10 Month Follow-Up," *International Journal of Obesity* 24 (11): 1445–53.
Gately, Paul J., Cooke, Carlton B., Barth, Julian H., Bewick, Bridgette M., Radley, Duncan and Hill, Andrew J. (2005) "Children's Residential Weight-Loss Programs Can Work: A Prospective Cohort Study of Short-Term Outcomes for Overweight and Obese Children," *Pediatrics* 116: 73–7.
Hembry, Phyllis M. (1997) *The British Spa from 1815 to the Present: A Social History*, London: Athlone Press.
Hicks, Frederick C. (1945) *William Howard Taft*, New Haven, Conn.: Yale University Press.
Holt, N.L., Bewick, B.M. and Gately, P.J. (2004) "Children's Perceptions of Attending a Residential Weight-Loss Camp in the UK," *Child: Care, Health & Development* 31 (2): 223–31.
Jirapinyo, Pipop, Limsathayourat, N., Wongarn, R., Bunnag, A. and Chockvivatvanit, S. (1995) "A Summer Camp for Childhood Obesity in Thailand," *Journal of the Medical Association of Thailand* 78 (5): 238–46.
Johnston, Craig A. and Steele, Ric G. (2006) "Treatment of Pediatric Overweight: An Examination of Feasibility and Effectiveness in an Applied Clinical Setting," *Journal of Pediatric Psychology* 32 (1): 106–10.
Jones, Billy M. (1967) *Health Seekers in the Southwest, 1817–1900*, Norman, Okla.: University of Oklahoma Press.
Millman, Marcia (1980) *Such a Pretty Face: Being Fat In America*, New York: Norton.

MSNBC (2006) "Last Resort School for Overweight Teens." Available online at <http://www.msnbc.msn.com/id/8985097> (accessed October 6, 2006).

National Center for Health Statistics (2003–4) "Prevalence of Overweight Among Children and Adolescents: United States, 2003–4," Centers for Disease Control and Prevention, available online at <http://www.cdc.gov/nchs/products/pubs/pubd/hestats/obese03_04/overwght_child_03.htm> (accessed December 20, 2006).

Ogden, Cynthia L., Carroll, Margaret D., Curtin, Lester R., McDowell, Margaret A., Tabak, Carolyn J. and Flegal, Katherine M. (2006) "Prevalence of Overweight and Obesity in the United States, 1999–2004," *Journal of the American Medical Association* 295 (13): 1549–55.

Schwarz, Richard W. (1970) *John Harvey Kellogg, MD* Nashville, Tenn.: Southern Publishing Association.

Snethen, Julia A., Broome, Marion E. and Cashin, Susan E. (2006) "Effective Weight Loss for Overweight Children: A Meta-Analysis of Intervention Studies," *Journal of Pediatric Nursing* 21 (1): 45–56.

Stein, Jeannine (2006) "Camp—with salads," *Los Angeles Times*, August 14, F1.

Sterns, Peter (1997) *Fat History: Bodies and Beauty in the Modern West*, New York: New York University Press.

Walker, L.L.M., Gately, P.J., Bewick, B.M. and Hill, A.J. (2003) "Children's Weight-Loss Camps: Psychological Benefit or Jeopardy?" *International Journal of Obesity* 27 (6): 748–54.

Wellspring Camps (2006) "Healthy Living Academies." Available online at <http://www.wellspringcamps.com> (accessed December 20, 2006).

# Fat-Positive

In a culture where thin bodies are idolized, thought beautiful and healthy, and sought for at the cost of women's (and increasingly men's) time and money and sometimes health, some people don't want them. There is an ever-growing movement variously referred to as "size acceptance," "fat acceptance," "fat positive," and "body positive." This movement has its forerunners in nineteenth- and early twentieth-century physicians such Hutchinson Woods, who critiqued the dieting culture as it became established. While both women and men are involved, many organizations have a decidedly feminist take on the perils of dieting culture and its celebration of a narrow standard of beauty.

The NAAFA (originally the National Association to Aid Fat Americans, later changed to National Association to Advance Fat Acceptance) was founded in 1969 to "eliminate discrimination based on body size and provide fat people with the tools for self-empowerment through public education, advocacy, and member support." It splintered in 1973, and members of the Los Angeles chapter founded the Fat Underground, a collective of fat activists with strong ties to the radical therapy, lesbian, and feminist communities. They published the "Fat Liberation Manifesto," a document outlining the collective's political ties to other oppressed groups, its antidiet stance, and its demand for equality in all areas of life for fat women. They argue, as does the International Size Acceptance Association (ISAA), that a person can be healthy at any size. They condemn the use of fear, guilt, and misinformation by the diet industry to sell (at best useless and at worst dangerous) products to consumers of all sizes. In their official position statement on dieting and the diet industry, the NAAFA emphasizes that the suffering of fat people is due to the stereotypes perpetuated by the diet industry. The various permutations of NAAFA, such as the Chicago Size Acceptance Group, have turned the tables, it is claimed, on the diet culture by allowing women to take pride in their size.

Their position paper includes the following recommendations:

- That local, state, and federal legislatures introduce, pass, enact, and enforce legislation which protects consumers against dangerous or ineffective diets and misleading diet advertising.

- That state and federal regulatory agencies, such as the Food and Drug Administration (FDA) and the Federal Trade Commission (FTC), adopt regulations based on NAAFA's "Guidelines for the Diet Industry" and closely monitor and control all aspects of the multi-billion-dollar diet industry.
- That all commercials for weight-loss diets and diet products be banned from radio and television because of lack of product success, negative health consequences, and the extreme negative impact of anti-fat propaganda on the self-esteem and quality of life of fat people.
- That federal regulations require all diets and weight-loss products to clearly display a health warning (similar to those found on cigarettes) regarding possible hazards and side effects.
- That regulations be adopted that require the diet industry to publish five-year (minimum) follow-up studies and "success" rates. All such statistics must be verifiable by objective outside researchers and clearly displayed on all diet products and advertising.
- That the Centers for Disease Control track morbidity and mortality caused by dieting and make the findings available to the public.
- That the National Institutes of Health (NIH) include input from consumer advocacy groups in establishing public health policy about dieting and obesity.
- That consumer-protection agencies, such as Consumers Union, conduct biannual studies on the efficacy of diet products and programs.
- That institutions such as the military, hospitals, schools, mental institutions, or prisons provide adequate food and not force anyone to diet against their will.
- That employers, schools, and judges never use weight loss or dieting as a condition for employment, promotion, admission, or avoiding incarceration.
- That healthcare professionals and medical institutions never deny other medical treatment to patients who choose not to diet.
- That the diet industry refrain from creating or perpetuating negative stereotypes about fat people in its marketing strategies.
- That diet companies and diet industry trade organizations voluntarily comply with NAAFA's "Guidelines for the Diet Industry."

- That individuals considering dieting study available literature on long-term results and side effects and carefully weigh dieting's possible benefits and risks.
- That dieters refuse to feel guilty or blame themselves for presumed lack of willpower if a diet fails.
- That no one allow themselves to be coerced into dieting against their will.
- That no one make assumptions or judge another person on the basis of body size or dietary preferences.

The ISAA, founded in 1997, has similar goals, with an international scope. They have active chapters in the U.S.A., U.K., France, Norway, Russia, Brazil, Australia, and the Philippines. Much of their work is internet-based, including downloadable literature, electronic magazines, and health and other resources on their site. They are currently focusing attention on "the obesity epidemic." They provide a link, for example, to a study at Yale that found anti-fat bias among health specialists working on obesity. The ISAA also provides an official position denouncing research on the "obesity virus" as "quackery." They therefore do not support the public health interventions trying to reduce obesity. In the past decade there has been a "celebrity" movement that paralleled the "plus size" movement in fashion.

SLG/ANGELA WILLEY

*See also* Anorexia; Imes-Jackson; Infectobesity; Manheim; Obesity Epidemic

## References and Further Reading
Brown, Laura S. and Esther D. Rothblum (1989) *Fat Oppression and Psychotherapy: A Feminist Perspective*, Binghamton, NY: Haworth Press.
Body Positive "Boosting Body Image at Any Weight." Available online at <http://www.bodypositive.com> (accessed April 28, 2006).
Frater, Lara (2005) *Fat Chicks Rule! How to Survive in a Thin-Centric World*, Brooklyn, NY: IG Publishers.
Gaesser, Glenn A. (2002) *Big Fat Lies: The Truth About Your Weight and Your Health*, Carlsbad, Calif.: Gurze Books.
International Size Acceptance Association (ISAA), available online at <http://www.size-acceptance.org> (accessed April 28, 2006).
Lebesco, Kathleen (2004) *Revolting Bodies: The Struggle*

to *Redefine Fat Identity*, Boston, Mass.: University of Massachusetts Press.
National Association to Advance Fat Acceptance (NAAFA), available online at <http://wwwnaafa.org> (accessed April 28, 2006).
Schwartz, Marlene B., Chambliss, Heather O'Neal, Brownell, Kelly D., Blair, Steven N. and Billington,

Charles (2003) "Weight Bias Among Health Care Professionals Specializing in Obesity," *Obesity Research* 11 (9): 1033–9.
Wann, Marilyn (1999) *Fat!SO? Because You Don't Have to Apologize for Your Size*, Berkeley, Calif.: Ten Speed Press.

# Fat Tax

American health policy has for the past decade acknowledged that an obesity problem exists in all strata of U.S. society. Approximately 127 million adults in the U.S.A. are now labeled overweight, 60 million obese, and 9 million severely obese. The common public-health answers to the causes of obesity are oversized portions and the vast availability of fast food and junk food. There is no doubt that America has a taste for nonnutritious fast and junk food, but the price discrepancy between this and nutritious, "healthy" food could also be to blame. When choosing what to eat, a consumer must weigh the accessibility, caloric content, and monetary cost of a meal against its nutritional value, taste, and the satisfaction or feeling of fullness it provides. Though this rough model is not meant to be sophisticated or necessarily complete, it makes a few important issues evident. The first is that caloric content and nutritional value must be understood as concepts and consciously considered each time in order to factor into the decision process. The current obesity rates tell us that Americans are making poor dietary choices that are leading to a detrimental aggregate weight gain. It has been argued that, from an evolutionary standpoint, our palates are wired to prefer calorie-dense foods, most of which are high in sugar and fat. When food was scarce, this made sense. With food more available than ever, it works against us, tempting us every time to choose the food and drink that will allow us to store energy in the form of fat. With high-fat and sugar-filled junk and fast food readily accessible, cheap, and tasty, it is no wonder America overdoses on it.

If there were a way to alter a consumer's attitude and therefore dietary preferences by either increasing the price of nonhealthy, fattening foods, decreasing the price of nutritious foods, or both, the Government might be able to evaluate the claim that poor dietary practices are at the center of the obesity problem.

The idea of a "fat tax" or a "Twinkie® tax" is not new. It was pioneered in the mid 1980s by Kelly D. Brownell, a psychologist at Yale University. Brownell proposed that a very small percentage tax be placed on junk and snack foods in order to generate revenue. The objective with a small tax, however, would not be to change dietary choices directly but to use this revenue for specific programs aimed at changing the public's dietary choices and promoting exercise. According to Brownell, the "toxic environment" is at the heart of the rise of obesity. The Federal Government should tax foods with little nutritional value. The less healthy, the higher the tax (as has been proposed for the taxation of the most fuel-inefficient automobiles). The highest taxed foods would quickly become too expensive for consumption, and the revenue generated could be used for "public exercise facilities—bike paths and running tracks" (Brownell and Horgan 2004). This fantasy of the nanny state providing the "positive democracy" (according to Sir Isaiah Berlin's critique) to force the ignorant or misled consumer on to the paths of health and longevity through the destruction of the toxic environment in which they live is seen by many as intrusive and ineffectual. Why assume that supplying exercise facilities is a necessary function of the state rather than full employment and a living wage?

"Fat tax" proposals have been met with general disapproval by the American public though advocated by those involved in public health lobbying, such as Marion

Nestle (Nestle 2003). Though these taxes have the potential to combat the current obesity problem, there are several drawbacks as well. Unlike cigarette taxes for instance, which only tax the demographic at risk (smokers), a fat tax would also tax healthy people who are able to avoid excessive consumption of junk and snack foods. On the other hand, if a fat tax were compensated with a subsidy on certain healthy foods, the only net monetary loss would be the administrative costs of the program itself. These would hopefully be offset by the increased welfare of the general public due to improved health. Another potential problem with a fat tax is that it would disproportionately affect people of lower socioeconomic status. However, this problem would be minimized with the tax/subsidy combination. In conclusion, the potential benefits of a "fat tax" are all merely speculation and there are many potential problems with it. For this reason, the initiative for such a program has been met with great disapproval.

SLG/Jason Weinstein

*See also* Developing World; Obesity Epidemic

### References and Further Reading

American Obesity Society (2005) "Obesity in the U.S. 2001." Available online at <http://www.obesity.org/subs/fastfacts/obesity_US.shtml> (accessed March 1, 2007).

Brownell, Kelly D. and Horgan, Katherine Battle (2004) *Food Fight: The Inside Story of the Food Industry, America's Obesity Crisis and What We Can Do About It*, New York: McGraw-Hill.

Mokdad, A.H., Marks, J.S., Stroup, D.F. and Gerberding J.L. (2004) "Actual Causes of Death in the U.S. 2000," *Journal of the American Medical Association* 291 (10): 1238–45.

Nestle, Marion (2003) *Food Politics: How the Food Industry Influences Nutrition and Health*, Berkeley, Calif.: University of California Press.

# Fletcher, Horace (1849–1919)

**B**etter known as "The Great Masticator," Fletcher was a popular and prominent food and health faddist of early twentieth-century North America. From 1895 to 1919, Fletcher devoted a majority of his time and energy to keenly distributing his doctrine of "Fletcherism." He wrote, "The most important part of nutrition is the right preparation of food in the mouth for further digestion" (Fletcher 1899: 15). This dogma put forward the idea that each mouthful of food should be completely masticated until it turns to liquid which can be done by precisely chewing each mouthful thirty-two times (once for each tooth), or ideally until liquefied, before swallowing. If food could not be liquefied (like fiber), then it should not be eaten in the first place; even "soup, wines, spirits, and other liquids" should be masticated. The reason is that this "is absolutely necessary to protection [*sic*] against abuse of the stomach and possible disease" (Fletcher 1899: 19). "Infallible evidence" that such an approach worked was that "the excreta [showed] . . . that the results of nutrition are observable" (Fletcher 1899: 56). Indeed, such rigorous chewing could even eliminate the great scourge of alcoholism: "No Fletcherite can be intemperate in the use of alcoholic stimulants" (Fletcher 1913: 36). It is no wonder that Fletcher's method was hailed and adopted by J.H. Kellogg who acknowledged in a letter to Fletcher that it was his work that made him aware of the "possible excess or the careless manner" by which foods were consumed (Fletcher 1903: xxxiv).

While Fletcher did not have any experience in medicine, nutrition, or health, his dogma about health and longevity rose in popularity during the Victorian era. It came to be a part of a culture that rejected obesity as a "disease of the will" and placed control firmly in the hands (or mouth) of the individual: "I argued that if Nature had given us personal responsibility for [nutrition] it was not hidden away in the dark folds and coils of the alimentary canal where we could not control it. The point was, then, to study the cavity of the mouth" (Fletcher 1913: 5). Self-control was in the form of chewing.

"Nature will castigate those who don't masticate," said Horace Fletcher. Chew your food thirty-two times and you will have a healthier body and a happier soul. This regimen was followed by celebrities such as John D. Rockefeller who advised "Don't gobble your food. Fletcherize, or chew very slowly while you eat" (Fletcher 1913: iii). Even the intelligentsia followed: Novelists Upton Sinclair and Henry James and Henry's brother, the philosopher and psychologist William James, by then a professor at Harvard, all regularly Fletcherized. Franz Kafka's father hid behind the newspaper at the dinner table, not wanting to watch his son compulsively chew.

Fletcher's evidence for his methods was purely anecdotal and experiential. He was denied health insurance in the 1880s due to his weight. "I weighted two hundred and seventeen pounds (about fifty pounds more than I should have for my height of five foot six inches) . . . I was an old man at forty, on the way to rapid decline" (Fletcher 1913: 1). Fletcher applied his technique of continuous chewing and claimed that he went down to 163 pounds. He invented complex validations for his claim,

expressing that lengthened chewing would reduce overeating, leading to improved bodily system functions, helping to reduce food intake, and therefore reducing monetary expenses. Fletcher also advised people to eat when they were "good and hungry," not when they were upset or worried. People could eat any type of food as long as it was chewed until the "food swallowed itself."

SLG/RAKHI PATEL

*See also* Aboulia; Kellogg

### References and Further Reading

Fletcher, Horace (1899) *Glutton or Epicure*, Chicago, Ill.: Herbert S. Stone.
—— (1903) *The A.B.Z. of Our Own Nutrition*, London: William Heinemann.
—— (1913) *Fletcherism: What It Is; or How I Became Young at Sixty*, London: Ewart, Seymour & Co.
Schwartz, Hillel (1986) *Never Satisfied: A Cultural History of Diets, Fantasies, and Fat*, New York: The Free Press.
Stearns, Peter N. (1997) *Fat History: Bodies and Beauty in the Modern West*, New York: New York University Press.

# Flockhart, Calista (1964–)

American actress who is best known for her starring role on the television show *Ally McBeal*, which aired between 1997 and 2002. In 1998, Flockhart won a Golden Globe for her portrayal of the quirky, temperamental lawyer—the self-titled protagonist Ally McBeal. In the late 1990s, because of the actress's wafer-thin appearance, she was rumored to have an eating disorder. Her extremely frail-looking body alarmed viewers and the media worldwide. Yet, Flockhart fervently denied these allegations. When asked whether she was "Karen Carpenter all over again," she replied that her thinness was an ideal, which made everyone else unhappy.

"So if you're thin, you somehow have it together, and that makes people mad. There's the ambiguity of this disease. It's twisted. Just because you're thin, and you're healthy, doesn't mean you're diseased. If you're thin, and you're healthy, there are certain people in the world who are going to be pissed off about it. It's discrimination. There's a double standard. In my life, a lot of people have said, 'Uchhhh! You're skinny!' As if they're just disgusted by it. But nobody would walk up to someone who's overweight and say, 'Ughhh! You're so fat!' It would never happen. It's a pathology."

(Snowden 1999)

She insisted that her skeletal stature was the result of the fact that "I was born with very tiny bones." Yet, the interview goes on to note her diet "consists almost entirely of low-fat, high-fibre foods, such as spinach and egg whites for breakfast" (Churcher 1999). The June 29, 1998 cover of *Time* magazine demonstrated what they called the "devolution" of the feminist movement into the "silly." It illustrated feminism beginning with Susan B. Anthony devolving into Ally McBeal.

Interestingly, Ally McBeal, a fictional character, is revered in many circles within American society as a feminist icon due to the way she portrayed both strength and softness. Moreover, "while Ally McBeal has been constructed in the media as the feminist 'ideal,' similarly Calista Flockhart . . . has been constructed-represented as the culture's 'beauty ideal' " (Leavy 2000). However, recently Flockhart has publicly admitted to having an eating disorder, although she does not specify exactly which one. According to the London *Daily Mirror*, the television starlet confessed: "I started under-eating, over-exercising, pushing myself too hard and brutalizing my immune system. I guess I just didn't find the time to eat. I am much more healthy these days" (Robertson 2006).

Flockhart is now considered one of the celebrity icons of eating disorders instead of beauty.

SLG/Jessica Rissman

*See also* Anorexia; Celebrities

## References and Further Reading
Churcher, Sharon (1999) "Calista a Picture of Poor Health," *Sunday Telegraph*, February 7, p. 36.
Leavy, Patricia (2000) "Feminist Content Analysis and Representative Characters," *The Qualitative Report* 5, available online at <http://www.nova.edu/ssss/QR/QR5–1/leavy.html> (accessed August 23, 2006).
Robertson, Cameron (2006) "Calista Flockhart Exclusive: I Did Have an Eating Problem," *London Daily Mirror*, April 7, available online at <http://www.mirror.co.uk/news/showbiz/tm_objectid=16914957%26method=full%26siteid=94762-name_page.html> (accessed April 25, 2006).
Snowden, Lynn (1999) "Flockhart Fights Back: Does the Star of Ally Mcbeal Accept That She's the Failure of Feminism, the Poster Girl for Anorexia? Fat Chance," *Ottawa Citizen*, May 1, 11.

# Fogle, Jared (1978–)

**A**lso known as "Jared the Subway Guy," Fogle, at 6 foot 2 inches, lost 245 pounds from an original 425 pounds while on a diet consisting of Subway sandwiches. He is now a spokesperson for Subway, starring in commercials and speaking across the U.S.A. about proper diet and exercise. He has also taken part in "Jared & Friends School Tour" and Subway's "FRESH (Feel Responsible, Energized, Satisfied and Happy) Steps" campaign, speaking to schoolchildren about having a healthy lifestyle with an effort to help overweight and obese kids.

While a college student at Indiana University, Fogle moved into an apartment next to a Subway store and began his diet in March 1998. His famous Subway diet excluded cheese and condiments and included sand-

wiches from the "6 grams of fat or less" menu. More specifically, his diet consisted of coffee for breakfast, a 6-inch turkey sub, Baked Lays potato chips, and diet soft drink for lunch followed by a foot-long veggie sub for dinner. As he started losing weight, he began exercising by walking to classes instead of riding the bus. A year later, he had lost 245 pounds, and now his diet has more calories but is still low in fat. He credits a friend who was a pre-med student with helping him realize that his morbid obesity was endangering his health by telling him that he had sleep apnea and that his edema (swelling) was linked to diabetes. At his father's recommendation, he visited an endocrinologist whom he was afraid to see for fear of stepping on the scale. However, the endocrinologist's advice did not help Fogle lose weight, so he tried many other diets until he began the Subway diet. "I had no intention of anyone ever finding out what I had done," he said.

However, after being featured in a friend's article in Indiana University's student newspaper and later in *Men's Health* magazine, Subway picked him up to help advertise, playing the part of a "regular guy," at a time when sales were already on the rise. Unlike Morgan Spurlock (*Super Size Me*), who denounced fast food for being unhealthy, Fogle gained prominence for supporting this healthy fast food chain. According to Patricia Dailey, editor-in-chief of *Restaurants and Institutions* magazine, the timing of Subway's advertising campaign as healthy fast food was advantageous as a national focus on the issue of obesity was just beginning to gain prominence. Subway also became the first sponsor of the American Heart Association's Jump Rope for Heart program, which is targeted at schoolage children.

Besides being recognized by people, and even by celebrities, Fogle's image has been mentioned or spoofed by Seinfeld, Jay Leno, David Letterman, *Saturday Night Live*, *South Park*, and *Austin Powers*. He has also been featured on *Oprah*, *Larry King Live*, and *48 Hours*. There were even rumors on the Internet that he lost the weight from AIDS or that he had since gained the weight back. According to Subway's website, Jared's fan letters, emails, and photos indicate that he has helped thousands of people lose a total of 160,000 pounds. Fogle's role is a prime example of the effect of celebrities in promoting diets and the creation of celebrities thanks to their diets.

SLG/DOROTHY CHYUNG

*See also* Spurlock; Winfrey

**References and Further Reading**
Subway Restaurants "All about Jared." Available online at <http://www.subway.com/subwayroot/menunutrition/jared/index.aspx> (accessed February 26, 2006).

CNN.com (2003) "Jared the Subway Guy, Superstar," Cable News Network, November 17, available online at <http://www.cnn.com/2003/SHOWBIZ/TV/11/17/subway.guy.ap> (accessed February 26, 2006).

Morgan, John and Shoop, Stephen A. (2004) "Jared Takes Steps to Help Kids Fight Fat," *U.S.A. Today*, July 15, available online at <http://www.usatoday.com/news/health/spotlighthealth/2004-07-15-jared_x.htm> (accessed February 26, 2006).

# Fonda, Jane (1937– )

Academy Award-winning actress, Jane Fonda, nicknamed "Hanoi Jane" in the 1970s for her controversial anti-war activism, has also battled a variety of body-image related issues in private. She "came out" about her struggles with bulimia and binge-eating in her 1981 book *Jane Fonda's Workout Book*. In publicizing it, she critiques the "thin is better, blonde is beautiful and buxom is best" feminine beauty ideal and recommends a series of exercises and dietary measures to forge strong healthy bodies that are also esthetically pleasing. In addition to her workout book, she was at the forefront of the exercise-video craze of the 1980s, a phenomenon that allowed people to experience celebrity workouts from their own homes. The ability to "see" celebrities undertake a program of exercise created a new commodity that could be sold in addition to the diet book. Contrary to her pacific stance on world issues, her workout video was very aggressive and contained famous phrases such as "feel the burn" and "no pain no gain." Upon viewing the financial success of the *Jane Fonda Workout*, many other celebrities made exercise videos to help people find fitness from their homes.

In her 2005 autobiography, Fonda constructs a pathologizing narrative around her obsession with weight. She speculates that the negative feelings she harbored about her body were possibly the result of her mother's suicide when she was thirteen. Her extreme dieting and bingeing at this time constituted an effort to ward off womanhood through a period of enforced "androgyny." She felt that maturation was associated in some oblique way with her mother's fate. She also counts her estranged relationship with her father as another contributing factor. If and when he commented on her appearance, it was to tell her she was fat. Her conflicting feelings about her body continued to define her life in different ways—from anxiety around food and weight to feeling like she was not fully "in her body." It is only now, in her sixties, that Fonda feels that she completely owns "her own womanhood" (Fonda 2005).

SLG/SHRUTHI VISSA

See also Binge-Eating; Celebrities

**References and Further Reading**
Fonda, Jane (1981) *Jane Fonda's Workout Book*, New York: Simon & Schuster.
—— (2005) *My Life So Far*, New York: Random House.

# Food Choice

Dieting seems to be largely about choosing what to eat. We believe that we determine which foods are the tastiest, most nutritional, filling, best for the environment, and cheapest. It is a complicated task, and yet there is still more to it. The categories change frequently, over years and sometimes days. If salmonella is discovered on spinach in one restaurant that receives its produce from a large corporation, then it is possible that any of the other ones might have it too. This causes spinach sales to drop, a short-lasting phobia of green leafy vegetables may develop, and what was yesterday a healthy lunch choice is now a host to a potentially deadly bacterium. Also, there are discrepancies within the qualifying categories for foods. What some claim to be a healthy food, others suggest never to eat, like fish, which has healthy fat but can have high levels of mercury. However, from the inconsistency and chaos that is our understanding of food, concrete feelings and ideas about health and nutrition can emerge.

The latter decades of the twentieth century focused on the differences between tasty, inexpensive food and healthy food, as seen in popular works such as *Fast Food Nation* and *Super Size Me*. This discrepancy is stereotyped as a problem of the industrialization of food, from restaurant food like the Big Mac™ to the store bought Twinkies®, which are inexpensive and easy to obtain because they are produced in mass quantity. The effect that such industrialized fast food has had on our world is significant. It is claimed that it has drastically altered eating habits and is labeled as the primary cause of widespread weight gain. In addition, it is often described as part of a food-industrial conspiracy with innumerable connections to both economical and structural development. Eric Schlosser's *Fast Food Nation* (2002) is perhaps the best representation of the Industrial Food Machine, from giant slaughterhouses that process thousands of cattle a day to the transformation of corn into high-calorie corn syrup—all of which ends up in the McDonald's menu (Schlosser 2002: 169). *Fast Food Nation* embodies a popular feeling that corporations lower quality standards in order to turn a profit. The health results are, according to this view, that people become obese, lead ever-unhealthier lives, and, on top of all that, damage the environment. Obesity becomes a metaphor for the overall destruction of the human and geographic environment by the industrial food conspiracy. Individuals lack any self-awareness, as such a conspiracy manipulates them into self-destructive acts, such as eating at McDonald's. These views are prefigured in the work of Kelly Brownell and Marion Nestle.

Michael Pollan, who regularly writes on such topics for the *New York Times Magazine*, has answered this lack of autonomy in food choice. Pollan, in his *The Omnivore's Dilemma* (2006), assesses our "national eating disorder," pointing out that Americans (and he could have added global society) are "a notably unhealthy people obsessed by the idea of eating healthily" (2006: 1, 3). Our national eating disorder lies in the "violent . . .

change(s) in our culture's eating habits" (Pollan 2006: 2). Focusing, like Schlosser, initially on corn and its importance in the American economy, Pollan sees the problem faced is not so much an industrial food conspiracy centered about fast food but the very nature of food choice. As we are intelligent and therefore autonomous individuals capable of raising nearly all types of foods, and because we are omnivorous, possessing the biological structures to metabolize them, we must learn which of those foods are healthy (and which unhealthy) for us. Even though virtually all food often comes to us in the form of fast and industrialized food, as most of us are alienated from food production, we do not know intuitively what not to eat. Our confusion over what to eat is to blame for our unhealthiness (Pollan 2006: 4, 5). And the fault in our modern world (again a new conspiracy theory) lies in the control of information by the nutritionists, who are concerned with our health as well as with selling dieting with all its proliferation of pills and potions. What Schlosser sees as a vast conspiracy of food manufacturers (and the entire system of modern capitalism) is seen by Pollan as a result of consumer ignorance. To be accurate, it is the nutritionists, concerned both with our health and with selling diet pills, who are at fault for our lack of knowledge about what is good to eat. Their desire, Pollan argues, is to perpetuate unhealthy eating so as to maintain their population of unhealthy, fat clients. They provide both bad and contradictory information, such as the Food Pyramid, which are at fault for our inability to know what is healthy to eat. Obesity, Pollan argues, is the result of the primacy of the professional and amateur nutrition culture, not the means of food production.

This argument about whether we should blame production or consumption for the problems of modern life is an old one. Yet, it continues to figure in debates about dieting as part of the explanation for the "lack of will" on the part of the dieters. If they are the subjects of "brain washing" by the food industry that explains their inability to choose; if they are ignorant of healthy eating choices because of the advocates for nutritional science, that too places their actions beyond personal choice.

For these views also depend on the claim that human beings are alienated from the "natural" world. The inherent claim that "natural man" did it better, lies at the core of a view of modernity as a degenerate deviation from the norm of health. Alienation in one form or the other, either through the self-serving industrialization of food production or the self-serving professionalization of health information lies at the core of the dilemma.

SLG/Benjamin D. Archer

*See also* Aboulia; Enlightenment Dietetics; Fast Food; Fat Tax; Food Pyramid; Natural Man; Professionalization of Dieting; Spurlock

## References and Further Reading

Brownell, Kelly D. and Michael Jacobson (2000) "Small Taxes on Soft Drinks and Snack Foods to Promote Health," *American Journal of Public Health* 90, 6: 854-857.

Brownell, Kelly D. and Katherine Battle Horgan (2004) *Food Fight: The Inside Story of the Food Industry, America's Obesity Crisis and What We Can Do About It,* New York: McGraw-Hill.

Nestle, Marion (2000) "Soft Drink 'Pouring Rights': Marketing Empty Calories to Children," *Public Health Reports* 115, 4: 308-19.

—— (2002) *Food Politics: How The Food Industry Influences Nutrition and Health*, Berkeley: University of California Press.

Pollan, M. (2006) *The Omnivore's Dilemma: A Natural History of Four Meals*, New York: Penguin.

Schlosser, E. (2002) *Fast Food Nation: The Dark Side of the All-American Meal*, New York: Harper.

# Food Pyramid

The original food guide pyramid was developed in 1992 by the United States Department of Agriculture (USDA) as a nutrition guide for Americans. The pyramid was separated into food groups; these categories constituted an ideal average daily diet.

Each category stipulated the recommended number of

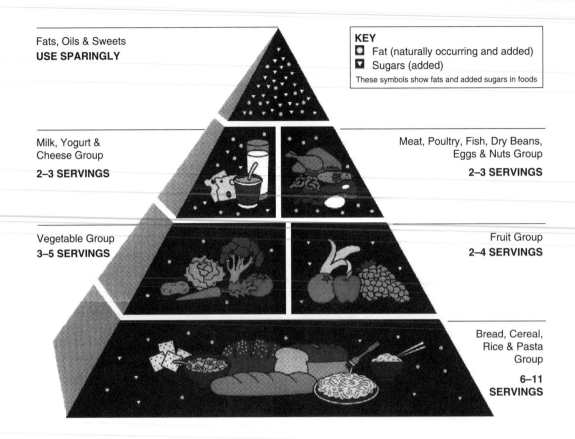

Fats, Oils & Sweets
**USE SPARINGLY**

**KEY**
☐ Fat (naturally occurring and added)
▼ Sugars (added)
These symbols show fats and added sugars in foods

Milk, Yogurt &
Cheese Group
**2–3 SERVINGS**

Meat, Poultry, Fish, Dry Beans,
Eggs & Nuts Group
**2–3 SERVINGS**

Vegetable Group
**3–5 SERVINGS**

Fruit Group
**2–4 SERVINGS**

Bread, Cereal,
Rice & Pasta
Group
**6–11
SERVINGS**

servings; for example, the USDA suggested two to four daily servings of fruits and three to five of vegetables. However, they failed to indicate what made up a serving. For instance, was one piece of broccoli considered a serving, or was a bushel of broccoli a serving? As there were no actual measurements indicated as a basis of serving size, this was mostly left to the interpretation of the consumer.

The food guide pyramid was used as a technique to teach nutrition to children as early as the 1950s in Australia. At an international conference in 1988, Helen Denning Ullrich, one of the primary founders of the Society for Nutrition Education in 1967, introduced it as a popular teaching tool for daily dietary needs. In the audience were scientists from the USDA who asked for copies. In 1992, this food guide pyramid was adopted as a replacement for the "four food groups" scheme in most school districts' health curriculums. These had been introduced as part of the war effort and food rationing in 1941 as the "basic seven groups" (green and yellow vegetables; oranges, tomatoes, and grapefruit; potatoes and other vegetables and fruit; milk and milk products; meat, poultry, fish, eggs, and dried peas and beans; bread, flour, and cereals; and butter and fortified margarine). In

1946 the "recommended daily servings" were suggested for the groups. The food groups were simplified to four in 1956 by the United States Department of Agriculture, and then, in the 1970s, a fifth group (fats, sweets, and alcoholic beverages in moderation) was added.

American students from the 1990s should have vivid memories of memorizing and drawing the food pyramid as part of a health class. But the tradition is actually much older. The USDA published its first dietary recommendations in 1894; in 1916, Caroline Hunt published her *Food for Young Children*, which divided food into five groups: milk/meat, cereals, vegetables/fruits, fats/fatty foods, and sugars/sugary foods. Over and over again the Government has attempted to define the basic food needs; each redefinition reflects the food ideologies of the day.

Health educators' insistence on considering the food pyramid as a guarantee of a healthy diet is the result of the USDA's influence via its "authoritative advice." Images of the food pyramid were so widespread that, according to the Harvard School of Public Health, the Pyramid was not only taught in schools, but it "appeared in countless media articles and brochures, and was plastered on cereal boxes and food labels" (Harvard School

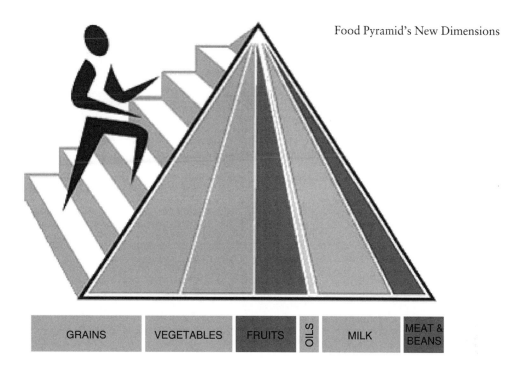

Food Pyramid's New Dimensions

GRAINS    VEGETABLES    FRUITS    OILS    MILK    MEAT & BEANS

of Public Health 2006). Moreover, the USDA collaborates with the Department of Health and Human Services in publishing a document—every five years since 1980—called *Dietary Guidelines for Americans*. According to the USDA's website, "the *Guidelines* provide authoritative advice for people two years and older about how good dietary habits can promote health and reduce risk for major chronic diseases. They serve as the basis for Federal food and nutrition education programs." The main aim of the guidelines is to establish the means to achieve "good health" for American citizens. Therefore, they include not only recommendations on food but also on exercise and unhealthy behaviors such as smoking. Ultimately, these suggestions seek to reduce the intake of substances that cause obesity, which the document notes is of "great public health concern" because of the deterioration of the body via an onslaught of diseases (Thompson and Venema 2005).

According to the Harvard School of Public Health, the *Dietary Guidelines for Americans* is not only a theoretical advocacy of health, it actually impacts how billions of dollars are spent each year (Harvard School of Public Health). The guidelines set the standards for all federal nutrition programs, including the school lunch program, and help determine what food products Americans buy. Thus, the food industry takes a great interest in what is included as "healthy" and what is not because their sales can be greatly impacted.

In the 2005 version of the Guidelines, the USDA altered the existing pyramid in order to better address portion control and health standards. The old pyramid did not adequately represent healthy eating. "Why not? Its blueprint was based on shaky scientific evidence, and it barely changed over the years to reflect major advances in our understanding of the connection between diet and health" (Harvard School of Public Health). The new food pyramid is laid out completely differently from the old. Instead of upwards layers, which visually provided an estimate of portions per food group, the new pyramid is composed of a series of vertical lines that siphon off the different categories. Each food group is color-coded, and its size depends upon how much of it you should eat. However, while the original pyramid was self-explanatory, this pyramid requires a lot of effort to understand. Its abstract nature may subtract from the intended message. If the average citizen cannot understand such an image with a glance, then it is arguably ineffective.

However, dieticians champion the new pyramid. They are now using it to promote healthy individual-based diets to their clients seeking weight loss. According to nutritionist Anne Collins, who offers weight-management strategies to her customers, the U.S. Department of Agriculture's 2005 *Dietary Guidelines* are centered upon helping citizens understand and achieve a "balanced diet, healthy eating, and healthy weight management" (Collins 2006). Collins believes in the integrity of the new guidelines to the point that her website even offers a strategy of how to adapt the USDA's new food pyramid into specific diets based on caloric intake levels. The new USDA 2005 pyramid, with its portion control recommendations, is a state-of-the-art government-sponsored balanced diet. Yet the critics have attacked it as advocating the consumption of certain fish labeled as dangerous because of contamination by the FDA. Today, one can go on the USDA website to *MyPyramid* and enter in their personal information (sex, age, weight, height), and the pyramid can suggest how many servings—which are broken down into ounces and actual amounts—a person should have in their day (Collins 2006).

SLG/JESSICA RISSMAN

*See also* Peters; Smoking

## References and Further Reading

Anon. "Food Pyramid," *Columbia Encyclopedia*, 6th edn, available online at <http://www.bartleby.com/65/fo/foodpyr.html> (accessed May 4, 2006).

Callaway, C.W. (1997) "Dietary Guidelines for Americans: An Historical Perspective," *Journal of the American College of Nutrition* 16 (6): 510–16.

Collins, Anne (2006) "What is a Balanced Diet?" Anne Collins Weight Loss Program, available online at <http://www.annecollins.com/nutrition/balanced-diet.htm> (accessed May 4, 2006).

Harvard School of Public Health (2006) "Food Pyramids." Available online at <http://www.hsph.harvard.edu/nutritionsource/pyramids.html> (accessed May 4, 2006).

Hunt, Caroline (1916) *Food for Young Children*, Washington, DC: U.S. Dept. of Agriculture.

Thompson, Tommy G. and Venema, Ann M. (2005) "Dietary Guidelines for Americans 2005." United States Department of Agriculture, January 12, available online at <http://www.healthierus.gov/dietaryguidelines> (accessed May 4, 2006).

# Franklin, Benjamin (1706–90)

Though more popularly noted for his role in the American Revolution and early American politics, in his personal life, Franklin expressed a continuous interest in food and the particular ways in which one could eat. Franklin, a man of simple tastes, most definitely enjoyed food (Franklin 1964: 55). His later tastes for simple foods can be accredited to the simple foods he was served as a young boy. In addition to the attainment of simple tastes, Franklin's childhood taught him to consider meals and eating to be a social function. Throughout his life, Franklin, as often as he could, continued this family tradition (Chinard 1958: 7).

At age sixteen, Franklin read Thomas Tyron's *The Way to Health, Long Life and Happiness* (1683), which recommended "temperance in eating and drinking, and moderation in their sleep and exercise. By such methods as these the seeds of vice might more easily . . . be subdued and a foundation laid for the building upon an excellent and accomplished person" (Tyron 1683: 34). It is the morality of good diet that appealed to Franklin. He strictly followed this vegetable diet for a short while, and soon started eating fish, reasoning that, "when the Fish were opened, I saw smaller Fish taken out of their stomachs: Then thought I, if you eat one another, I don't see why we mayn't eat you" (Zall 2005: 163). The philosophy Tyron expressed in his book pervaded Franklin's moral virtues, which he included in his writing of *Poor Richard's Almanac*. While Franklin did enjoy both eating and drinking, he tried not to overdo either one, as he stated in *Poor Richard's Almanac*, "Eat not to dullness. Drink not to elevation" (Chinard 1958: 12). Also included in one of Franklin's many versions of *Poor Richard's*, was the instruction to his fellow countrymen, "to supply our selves from our own Produce at home" (Chinard 1958: 12).

As an avid traveler, Franklin enjoyed tastes and recipes

from abroad; yet, he still remained true to American food and flavors. In his 1742 version of *Poor Richard's*, the section, "Rules of Health and Long Life, and to Preserve from Malignant Fevers, and Sickness in General," demonstrates Franklin's dedication to eating for health. Franklin was also an advocate of the strenuous life. His belief in swimming as a sport made it popular in England, where William Wyndham offered to fund Franklin's creation of the first swim club. As with diet, it was a book that Franklin had read, Melchisedec Thevenot's *The Art of Swimming and Advice for Bathing* (1696), that persuaded him of the health benefits of exercise. With all of this said, and while Franklin did avidly believe in eating for health, he no doubt enjoyed his food, as he was over 300 pounds at the time he died.

SLG

## References and Further Reading

Chinard, Gilbert (ed.) (1958) *Benjamin Franklin on the Art of Eating: Together with the Rules of Health and Long Life and the Rules to Find Out a Fit Measure of Meat and Drink, with Several Recipes*, Princeton, NJ: Princeton University Press.

Coveney, John (2000) *Food, Morals and Meaning: The Pleasure and Anxiety of Eating*, New York: Routledge.

Franklin, Benjamin (1964) *The Autobiography of Benjamin Franklin*, ed. Leonard W. Labaree, Ralph L. Ketcham, Helen C. Boatfield, and Helene H. Fineman, New Haven, Conn.: Yale University Press.

Tyron, Thomas (1683) *The Way to Health, Long Life and Happiness*, London: Andrew Sowle.

Zall, Paul M. (2005) *Ben Franklin's Humor*, Lexington, Ky.: The University Press of Kentucky.

# Friedman, Jeffrey (1954–) MD, Ph.D.

Friedman led the team that discovered the obesity hormone, Leptin, by studying genetic mechanisms of weight regulation in mice. The fat mouse had been "discovered" at the Jackson Laboratory in Bar Harbor, Maine in the early 1950s. This mutant mouse was so huge that researchers assumed that it was pregnant, until it was discovered that it was a male mouse. Friedman was inspired by the work of Ethan Allen Sims, a physician at the University of Vermont College of Medicine who had been exploring the link between obesity and diabetes using male inmates at the Vermont state prison. Allen found that only very few inmates could easily put on weight, and these found it the most difficult to lose it.

In late 1994, Friedman's research had received national recognition after the isolation of the obesity gene (ob) and its human homologue had been publicized (Zhang et al. 1994). This was a key paper for any further research in the field of obesity and dieting because it specified the exact code of this gene. Its central importance and credibility in this particular field of research is that any researcher wanting to study this gene in ob mice must have information about the gene itself. Knowing the exact code allows hypotheses to be set up about whether the physiological problem is a defect in the protein that the ob gene makes, or whether it is the perhaps defective receptor of ob that is the problem.

In this case, as subsequent studies were able to confirm, there are in fact multiple ways of having an obese phenotype (i.e., a fat mouse). In some cases, the ob gene itself is defective, and in others, the receptor gene is defective (a different gene, called db). Of course, other genes entirely can also cause obesity. This paper was the starting point for any closer examination of what the gene products resulting in obesity are, and how they interact. Their paper is credible as the techniques used to determine this sequence are standard, universally accepted genetic methods for finding genes. It was done as follows: First, recombination studies are done. This means that researchers allow mice to breed in large numbers and then look for inheritance patterns that do not necessarily follow Mendelian patterns. By comparing numbers of fat to lean offspring in relation to some other genetically related trait (molecular markers), it is possible to determine approximately where on a chromosome (and on which chromosome) a mutation is.

The chromosome and the gene's approximate location

were already known to Friedman and his colleagues. The next step was to continue to narrow down where on the chromosome ob is by comparing it to other genes close to it (by making a genetic map, which gets increasingly specific). After this, they had a very small (comparatively) region of DNA which they know contains the gene, and by insetting the region via recombinant techniques in bacteria and growing them, they can see which parts are expressed, and are therefore part of the gene. Furthermore, the sequences are compared to standard DNA libraries to see if homology to other genes exists. In the case of Friedman's work, this technique worked because the product of the gene, a protein called Leptin, was already known, and so they only had to compare the region of DNA and its putative gene product to the protein Leptin to see whether they had the right region. These methods are entirely standard, and there is no reason to doubt the report's veracity. Thus, this paper is central because not only is it entirely within the bounds of standard genetic research, but it is also the starting point for any further work. However, its genetic credibility does not absolve its scientific weaknesses, namely that it equates obesity with bad health and considers obesity the cause rather than the symptom of other illnesses.

But Friedman's hypothesis did not rest with the explanation of where the genetic key to obesity in mice lay. He concludes with the evolutionary biological explanation that "heterozygous mutations at ob may provide a selective advantage in human populations subjected to caloric deprivation. Identification of ob offers an entry point into the pathways that regulate adiposity and body weight and should provide a fuller understanding of the pathogenesis of obesity" (Zhang et al. 1994: 431). At that point, the meanings associated with obesity shifted radically from psychological to genetic explanations. However, the genetic explanations were given an evolutionary meaning to explain their "function" (Shell 2001). Fat had to have purpose if it were an inherent part of the genome. It could not be a random or a secondary effect. It had "meaning" in the past when entire populations starved to death. Actually, a counter "just-so-story" could be told about the fat members of prehistoric populations who were the favorite prey of saber-tooth tigers as they ran much slower.

The notion of giving meaning to fat in the evolutionary past made it "natural" rather than pathological. As Friedman later wrote:

In their efforts to lose weight, obese individuals may be fighting a powerful set of evolutionary forces honed in an environment drastically different from that of today. . . . Twin studies, adoption studies, and studies of familial aggregation confirm a major contribution of genes to the development of obesity. Indeed, the heritability of obesity is equivalent to that of height and exceeds that of many disorders for which a genetic basis is generally accepted. It is worth noting that height has also increased significantly in Western countries in the 20th century; for example, the average U.S. Civil War soldier was 5′4″ tall. Yet, in contrast to the situation with obesity, most people readily accept the fact that genetic factors contribute to differences in stature.

(Friedman 2003: 856)

Strangely, this is precisely the argument that Francis Galton (1822–1911), Charles Darwin's cousin and the creator of "eugenics," made concerning the inheritability of physical characteristics (Galton 1869). He wanted to prove that the British working class was stupid, small, and puny because of their inheritance following his dictum that "nature" outweighed "nurture" (a phrase that he coined). Even his contemporaries dismissed this, noting the radical difference in nutrition between the working class and Galton's ideal upper-middle-class Englishman (Constable 1905).

Subsequent to defining the ob gene, Friedman's laboratory found that injecting leptin into mice decreased their body weight because food intake was reduced and energy expenditure increased. As a result of Friedman's discovery, current research has been aimed at trying to understand the genetic basis of obesity in humans and the role Leptin plays in transmitting its weight-reducing signal.

Currently, Friedman is a professor at the Rockefeller University in New York City and an investigator at the Howard Hughes Medical Institute. Research in progress involves the regulatory mechanisms controlling body weight, Leptin's mechanism of action, and its importance to the pathogenesis of obesity. Other studies try to clarify the mechanism by which Leptin controls feeding. Lastly, efforts to investigate the genetic basis of the high incidence of obesity on the Pacific Island of Kosrae are also in progress (Bonnen et al. 2006). Through Friedman's continued studies of Leptin and his search for other genes that influence weight in humans, he hopes to lay the foundation for developing treatments to fight the global epidemic of obesity.

SLG/Rakhi Patel

*See also* Genetics

## References and Further Reading

Bonnen, P.E., Pe'er, I., Plenge, R.M., Salit, J., Lowe, J.K., Shapero, M.H., Lifton, R.P., Breslow, J.L., Daly, M.J., Reich, D.E., Jones, K.W., Stoffel, M., Altshuler D. and Friedman, J.M. (2006) "Evaluating Potential for Whole-Genome Studies in Kosrae, an Isolated Population in Micronesia," *Nature Genetics* 38 (2): 214–17.

Constable, Frank Challice (1905) *Poverty and Hereditary Genius: A Criticism of Mr. Francis Galton's Theory of Hereditary Genius*, London: A.C. Fifield.

Friedman, J.M. (2002) "The Function of Leptin in Nutrition, Weight, and Physiology," *Nutrition Reviews* 60 (10, part 2): S1–14, S68–84, and S85–87.

—— (2003) "A War on Obesity, Not the Obese," *Science* 299 (5608): 856–8.

—— "Heads of Laboratories," The Rockefeller University, available online at <http://www.rockefeller.edu/research/abstract.php?id=41> (accessed April 18, 2006).

—— Howard Hughes Medical Institute, available online at <http://hhmi.org/research/investigators/friedman_bio.html> (accessed April 12, 2006).

Galton, Francis (1869) *Hereditary Genius: An Inquiry into Its Laws and Consequences*, London: Macmillan.

Kolata, Gina (2007). *Rethinking Thin: The New Science of Weight Loss—and the Myths and Realities of Dieting*, New York: Farrar, Straus and Giroux.

Shell, Ellen Ruppel (2001) *The Hungry Gene: The Science of Fat and the Future of Thin*, New York, Atlantic Monthly Press.

Zhang, Y., Proenca, R., Maffei, M., Barone, M., Leopold, L. and Friedman, J.M. (1994) "Positional Cloning of the Mouse Obese Gene and Its Human Homologue," *Nature* 372 (6505): 425–32.

# G

## Gandhi, Mohandas Karamchand (1869–1948)

Born on October 2, 1869 in Porbandar, India to a family of the Vaisya, or merchant, caste, Gandhi's childhood ambition was to study medicine, but because this was considered "defiling: to his caste, his father persuaded him to study law instead" (Anon. 1998). Gandhi's religious background influenced his eating habits throughout his life. Ironically, he did not at first trust the connection between his religion and his family's diet, but, according to his autobiographical account, it was through his experimentation with his eating habits that Gandhi found his religious and moral mission in life.

Gandhi's family followed the Vaishnava version of Hinduism and was rigorously opposed to meat-eating. For the young Gandhi, raised in British colonial India, Indian subservience to the British was understood in terms of a superior British diet. One of Gandhi's friends and even his own older brother had begun to eat meat and argued with Gandhi on behalf of their own lifestyle:

> We are a weak people because we do not eat meat. The English are able to rule over us, because they are meat-eaters. You know how hardy I am and how great a runner too. It is because I am a meat-eater. Meat-eaters do not have boils or tumours, and even if they sometimes happen to have any, these heal quickly. Our teachers and other distinguished people who eat meat are no fools. They know its virtues. You should do likewise. There is nothing like trying. Try, and see what strength it gives.
>
> (Gandhi 1939: 17 and 19)

Meat makes one healthy, stronger, and able to cope with the exigencies of the world. As Gandhi noted: "I certainly looked feeble-bodied by the side of my brother and this friend. They were hardier, physically stronger, and more daring" (1939: 17).

But Gandhi also understood the political implications of health and strength: "A doggerel of the Gujarati poet Narmad was in vogue amongst us schoolboys, as follows":

> Behold the mighty Englishman
> He rules the Indian small,
> Because being a meat-eater
> He is five cubits tall.
> (Gandhi 1939: 18)

His friends urged Gandhi to see that many of his teachers were meat-eaters and those who ate meat were both "hardier, physically stronger, and more daring" (Jack 1956: 10). Also, they convinced him into believing that "if the whole country [India] took to meat-eating, the English could be overcome" (Jack 1956: 11). With these arguments, Gandhi decided to eat meat. Immediately after he first tried it, he had nightmares of animals inside him and was full of remorse. However, this new diet was an experiment to teach him about the strength that meat provided and thus he "would remind myself that meat-eating was a duty and he became more cheerful" (Jack 1956: 12).

With this realization, Gandhi came to use dieting practices, mainly abstinence from food, to further the objectives of his missions. His physical emaciation as a result of these practices came to be viewed as a symbol of strength and protest, rather than one of malnutrition often associated with extraordinarily thin individuals in third-world countries.

Gandhi recognized that he was lying constantly to his parents about his new eating habit. He acknowledged that "though it is essential to eat meat, and also essential to take up food reform in the country, yet deceiving and lying to one's father and mother is worse than not eating meat" (Jack 1956: 13). In their lifetime, therefore, meat-eating was beyond the pale. He stated that he decided to pursue vegetarianism at least until his parents passed away. But part of the reason he gives as an adult is the image of the "meat-eater," not as the ruling Englishman in Rudyard Kipling's image but rather as the crude and hypocritical Indian avatar, the convert to Christianity as the meat-eating parvenu:

In those days Christian missionaries used to stand in a corner near the high school and hold forth, pouring abuse on Hindus and their gods. I could not endure this. I must have stood there to hear them once only, but that was enough to dissuade me from repeating the experiment. About the same time, I heard of a well-known Hindu having been converted to Christianity. It was the talk of the town that, when he was baptized, he had to eat beef and drink liquor, that he also had to change his clothes, and that thenceforth he began to go about in European costume including a hat. These things got on my nerves. Surely, thought I, a religion that compelled one to eat beef, drink liquor, and change one's own clothes did not deserve the name. I also heard that the new convert had already begun abusing the religion of his ancestors, their customs and their country. All these things created in me a dislike for Christianity.

(Gandhi 1939: 29)

And, one can add, eating meat.

While in England attending law school, Gandhi reaffirmed his commitment to vegetarianism and rather than abstaining from meat for the sake of his parents, he did so as a personal choice (Jack 1956: 18). In England, he actively searched for vegetarian restaurants and would often "trot 10 or 12 miles each day" in order to find one of these restaurants. During one of these searches, Gandhi found a vegetarian restaurant in Farringdon Street, London and believed "God had come to my aid" (Jack 1956: 18–19). At this restaurant, he purchased a book by Henry Stephen Salt entitled *A Plea for Vegetarianism* (1886) and now claimed to have become a

vegetarian by choice. That day, he made the choice "in favor of vegetarianism, the spread of which forward became my mission" (Jack 1956: 18–19). But, like his hated Hindu convert, it was within the realm of British vegetarian practice that Gandhi found an acceptable Western scientific and therefore moral rationale for avoiding meat:

I saw that the writers on vegetarianism had examined the question very minutely, attacking it in its religious, scientific, practical and medical aspects. Ethically they had arrived at the conclusion that man's supremacy over the lower animals meant not that the former should prey upon the latter, but that the higher should protect the lower, and that there should be mutual aid between the two as between man and man. They had also brought out the truth that man eats not for enjoyment but to live.

(Gandhi 1939: 46)

The Christian underpinnings of this view, so obvious even in the high Victorian period, the 1880s, when Gandhi studied in England, are part of his account.

While at a vegetarian boarding house in Manchester, Gandhi met a vegetarian Christian who persuaded him to read the Bible (Jack 1956: 22). While reading the New Testament, Gandhi reconciled the Sermon on the Mount with the teachings of the Gita and the Light of Asia (Jack 1956: 23). He wrote that the Sermon "went straight to my heart." The verses read, "But I say unto you, that ye resist not evil: but whosoever shall smite thee on thy right cheek, turn to him the other also" (Jack 1956: 23). These teachings promoted the ideas of nonviolent protest. In 1904, while in South Africa and writing news columns, he met Henry S.L. Polack in a vegetarian restaurant, who introduced him to the writings of John Ruskin, by lending Gandhi the book *Unto this Last* (Jack 1956: 56). Gandhi claimed that the book "gripped me ... I discovered some of my deepest convictions reflected in this great book" (Jack 1956: 56). He believed the teachings of that book centered on the good of the individual being determined by the good of the community, the work of any man is as good as that of any other, and the life of labor is worth living. After this reading, Gandhi claims that "he arose with the dawn, ready to reduce these principles to practice" (Jack 1956: 56). He considered his religious disciplinary "conclusions" to include "chiefly vegetarianism, abstinence from stimulants, and self-control in general" (Jack 1956: 471).

According to his account, Gandhi had only remained a vegetarian "in the interests of truth and the vow I had taken [in front of my mother], but had wished at the same time that every Indian could be a meat-eater, and had looked forward to being one myself freely and openly someday, and to enlisting others to the cause" (Jack 1956: 19). But suddenly being a "good" British subject meant following a new (yet old) dieting practice.

Vegetarianism becomes the space in which all Indians can be reconciled, as in Gandhi's account of the establishment of the "Tolstoy Farm" in 1904.

> We were all vegetarians on Tolstoy Farm, thanks, I must gratefully confess, to the readiness of all to respect my feelings. The Musalman youngsters must have missed their meat during ramzan, but none of them ever let me know that they did so. They delighted in and relished the vegetarian diet, and the Hindu youngsters often prepared vegetarian delicacies for them, in keeping with the simplicity of the Farm.
>
> (Gandhi 1939: 276)

Later in his life, Gandhi became a greater figure of political, cultural, and economic protest. His eating habits became part and parcel of his politics. Gandhi first protested in attempt to eradicate race prejudice in South Africa in 1893. Later, after years of civil protest in South Africa, he returned to his homeland, India, where he spoke of a new India in which Indians could be free of class constraints. Following the passage by the English ruling government of India of the repressive Rowlatt Act of 1919, Gandhi called for a general strike against Englishmen throughout the country, and, after 400 Indians were killed in the Amritsar Massacre that year, he called for non-cooperation with British courts, stores, and schools. In 1921, the Congress Party, a coalition of various nationalist groups, voted again for a nonviolent disobedience campaign. After England's entry into World War II, Gandhi proposed non-cooperation, and, as a result, he was imprisoned along with other members of the Congress Party.

When the British attempted to blame Gandhi, he fasted for about three weeks while in jail. The politics of fasting always maintained an ethical dimension well learned as a student in Britain:

> Fasting and restriction in diet now played a more important part in my life. Passion in man is generally co-existent with a hankering after the pleasures of the palate. And so it was with me. I have encountered many difficulties in trying to control passion as well as taste, and I cannot claim even now to have brought them under complete subjection. I have considered myself to be a heavy eater. What friends have thought to be my restraint has never appeared to me in that light. If I had failed to develop restraint to the extent that I have, I should have descended lower than the beasts and met my doom long ago. However, as I had adequately realized my shortcomings, I made great efforts to get rid of them, and thanks to this endeavour I have all these years pulled on with my body and put in with it my share of work.... And if there was some occasion for penance or the like, I gladly utilized it too for the purpose of fasting. But I also saw that, the body now being drained more effectively, the food yielded greater relish and the appetite grew keener. It dawned upon me that fasting could be made as powerful a weapon of indulgence as of restraint.
>
> (Gandhi 1939: 267)

Gandhi believed that Hindu–Moslem unity was natural and undertook a twenty-one-day fast to bring the communities together. He also fasted in a strike of mill workers in Ahmedabad. Later, in 1946, after he emerged from being imprisoned by the British, he looked to create a united India with a federal parliament. He objected to the separate Muslim state of Pakistan that Muhammad Ali Jinnah demanded. However, Jinnah refused to compromise and instead commanded communal killings that left 5,000 dead and 15,000 wounded in Calcutta, and this violence spread throughout India. As a result, in Bengal, Gandhi declared that he would fast until his death unless Hindus and Muslims could learn to live peacefully together. The situation calmed in Bengal, but riots continued in other parts of India. Gandhi did not participate in his nation's celebration of their independence from England in 1947, for he despaired his nation's lack of unity. On September 1, 1947, he began another fast for Indian unity, after an angry mob broke into the residence he stayed at in Calcutta. His fast ended when both Hindu and Muslim leaders agreed that there would be no more killings. On January 13, 1948, in Delhi, he began his last fast, praying for Indian unity. That day, he was assassinated by Nathuram Godse, a Hindu extremist, as he fasted.

Gandhi changed the emaciated image from one of victim of Third World hunger, to that of strength to abstain from food for moral aims. Likely, it was his extreme practice and unusual motivation that garnered Gandhi attention and respect during his protests. Through the success of such spectacular displays of food abstinence, Gandhi inevitably was an essential figure in setting the forefront for more modern-day fasters.

SLG/CAROLINE A. BUGG

*See also* Emaciated Body Images; Religion and Dieting; Vegetarianism

**References and Further Reading**

Anon. (1998) "Gandhi, Mohandas Karamchand," in Paula K. Byers (ed.), *Encyclopedia of World Biography*, 2nd edn, Vol. XVII, Detroit, Mich.: Gale Research Group.

Gandhi, Mahatma (1939) *Gandhi: An Autobiography— the Story of My Experiments with Truth*, trans. Mahadev Desai, London: Pheonix Press.

—— (1949) *Diet and Diet Reform*, Ahmedabad: Navajivan Publishing House.

—— (1959) *The Moral Basis of Vegetarianism*, Ahmedabad: Navajivan Publishing House.

Jack, Homer Alexander (ed.) (1956) *The Gandhi Reader: A Source Book of His Life and Writings*, Bloomington, Ind.: Indiana University Press.

Salt, Henry Steven (1886) *A Plea for Vegetarianism*, Manchester: Vegetarian Society.

Walters, Kerry S. and Portmess, Lisa (2001) *Religious Vegetarianism: from Hesiod to the Dalai Lama*, Albany, NY: State University of New York Press.

Wolpert, Stanley A. (2001) *Gandhi's Passion: The Life and Legacy of Mahatma Gandhi*, Oxford: Oxford University Press.

# Genetics

The field of genetics has evolved rapidly since 2000. New technology has allowed researchers to identify genes, which provide the blueprint necessary for the body to manufacture specific hormones like insulin and estrogen. These hormones tell the body to store or burn fat, carbohydrates, and protein. Additionally, hormones maintain body temperature, regulate digestive rate, tell the body to stop or start eating, and initiate growth in children and adolescents. When a person does not have a gene that is essential for the production or activation of a hormone, a disease usually develops. For example, a person who lacks the gene to manufacture growth hormone (pituitin) will not be able to grow to normal height. People can carry a gene without having the disease, which means that a child can inherit a disease that neither parent has.

As scientists discovered genes that seemed to trigger diseases such as cancer and diabetes, they began searching for genes that cause weight gain or loss as well. Genes in animals are very similar to those in humans, thus animals are frequently used to find new genes and to understand their function. In the 1940s, a gene in mice was discovered that was the blueprint for a hormone called leptin (Kalra et al. 2003). Leptin is secreted in response to the amount of fat in the body of the animal. The release of leptin decreases appetite and tells the mouse to stop eating. If the gene producing leptin is missing, the mouse will not stop eating and will gain significant amounts of body fat. When the animals are injected with leptin, they will stop eating and return to normal weight (Stipanuk 2000: 443–4).

The discovery of the function of leptin led researchers to predict that if leptin was administered to obese individuals, they would lose weight. Despite unsuccessful clinical trials, drug companies began to market leptin in the form of over-the-counter dieting supplements like Leptoprin. The problem with these supplements is that leptin is minimally effective in controlling weight when injected and completely ineffective when taken orally. As of 2007, leptin had not yet been shown to be a useful treatment for weight loss, but the research is still ongoing. A very few families have been identified who possess copies of the ob gene from both parents; their obesity was indeed treatable through the use of leptin (Small and Bloom 2004: 117).

Although leptin was not the answer to weight loss that scientists had hoped, research to locate a gene responsible for fat gain continued. As with leptin, if a hormone could be discovered that reduces body weight, the pharmaceutical industry could potentially manufacture and distribute the hormone as a drug or supplement to aid in weight loss. Two hormones of interest are ghrelin (Small and Bloom 2004), discovered in 1996, and obestatin (Zhang et al. 2005), discovered in 2005. The role of ghrelin in obesity is not fully understood, yet obese individuals tend to have lower levels of this hormone compared with nonobese people. Additionally, people suffering from anorexia nervosa tend to have higher ghrelin levels than people of normal weight (Gale et al. 2004). These two findings have led researchers to believe that ghrelin is an important hormone for controlling appetite. Obestatin decreases the appetite of mice and could possibly do the same in humans (Zhang et al. 2005).

There are also pathological explanations for the inheritance of obesity. There are over forty different complex syndromes listed in the on-line "Mendelian Inheritance in Man" database that include "obesity" as one of their diagnostic criteria. Yet each may well be triggered by different combinations of genes for different reasons (Bray and Allison 2001: 9). The discovery of these and other hormones could provide a scientific basis to treat individuals who have high body fat in the same way that doctors treat high blood pressure or cholesterol (Scharf and Ahima 2004; Orr and Davy 2005). Furthermore, such genetic anomalies could also be detected by genetic screening in analogy to Downs Syndrome and identify high-risk individuals.

SLG/Suzanne Judd

*See also* Anorexia; Friedman; Hormones Used in Dieting

## References and Further Reading

Bray, M.S. and Allison, D.B. (2001) "Obesity Syndromes," in John B. Owen, Janet Treasure, and David A. Collier (eds), *Animal Models: Disorders of Eating Behavior and Body Composition*, Dordrecht: Kluwer, pp. 1–18.

Gale, S.M., Castracane, V.D. and Mantzoros, C.S. (2004) "Energy Homeostasis, Obesity and Eating Disorders: Recent Advances in Endocrinology," *Journal of Nutrition* 134 (2): 295–8.

Kalra, S.P., Bagnasco, M., Otukonyong, E.E., Dube, M.G. and Kalra, P.S. (2003) "Rhythmic, Reciprocal Ghrelin and Leptin Signaling: New Insight in the Development of Obesity," *Regulatory Peptides* 111 (1): 1–11.

Orr, J. and Davy, B. (2005) "Dietary Influences on Peripheral Hormones Regulating Energy Intake: Potential Applications for Weight Management," *Journal of the American Dietetic Association* 105 (7): 1115–24.

Scharf, M.T. and Ahima, R.S. (2004) "Gut Peptides and Other Regulators in Obesity," *Seminars in Liver Disease* 24 (4): 335–47.

Shell, Ellen Ruppel (2001) *The Hungry Gene: The Science of Fat and the Future of Thin*, New York: Atlantic Monthly Press.

Small, C.J. and Bloom, S.R. (2004) "Gut Hormones and the Control of Appetite," *Trends in Endocrinology and Metabolism* 15 (5): 259–63.

Stipanuk, M.H. (2000) *Biochemical and Physiological Aspects of Human Nutrition*, Philadelphia, Pa.: Saunders.

Zhang, J.V., Ren, P.-G., Avsian-Kretchmer, O., Luo, C.-W., Rauch, R., Klein, C. and Hsueh, A. (2005) "Obestatin, a Peptide Encoded by the Ghrelin Gene, Opposes Ghrelin's Effects on Food Intake," *Science* 310 (5750): 996–9.

# Globalization

Though there has been much speculation about the origins of globalization, with some historians arguing that it dates back to the fifteenth century and the spread of European colonialism, there is an understanding that both in terms of scope as well as in terms of historical specificity, globalization is a uniquely "modern" phenomenon. Globalization in the twentieth century, which can be broadly defined as the transnational movement of goods, people, and capital across national borders, boasts characteristics that mark it as peculiarly contemporary. Politically speaking, academics argue that the nation-state is growing increasingly redundant, while economically one has seen a paradigm shift in the realm of production and consumption from Fordism to Post-Fordism, which incorporates technological advances like computers and the internet (Thompson, n.d.). There have been changes in culture and, as mentioned, patterns of consumption that have articulated these larger structural changes. Another change is the feminization of the work force—the appearance of more women in the formal economy—as well as the growing emergence of a white and what is also known as a "pink" collar workforce in developing countries (Freeman 2000; Littlewood 2004). These have led to the burgeoning of a transnational dieting culture accompanied by, according to certain social scientists, a rise in eating disorders.

In May 2004, the Fifty-Fifth World Health Assembly called for the development of "a global strategy on diet, physical activity and health" based on reports such as *Obesity: Preventing and Managing the Global Epidemic* (2001) which argued that the majority of the world's deaths are caused by noncommunicable diseases (NCDs), such as cancer, diabetes mellitus, cardiovascular conditions, and obesity. The reasons behind this phenomenon: "industrialization, urbanization, economic development and increasing food market globalization," which manifest as a lack of well regulated diet and appropriate levels of physical activity (World Health Organization 2001). Dubbed "Globesity" by some, globalization is seen as the key engine powering the unsavory new "pandemic" of worldwide obesity which is considered both a disease in its own right as well as a contributory factor in most NCDs.

An important manifestation of this increased transnationalism is the shared pathologization of fat/overweight in various parts of the world, including among the upper classes in the developing world. There has been a corresponding boom in the weight-loss and weight-control industry, which ranges from "slimming centres" or "obesity clinics" to diet pills and drugs. In India, national centers such as VLCC (Vandhara Luthra Clinics) and regional ones such as La Belle specialize in "passive" and "active" weight loss approaches: Passive refers to the use of "fat redistribution machines" as well as liposuction, while "active" refers to exercise regimens that include yoga, weight training, and cardiovascular training. These clinics also come equipped with nutritionists and dieticians who advise women (and increasingly men) on how to reduce caloric intake and eat more healthily. Dieting could be said to consist of a spectrum of practices whose sole aim is weight loss in order to "look good" (and is indexical of a larger culture of body consciousness). It has manifested itself in many corners of the world, not in the form of fad diets, but in the use of specific weight-loss aids that need to be ingested.

Although most scientists agree that people from diverse backgrounds and classes engage in dieting practices and suffer from eating disorders, dieting and eating disorders, such as anorexia nervosa, are also seen as closely connected to the introduction of First World attitudes toward food consumption and body ideals among the educated middle and upper-middle classes in the Global South. However, scholars have also called for more qualitative research that will better elucidate the local articulations of phenomena that are phenomenologically the same. In one study of the incidence of anorexia nervosa in Hong Kong, the researcher found that though the women studied met all the diagnostic criteria for anorexia nervosa, "fat phobia" wasn't a feature of their condition (Becker 2004).

Globalization has also had a major impact on dieting. Everything from popular fad diets to exercise crazes to fast food have been exported from the U.S.A. to other parts of the world. At the same time, a variety of foods and practices are imported to the U.S.A. from various parts of the world. This is a phenomenon unique to modern times. It has made studying the diets of people around the world a bit more complicated because they are more homogenous than they once were. Since diets today are more similar than they are different, finding dietary factors that lead to diseases is a major challenge. In addition to food, Americans have become more exposed to Eastern medicine and dietary practices. For example, Hatha yoga, an ancient Indian form of exercise, has become very popular in the U.S.A. Although many people focus only on the economic consequences of globalization, it has affected much more than just commerce.

SLG/SHRUTHI VISSA

*See also* Alternative Medicine; Anorexia; Bariatric Surgery; Craig; Fat Camp; Food Choice; Spurlock

**References and Further Reading**

Becker, Anne E. (2004) "New Global Perspectives on Eating Disorders," *Culture, Medicine and Psychiatry* 28 (4): 433–7.
Freeman, C. (2000) *High Tech and High Heels in the*

*Global Economy: Women, Work and Pink-Collar Identities in the Caribbean*, Durham, Md.: Duke University Press.
Littlewood, R. (2004) "Commentary: Globalization, Culture, Body Image, and Eating Disorders," *Culture, Medicine and Psychiatry* 28 (4): 597–602.
Thompson, Fred (n.d.) "Fordism, post-Fordism and the flexible system of production," Willamette University, available online at <http://www.willamette.edu/~fthompso/MgmtCon/Fordism_&_Postfordism.html> (accessed February 18, 2007).
World Health Organization (2001) *Obesity: Preventing and Managing the Global Epidemic*. Report of a WHO consultation: Technical Report Series, No. 894.
—— "Global Strategy on Diet, Physical Activity and Health." Available online at <http://www.who.int/dietphysicalactivity/goals/en/index.html> (accessed February 18, 2007).

# Gold, Tracy (1969–)

Best known for her role as Carol Seaver on the sitcom *Growing Pains* (1985–92), Gold was one of the first child actresses to make a public confession about her battle with anorexia. According to Gold, she was first diagnosed with anorexia at age twelve, and while she recovered rather quickly from this particular bout of the disease, her battle was not over. At age nineteen Gold began another diet in order to attain her "ideal weight" of 113 pounds, but this diet spun out of control, eventually bringing the actress down to 90 pounds. Due to the seriousness of her disease, Gold was forced to take a sabbatical from the show. Gold's subsequent weight "yo-yoed"; at times she seemed to be recuperating and then got much worse. At its lowest, Gold's weight was reported to have dropped to 79 pounds. Eventually, Gold recovered, returned to her acting career, and then went public with a description of her "battle" with anorexia. Since then Gold has traveled widely, speaking to audiences about anorexia and the mental and physical dangers of the disorder. She has made a second career out of "conquering" her "battle" with anorexia.

As one of the first child celebrities to go public with her eating disorder in the age of television, Gold paved the way for future celebrities to do the same. In April 2005, Gold related how coming to terms with her other problems and situations, specifically her arrest for "drunk driving" on September 3, 2004, was similar to the way she came to terms with anorexia. She stated, "I've always been the person who's the people pleaser, the person who tries to make everybody else happy. I've come a long way and I've done a lot of work on myself, and I'm really proud of myself about that. But it's still a part of who I am" (Anon, 2005). All forms of asocial behavior can be explained by claiming a personality rooted in a socially acceptable form of mental illness, such as addiction. By this point, the proof of her claim is her position as a celebrity revealing her anorexia nervosa to the public.

SLG/LAURA GOLDSTEIN

*See also* Anorexia

## References and Further Reading

Anon. (2004) "Actress Warns Against Anorexia," *Arizona Daily Wildcat Campus News*, January 19, available online at <http://www.healthyplace.com/Communities/Eating_Disorders/Site/story_anorexia_warning.htm> (accessed April 30, 2006).

Anon. (2005) "Wake-Up Call," *The Oprah Winfrey Show*, April 4, Harpo Productions, details online at <http://www.oprah.com/tows/slide/200504/20050411/slide_20050411_101.jhtml> (accessed April 30, 2006).

# Graham, Sylvester (1794–1851)

## Presbyterian minister, social reformer, and early advocate of dietary reform in America

Graham was chronically ill as a young man, diagnosed with "consumption" (tuberculosis), which interrupted his studies at Amherst College. After one of his illnesses, he married his nurse. As a preacher, he was an advocate of the "temperance" movement. In 1830, while preaching in Pennsylvania against the dangers of drink, he met members of the Vegetarian Bible Christian Church and thereafter became an advocate of vegetarianism. After 1839, he withdrew from his public activities to devote himself to developing his system. Like many reformers of his day, Graham associated capitalism with moral decay (Nissenbaum 1980: 48). Responding in part to the advent of preprepared foods, Graham wrote his famous *Treatise on Bread and Bread-Making* (1837), in which he urged readers to make quality bread at home and eat it fresh. His Graham bread was made primarily with wholewheat and molasses, as opposed to white flour, and it contained neither yeast nor eggs. The ideal food came to be bread. It was plain, unadorned, and true to itself. As Catharine Beecher was to write a decade later of "Nourishing and Unstimulating Food,"

> wheat stands at the head, as the most nutritive, safe, and acceptable diet to all classes and in all circumstances. This can be used in the form of bread, every day, through a whole life, without cloying the appetite, and to an extent which can be said of no other food.
>
> (Beecher 1846: 234)

With food, American culture enters into what Amy Kaplan identifies as the "paradox of . . . imperial domesticity"

in which the work of the home "becomes the engine of national expansion" (Kaplan 1998).

Graham was also a staunch advocate of vegetarianism and apparently the first American to link a philosophy of vegetarianism to a physiological argument about health (Harris 1990). Others of his time shared his belief that to kill animals was barbaric and that a vegetarian diet reinforced better elements of human nature, but for Graham it was also medicalized, as he believed vegetarian diets led to longer life.

Graham's advocacy of a pure diet was very much linked to sexual reform. In his 1834 *Lecture to Young Men on Chastity* his motto is "beware the fleshly lusts, which war against the soul." Human beings, he notes, have "two grand functions . . . that are necessary for his existence . . . The first is NUTRITION; the second is REPRODUCTION" (Graham 1837a: 29). He condemns "self-pollution" as more dangerous even than the "illicit commerce between the sexes" (Graham 1837a: 16) as it "ruins the physical constitution" (1837a: 40). Sex should be treated as he imagines food must be: "when we eat and drink for the purpose of sustaining our bodies in the best condition with the ulterior view of promoting the healthiest and most vigorous state of our intellectual faculties" rather than merely "pandering to our appetites" (Graham 1837a: 60). It is the stomach that "more directly and powerfully fully sympathizes with the genital organs, in all their excitement and affections, than any other organ or portion of the body" (Graham 1837a: 92). Bread and pure foods would cure the ravages of masturbation as well as dampen sexual excess. His eccentric diet prohibited consumption not only of meat, but also of tea, alcohol, spices, and sweets because of their intensifying effects on the sexual drives of men, women, and children alike (Nissenbaum 1980: 34). For Graham, diet was essential. Without dietary reform, no reform or rehabilitation was possible.

In his *Lectures on the Science of Human Life* (1839), Graham argued for a divine self-awareness of man that led him to first eat of the fruits surrounding him. He rejects the argument of the scientists of his day, such as Georges-Louis Leclerc, Comte de Buffon (1707–88), that man is an omnivorous animal. For Graham, the very anatomy of the human being predisposes him to eating fruits and vegetables. Man is an herbivorous animal, whose teeth and digestive system are predisposed not to eat meat. He rejects, therefore, the common notion of the day that "animal food renders man strong and courageous" while vegetable diet "is . . . connected with weakness and cowardice" (Graham 1897: 115). The best of human society in history subsisted on vegetables and fruits—from the Spartans to the Romans—while "Natural Man," such as those humans ranked as on the lowest rung of humanity of the day, the inhabitants of Tierra del Fuego in Argentina, eat 15 to 20 pounds of barely cooked flesh a day which leads to their "indolence" (Graham 1897: 150). Modern man must be healthy and be able to work; this is possible only through a meatless diet.

SLG/ANGELA WILLEY

*See also* Beecher; Cornaro; Natural Man; Vegetarianism

## References and Further Reading

Beecher, Catharine (1846) *Miss Beecher's Domestic Receipt Book Designed As a Supplement to the Treatise on Domestic Economy*, New York: Harper.

Graham, Sylvester (1837a) *Lecture to Young Men on Chastity*, 2nd edn, Boston, Mass.: Light & Stearns.

—— (1837b) *A Treatise on Bread, and Bread-making*, Boston: Light & Stearns.

—— (1839) *Lectures on the Science of Human Life*, Boston: Marsh, Capen, Lyon & Webb.

—— (1897) *The Physiology of Feeding, Consisting of the Three Lectures on Diet from "the Science of Human Life,"* London: Ideal Publishing Union.

Harris, Neil (1990) *Cultural Excursions: Marketing Appetites and Cultural Tastes in America*, Chicago, Ill.: University of Chicago Press.

Kaplan, Amy (1998) "Manifest Domesticity," *American Literature* 70 (3): 581–606.

Nissenbaum, Stephen (1980) *Sex, Diet, and Debility in Jacksonian America: Sylvester Graham and Health Reform*, Westport, Conn.: Greenwood Press.

Roe, D.A. (1986) "History of Promotion of Vegetable Cereal Diets," *Journal of Nutrition* 116 (7): 1355–63.

Schwartz, Hillel (1986) *Never Satisfied: A Cultural History of Diets, Fantasies, and Fat*, New York: Free Press.

Shryock, Richard H. (1931) "Sylvester Graham and the Popular Health Movement, 1830–1870," *Mississippi Valley Historical Review* 18 (2): 172–83.

# Greek Medicine and Dieting

In ancient Greek medicine, as the Hippocratic author of *On Ancient Medicine* famously claimed, it is physicians and not philosophers who understand best the nature of man. In ancient Greece, fat as a pathological category appears in texts ascribed to Hippocrates (440–340 BCE). Hippocrates, or at least as attributed to him in the approximately sixty texts of the Hippocratic corpus, based his notion of health and illness on the balance of the humors, the *chymoi*. According to this view, these four crucial bodily fluids—blood, yellow bile, black bile and phlegm—were found in all individuals and produced health when in balance and illness when one dominated over the others. They also produced the visible aspects of the body that could be measured by the physician: Blood made the body hot and wet, choler hot and dry, black bile cold and dry and phlegm cold and wet. They were also correlated to the four ages of man—infancy, youth, adulthood, and old age—and to the essential aspects of the world, air, fire, earth, and water. The physician could impact the domination of one or the other humors by intervening, often with lifestyle or regimen changes, which entailed changing the food or activities of the patient. But the humors were also the key to bodily shape and physique. Thus, if one had a natural predisposition to phlegm, it resulted in fat. Each humor also determined temperament: The phlegmatic person (who was also fat) was pale, lazy, inert, and cool in character—as well as, of course, phlegmatic. Phlegm was "naturally" of water and of old age.

In humoral theory, fat could either be a sign of indisposition with the domination of phlegm to be treated by hot and dry foods or a constitutional status (as in aging) in which one's phlegmatic nature could be mitigated but not altered. In the first case, one was a fat patient but not in the latter. Greek medicine was rooted in the practice of *diatetica*, the diet as the primary therapy or, to use a more modern phrase, "eating as healing." The Greek physicians therefore also believed that there was a one-to-one relationship between foods and their effects. Dionysus of Carystus (in Euboea), who practiced in the fourth century BCE and was known to the Athenians as the "younger Hippocrates," argued like Hippocrates for a completely causal relationship in dietetics (van der Eijk 2000: 246–9). Certain foods were not only healthful but also curative; just as a surfeit of others was the cause of illness, and central among those illnesses was obesity.

For the followers of Hippocrates, fat and thin could be either "natural" antitheses or signs of illness in terms of the balance and unbalance of the humors. Thus, fat reflects the pathological state of the body caused by imbalance. For the sufferer from fat as a sign of disease, there is also a clear distinction between fat men and fat women: "When unnaturally fat women cannot conceive, it is because the fat presses the mouth of the womb, and conception is impossible until they grow thinner" (Jones 1931: V, XLVI). But men "who are constitutionally very fat are more apt to die quickly than those who are thin" (Jones 1931: II, XLIV), abandoning their families and their role in society, both paramount responsibilities in the ancient world. In all cases, extreme fat falls in the realm of medicine: "Repletion too, carried to extremes, is perilous," he observes (Jones 1931: I, IV). Hippocrates does acknowledge that corpulence gave one a slight advantage against febrile diseases, but it was greatly outweighed by the pathological effects. The cure was eating after "exercise and while still panting from fatigue

and with no other refreshment before meals except wine, diluted and slightly cold. They should, moreover, eat only once a day and take no baths and sleep on a hard bed and walk naked as long as possible" (Shell 2001: 25). Quite literally a Spartan regime, as this was the way that the Spartan society deemed its citizens to act!

Greek medicine, in seeing the dominance of phlegm as pathology, also evolved the concept of *polysarkia*, too much flesh. This is a term reintroduced into Roman medicine by the North African Caelius Aurelianus in the fifth century CE in his *De morbis acutis et chronicis*. Polysarkia was the result of the imbalance of the humors but also a quality of temperament. Thus the lazy, phlegmatic person also consumes too much food. They live in a concomitant state of slothfulness and stupidity (Orth 1960). Such people violated the principle of constraint in all things. Constraint, Socrates frequently reminded his listeners, is the greatest good and in complex ways the obese male violates this dictum (Fox 1998).

The line that the Hippocratic corpus assumes between acceptable fat and excessive fat (extreme repletion) is the difference between life and death. In Aristotle's essay on longevity, fat is the quality that preserves warmth. Animals (including human beings) are "naturally moist and warm, and life too is of this nature, whereas old age is cold and dry, and so is a dead body" (Aristotle 1936: 403). He continues: "Fatty things are not liable to decay because they contain air . . . air like fire does not become corrupt" (Aristotle 1936: 403). Animals which are "bloodless" are protected by their fat: "In animals the fat is sweet; for this reason, bees are longer lived than other larger animals" (Aristotle 1936: 407). Here too the line is assumed between acceptable "fatness" and pathological obesity.

Strength, health, and beauty are the "virtues" of the classical Greek body. It is no accident that one of the most important commentators on diet of the ancient world was Herodicus of Selymbria, a trainer of athletes, who used gymnastics to cure his own fat body (Jaeger 1944: 3 and 34). Hippocrates had stressed that

in athletes a perfect condition that is at its highest pitch is treacherous. Such conditions cannot remain the same or be at rest, and, change for the better being impossible; the only possible change is for the worse. For this reason it is an advantage to reduce the fine embonpoint quickly, in order that the body may make a fresh beginning of growth.

(Jones 1931: I, III)

Here it is the professional *athletae*, who competed in the games, rather than the *agonistae*—those who sought health and strength through gymnastics—who need to be thin. And that cure for the fat body was diet and exercise.

SLG

*See also* Roman Medicine and Dieting; Sports

**References and Further Reading**

Aristotle (1936) "Aristotle: on Length and Shortness of Life," in W.S. Hett (trans.) *Aristotle: Volume VIII. On the Soul. Parva Naturalia. On Breath*, Cambridge, Mass.: Harvard University Press.

Fox, Matthew (1998) "The Constrained Man," in Lin Foxhall and John Salmon (eds), *Thinking Men: Masculinity and Its Self-Representation in the Classical Tradition*, Routledge: London and New York, pp. 6–22.

Grottanelli, Cristiano and Milano, Lucio, eds. (2004) "Food and Identity in the Ancient World," *History of the Ancient Near East Studies* 9. Padova: S.A.R.G.O.N. editrice e libreria.

Jones, W.H.S. (trans. and ed.) (1931) "Hippocrates. Aphorisms," *Nature of Man. Regimen in Health. Humours. Aphorisms. Regimen 1–3. Dreams. Heracleitus. On the Universe*, Vol. IV of *Hippocrates*. Cambridge, Mass.: Harvard University Press, pp. 97–222.

Jaeger, Werner (1944) *Paideia: The Ideals of Greek Culture*, 3 vols, trans. Gilbert Highet, New York: Oxford University Press.

Orth, H. (1960) "Die Behandlung der Fettleibigkeit in der griechisch-römische Antike," *Medizinischer Monatsspiegel* 9: 193–8.

Shell, Ellen Ruppel (2001) *The Hungry Gene: The Science of Fat and the Future of Thin*, New York: Atlantic Monthly Press.

van der Eijk, Philip J. (2000) *Diocles of Carystus: A Collection of the Fragments with Translation and Commentary*, Vol. I, Leiden and Boston, Mass.: Brill.

# Grunberger, George, MD

## Founder of a private practice called the Grunberger Diabetes Institute in Bloomfield Hills, Michigan

The Grunberger Diabetes Institute is a place where diabetes patients can receive quality care. Grunberger has also worked at the National Institutes of Health, Wayne State University, and the Detroit Medical Center.

Grunberger is one of the most vocal specialists in diabetes in the U.S.A. Working mainly with adults who have diabetes due to obesity, recently he has commented on the increasing number of adolescents who have diabetes also due to weight. His research is mostly focused on diabetes and its complications, and ranges from the function of insulin to studies on diabetes and how to manage it. His work also reflects the need for a nuanced approach to different ethic groups, such as African-Americans, because of their cultural location. Grunberger is a voice arguing that diabetes in children is increasing at an alarming rate, and he believes this increase is directly linked to obesity. He argues that parents need to start teaching their children to eat more healthily and take on more physical activity. In addition, he stresses the role of society in taking on this issue of obesity by teaching its members to eat better and exercise more frequently.

In 2005, Grunberger became the public advocate for a "quick" cure for obesity and, therefore, for the illnesses associated with it. He championed "FBCx," touted as "an all natural dietary fiber," from ArtJen Complexus Holdings Corp. in Windsor, Ontario, Canada that, to quote the publicity, "has the unique ability to complex and remove nine times its own weight in dietary fat with no side effects. Without changing their diet or lifestyle patients are removing 500 kcal per day from their diets and losing 1–1½ pounds per week." FBCx was developed at Wayne State University by two of Grunberger's colleagues. Grunberger conducted the first clinical studies on FBCx and in June 2005 presented his results at the American Diabetes Association annual meeting in San Diego. Joseph Artiss, one of the two inventors, said of his invention, "It's a Fat Binding Complexer, so we called it FBCx. FBCx appears to have effects on some hormones so that while you absorb fewer calories you still have the feeling of fullness or satiety" (PRWeb).

FBCx is the "newest" addition to the "natural food" cure for obesity and all of its attendant ills. It is the ultimate quick fix, parallel to Proctor and Gamble's introduction of "olestra" in 1996. The calorie-free "fat" flopped to no little extent because of the FDA label affixed to any product that used it: "Olestra may cause abdominal cramping and loose stools. Olestra inhibits the absorption of some vitamins and other nutrients." The experience of "anal leakage" was sufficient to cramp this product's general use as a weight-reduction method. Parallel to this was the introduction of Xenical in 1999. It causes about a third of the fat in foods consumed to pass through the digestive system unprocessed, with results similar to Olestra (Shell 2001: 142). Grunberger now argues that FBCx is a positive means to control weight and, therefore, to prevent Type 2 Diabetes.

SLG/MARY STANDEN

*See also* Kellogg

### References and Further Reading

Daniel, Kaniqua S. (2005) "Experts Say Childhood Obesity Not a Disease: It's an Epidemic." Available online at <http://www.theoaklandpress.com/stories/032705/loc_20050327025.shtml> (accessed April 11, 2006).

Fitzgerald, J.T., Anderson, R.M., Funnell, M.M., Arnold, M.S., Davis, W.K., Aman, L.C., Jacober, S.J. and Grunberger, G. (1997) "Differences in the Impact of Dietary Restrictions on African Americans and Caucasians with NIDDM," *Diabetes Educator* 23 (1): 41–7.

Fitzgerald, J.T., Anderson, R.M., Gruppen, L.D., Davis, W.K., Aman, L.C., Jacober, S.J. and Grunberger, G. (1998) "The Reliability of the Diabetes Care Profile for African Americans," *Evaluation and Health Profession* 21 (1): 52–65.

Grunberger Diabetes Institute (2006) "Our Team." Available online at <http://www.gdi-pc.com/dr_g.html> (accessed April 2, 2006).

Mayfield, Jennifer, and Havas, Stephen (2004) "Self-Control: A Physician's Guide to Blood Glucose Monitoring in the Management of Diabetes." Available online at <http://www.aafp.org/online/etc/medialib/aafp_org/documents/news_pubs/mono/afp/smbg.Par.0001.File.tmp/smbgmonograph.pdf> (accessed May 1, 2006).

PRWeb (2005) "Grunberger Diabetes Institute Introduces New Weapon in the War on Obesity," Press Release Newswire, October 4, available online at <http://www.prweb.com/releases/2005/10/prweb292738.htm> (accessed February 21, 2007).

Shell, Ellen Ruppel (2001) *The Hungry Gene: The Science of Fat and the Future of Thin*, New York, Atlantic Monthly Press.

# Gull, Sir William Withy (1816–90)

## Known for naming the disease anorexia nervosa in 1874

Many credit Gull with the discovery of the disorder, which he described as "emaciation as a result of severe emotional disturbance" and "a perversion of the ego." His article entitled "Anorexia Nervosa (Apepsia Hysterica, Anorexia Hysterica)" was published in the *Trans-actions of the Clinical Society of London* in 1874 and was based on a speech he gave at Oxford in 1868 (Gull 1896: 205–14). The formulation "anorexia nervosa," however, first appears in his 1874 essay. It is clear that there was a complex history of the disease that reached back to the seventeenth century. Gull's contemporaries, many of whom he acknowledged, also sharpened the diagnosis in the nineteenth century. The French neuropsychiatrist Charles Lasègue (1816–83) developed a diagnostic category very similar to that of Gull at the same time and is often acknowledged as one of the creators of anorexia (Vandereycken and van Deth 1989). Both built on older discussions of the pathologies of eating.

Gull's description was among the first to acknowledge the psychological factors involved in anorexia nervosa, although it focused on the physical symptoms (Madden 2004: 150). In fact, he was praised for "his powers of discernment, especially in distinguishing real disease from the troubles of nervous and hysterical people" (Anon. "Obituary: Sir William Gull" 1890: 261–2). Gull identified reduced food intake and hyperactivity as risk factors for anorexia nervosa, which are still among the current definitions of the disorder. He described patients as refusing to be treated and with such physical features as loss of menstrual period, decreased pulse, breathing and temperature, and binge-eating. Further, he found most patients to be female between the ages of sixteen and twenty-three. Unlike his peers, he viewed anorexia as a disease of the mind and not of the gastrointestinal system even, as he wrote, though "in the stage of greatest emaciation one might have been pardoned for assuming that there was some organic lesion" (Gull 1896: 307). Gull's recommendation for treatment was to administer food without "allowing the starvation-process to go on" (Gull 1896: 307). His paper presented two case studies, accompanied by "before and after" images. At the end of his life he presented one further case study of anorexia, again accompanied by "before and after" images proving that the return to a healthy state of mind from the "perversions of the 'ego' being the cause and determining the course of the malady" could literally be seen on the patient (Gull 1896: 311–14).

In addition to his role in defining anorexia nervosa, Gull also studied other diseases that impacted on bodily appearance such as the marked physiognomy and mental deficiency of hypothyroidism, known as "Gull's disease" (a term also applied by physicians in the early twentieth century to anorexia). He is credited with identifying the association between myxoedema and thyroid atrophy;

although Gull credited Dr. Hilton Fagge with this discovery. Gull was named a baronet after treating the Prince of Wales's (later Edward VII) typhoid. He was also the physician to Queen Victoria and, consequently, was one of many physicians of the time suspected to be "Jack the Ripper" because of the seemingly "medical" mutilation of "Jack's" victims.

His philosophy included the minimal use of drugs in treatment, focusing on diagnostics rather than disease and looking at large numbers of patients to identify health problems.

SLG/Dorothy Chyung

*See also* Anorexia; Binge-eating; Morton; Murray

## References and Further Reading

Anon. (1890) "Obituary: Sir William Withy Gull," *Lancet* 1: 324–26.

Anon. (1890) "Obituary: Sir William Gull," *British Medical Journal* 1: 256–63.

Bergh, Cecilia and Per Sodersten (1998) "Anorexia Nervosa: Rediscovery of a Disorder," *Lancet* 351 (9113) (May 9): 1427–9.

Enersen, O.D. (2002) "Sir William Withy Gull. Who Named It?" available online at <http://www.whonamedit.com/doctor.cfm/85.html> (accessed February 19, 2006).

Gull, William Withey (1896) *A Collection of the Published Writings of William Withey Gull*, Vol. II, London: New Sydenham Society.

Herman, Joseph (1999) "Setting the Record Straight: An Episode in the Life of Sir William Withy Gull," *Perspectives in Biology and Medicine* 42 (4): 507–11.

Madden, Sloane (2004) " 'Anorexia Nervosa': Still Relevant in the Twenty-First Century? A Review of William Gull's Anorexia Nervosa," *Clinical Child Psychology and Psychiatry* 9 (1): 149–54.

Silver, Anna Krugovoy (2002) *Victorian Literature and the Anorexic Body*, Cambridge: Cambridge University Press.

Vandereycken, Walter and van Deth, Ron (1989) "Who Was the First to Describe Anorexia Nervosa: Gull or Lesègue?" *Psychological Medicine* 19: 837–45.

# H

## Hauser, Bengamin Gayelord (1895–1984)

### Popular advocate of diet and nutrition

Born Helmut Eugene Benjamin Gellert Hauser in Germany, he was also known as Eugene Helmuth Hauser and legally changed his name in 1923. Described as a "youngish man with a flashy smile and a broken accent" (Anon. "Garbo's Gayelord," 1942) and a "handsome man who wears his hair in a permanent wave" (Fishbein 1938: 113), "Dr. Hauser" studied naturopathy and chiropractic medicine but dropped his claim to have an MD following an investigation by the American Medical Association. Hauser said that at the age of sixteen, after all his American doctors failed him, two weeks of lemon juice recommended by a foreign doctor cured him of tuberculosis of the hip.

Hauser's diets sought to cure both physical and psychological ailments, change body weight, and promote longevity. He argued very early that "health is nature, and disease is unnatural" and "no disease can exist in a chemicalized blood stream" (Hauser 1930: 33). Self-cure with foodstuffs, he claimed, especially acidic ones will eliminate "sickness and old age" (Hauser 1930: 38). Hauser's proof of this is the prison and orphanage studies undertaken by Dr. Joseph Goldberger in 1914, which determined that pellagra was a disease of poor diet rather than an infectious disease. Able to draw on the "real" science of vitamin deficiency diseases by the 1930s, Hauser cloaked his vegetarian diets in the model of the Goldberger study (Hauser 1934: 6–7).

Hauser's diets included "eliminative feeding system," "the mending diet," "the vitality diet," "the transition diet," "the cosmetic diet," and "the zigzag diet." "The cosmetic diet" recommended sulfur-rich foods and an iron-rich cocktail of spinach, parsley, and citrus juice for beautiful skin. The "zigzag diet" for weight loss involved a purge of Epsom salt in the morning and senna at night. He was a strong advocate of fortifying meals with "natural ingredients," such as dry brewer's yeast, wheat germ, yogurt, powdered skim milk, honey, blackstrap molasses, vegetable salt, vitamins, and minerals. The mass popularity of Hauser's "cures" was such that they became part of the routine of stand-up comics of the day. The great vaudeville and television comic Jimmy Durante joked that blackstrap molasses doesn't really make you live longer, it just seems longer.

Hauser developed a line of branded foods and supplements supporting his diets, which included products like Santay-Swiss, Anti-Diabetic Tea, and Nutro-Links. He also owned a restaurant in St. Petersburg, Florida, which featured his diet products on the menu. He encouraged his followers to open similar restaurants and sell his products. Virtually all of his books published in Great Britain suggest the consumption of foods available "direct from the manufacturers, Rational Diet Products, Chantry House, Grimsby" (Hauser 1939: 43). Three of his products, Slim, Correcol, and Hauser Potassium Broth, were seized by the FDA for fraudulent claims that violated the Pure Food and Drug Act.

Gayelord Hauser's advertising strategy largely relied on his personal image; that is, his physical attractiveness and glamorous social life added to his mass appeal, as did having media celebrity followers such as Cary Grant, Mae West, and Greta Garbo, whom he personally advised. As one critic commented recently about Hauser's importance in changing Hollywood's body image: "Hefty bodies and substantial meat-and-potatoes meals epitomized wealth and station—until the wraithlike Garbo slid narrowly on screen, and, off screen, ate salads and juices with her health-food guru lover, Gaylord Hauser" (Morrison 2006).

SLG/DOROTHY CHYUNG

*See also* Celebrities

### References and Further Reading

Anon. (1942) "Garbo's Gayelord," *Time Archive*, February 16, available online at <http://www.time.com/time/archive/printout/0,23657,766416,00.html> (accessed March 26, 2006).

Davies, Jill (1994) "Fad Diets: Health Implications," *Nutrition and Food Science* 94 (5): 22–4.

Fishbein, M. (1938) "Modern Medical Charlatans," *Hygeia* 16 (February): 113–14.

Hauser, Bengamin Gayelord (1930) *Food Science and Health*, New York: Tempo.

—— (1934) *Here's How to Be Healthy*, New York: Tempo.

—— (1939) *Eat and Grow Beautiful*, London: Faber and Faber.

—— (1950) *Look Younger, Live Longer*, New York: Farrar, Straus & Company.

Morrison, Patt (2006) "125 Years/Hollywood: The Pictures-Perfect City," *Los Angeles Times*, May 21: S3.

Spencer, M. (1990) "A Run-in with the Elusive Garbo Provides the Perfect Party Topic," *Los Angeles Times*, April 17: 5.

---

# Hay, William Howard, MD (1866–1940)

## Creator of the Hay Diet in 1911, the original inspiration for "food combining"

Hay's approach was based on the idea that eating certain foods together will yield improved digestion and that certain foods are simply "incompatible" with one another. He categorized foods as protein, neutral, or starch and urged people to eat proteins and starches separately, although neutral foods could be eaten with either group. Hay believed that, according to the "immutable laws of chemistry," mixing the food groups led to incomplete digestion, which would then lead to the accumulation of toxins (for which a daily enema was also recommended) and weight gain. Digestion would be affected because the action of ptyalin and pepsin would be stopped and because the environments for digestion differed (alkaline environment for starch and an acidic one for protein). Hay also advocated eating more vegetables and fruits instead of carbohydrates and proteins, believing that these acid-forming foods led to a chemical imbalance caused by decreasing alkaline reserves in the body.

Critics of the diet pointed to the fact that many naturally occurring foods already combined starches and protein and that the diet actually encouraged weight loss only by encouraging calorie reduction. To date, no scientific evidence has proven the theory of food combining; however, Hay's approach was very much in line with the general notion of food as a means of purifying the body. Like his contemporaries, he saw this purification as a return to the "natural" as well as a rejection of the mechanistic nature of contemporary life. His was, in this sense, a very American approach to food, "for we are becoming a nation of vegetable and fruit-eaters, while the Englishman is still content with his gooey puddings and his afternoon starchy teas" (Hay 1933: 34). This shift in diet was necessary for America to become great as many Americans are suffering from an "individual and national fatigue," which is "making us a near second class nation" (Hay 1933: 65). As "the causes of fatigue are the cause of disease," a new diet will eliminate much illness and increase longevity and productivity (Hay 1933: 69). Indeed, all death can be attributed to bad diet, "there is no natural death; all deaths are the end-point of acid accumulation" (Hay 1933: 71).

In his interest to improve national health and decrease mortality, Hay became more interested in natural medicine. He resolved, "to take such things as he believed were intended by nature as foods for men" after he cured himself of Bright's disease (now known as nephritis, or kidney disease) (Hay 1933: 13). He also lost weight by changing his diet, and "at the end of three months he was able to run long distances without distress. His weight decreased from 225 lbs. to 175 lbs; years seem to fall away from him, and he felt younger and stronger than before for many years" (Hay 1934: 14). He accomplished this all by eating foods in their natural, unprocessed state and not eating to excess: "Proportion the amounts to the real desire at the time; do not try to eat the whole because it is offered; a mistake that is often made by those following suggested diets" (Hay 1934: 158). In addition, he believed that exercise is needed "to keep us clean inside, and to enjoy all these periods as only one can do who is giving to each his due need" (Hay 1934: 174). He documented his belief in the necessity of exercise in widely popular publications, including *Health via Food* (1929) and *A New Health Era* (1933). In *Health via Food*, Hay picked up a thread of argument that has its roots in the very earliest reaches of Western dieting. Based on the experiences of World War I, he saw poor diet as the reason that "half of these young men [called to duty] . . . were unfit to serve her in an emergency." They had "poor teeth, poor eyesight, weak arches . . . deficient chest expansion . . . things that make a man unfit to . . . stand the rigors of a campaign" (Hay 1934: 20). Unhealthy young men were thus poor citizens and rather poorer examples of what "real men" should be, but he was also concerned about the poor health of women, who bear listless children and nurture them poorly as they themselves are deficient (Hay 1934: 62). His argument about the causes of poor health and high mortality was not those of the classic prohibitionists against "tobacco, whiskey, tea, coffee . . . [or] jazzy parties." Instead, he focused on poor nutrition and argued that the "compatibility" of foods will revive America and make for stronger men and women, each to fulfill their own role in a healthy society (Hay 1934: 25).

Hay pursued his diet through professional organizations and activities. He was a member of the American Association for Medico-Physical Research, and merchan-

dized his system when in 1927 he became director of the Sun-Diet Health Foundation (he would later become its president). After purchasing the Pocono Hay-ven resort in 1932, he became the Medical Director of Hay System, Inc. in 1935. As a result, the Hay diet was popular in the early 1930s, with Hay-friendly menus at many restaurants and followers of the system, including Henry Ford, who called themselves "Hayites."

Since then, there have been regular revivals in the Hay diet, resulting in publications by others about their advice and experiences regarding food combining. For example, the acid base diet, which claims to restore body chemistry to proper balance, is very similar to Hay's original diet. In addition, actors Koo Stark, Helen Mirren, Liz Hurley, Catherine Zeta-Jones, and Sir John Mills; television personality Jill Dando; and Princess Diana have all supported food-combining diets.

SLG/DOROTHY CHYUNG

*See also* Celebrities; Detoxification; Diana; Kellogg

## References and Further Reading

Anon. (2005) "Pioneers of the North American Natural Health Movement," Alive.com, available online at <http://www.alive.com/2541a8a2.php> (accessed February 19, 2006).

Anon. "What is the Hay Diet?" Vitamin U.K., available online at <http://www.vitaminuk.com/pages/articles/whatisthehaydiet.htm#WhatistheHayDiet> (accessed February 19, 2006).

Bailey, Eleanor (1998) "Have These Dieters Got Their Combinations in a Twist?" *Independent On Sunday*, January 11.

Fishbein, M. (1938) "Modern Medical Charlatans," *Hygeia* 16 (February): 113–14.

Hay, William Howard (1929) *Heath via food*, East Aurora, NY: Sun-Diet.

—— (1933) *A New Health Era*, New York: Hay System.

Jackson, Donald Dale (1994) "The Art of Wishful Shrinking Has Made a Lot of People Rich," *Smithsonian* 25 (8): 146.

McKeith, Gillian (2006) "Six 21st-Century Diets and What They Claim to Do," *The Independent*, February 9.

Thomson, Peter "Why Science and Medicine Support Food Combining: History of Food Combining." Available online at <http://www.peter-thomson.co.uk/

foodc/_why_science_and_medicine_support_food_combining.html> (accessed February 20, 2006).

Wolberg, Lewis Robert (1938) "Hay Food Fantasy," *Hygeia* 16 (April): 311–13 and 372.

# Homeostasis

Biological systems like the human body are designed to operate in harmony with the environment in which they live. The body is also designed to operate under very specific conditions; for example, body temperature is maintained at approximately 98.6 degrees Fahrenheit, and the heart rate is generally maintained around 70 beats per minute (Widmaier 2006: 408). These conditions or set points allow optimal function within the body. When something in the environment changes, the body has to make changes to bring itself back or near to that set point. The process of bringing the body back to its original set point is homeostasis. For example, when a person exercises, the muscles of the body require more oxygen. In order to maintain a steady stream of oxygen to the muscles, the heart rate will increase so that more blood, which contains oxygen, is delivered to the muscles.

In terms of diet, the human body is good at preserving energy from food so that periods of starvation do not end life (Stipanuk 2000: 385–407). When a person restricts food intake, as is the case when one is dieting, the body will adjust to the decreased intake in food by slowing down metabolism in order to maintain homeostasis. If the body cannot meet energy requirements by simply reducing metabolic rate, it will then pull energy from the fat and muscle within the body in order to maintain energy to all organs. Homeostasis is therefore widely studied in reference to diet. In fact, some people who have published dieting literature have created diets that claim to change metabolic set point so that as the body finds homeostasis, it will actually be burning greater amounts of fat and thus will change the shape.

SLG/SUZANNE JUDD

*See also* Atkins; Metabolism; Sugar Busters; Zone Diet

### References and Further Reading

Stipanuk, M.H. (2000) *Biochemical and Physiological Aspects of Human Nutrition*, Philadelphia, Pa.: Saunders.
Widmaier, E.P. (2006) *Vander's Human Physiology: the Mechanisms of Body Function*, New York: McGraw-Hill.

# Hopkins, Sir Frederick Gowland (1861–1947)

## Considered the founder of British biochemistry

Born in Sussex, England, as a child, Hopkins showed an exclusive interest in science, in particular chemistry, which continued for the rest of his life. Hopkins became the first Professor of Biochemistry at Cambridge in 1914. He pioneered the study and application of what he termed accessory food factors, which are now referred to as vitamins. In addition to his work on vitamins, Hopkins also pioneered the study of cell metabolism. One of his earliest contributions to biochemistry was the technique he used to detect the presence of uric acid in urine. He also studied the role of amino acids arginine and histidine in nutrition. This discovery showed him that it is the presence of differing amino acids, which creates the nutritional quality of proteins.

Through further experimentation with rats, Hopkins realized that accessory food factors (vitamins) were also playing a role in nutrition and growth. After isolating specific vitamins, Hopkins concluded that such diseases as rachitis, or rickets, and scurvy, occurred when food lacked certain vitamins. In 1912, Hopkins published, "Feeding Experiments Illustrating the Importance of Accessory Food Factors in Normal Dietaries," which is generally regarded as the most important piece of early literature on vitamins. Hopkins' nutritional theories were contested by colleagues until 1920, but since then have been considered indisputable. During the 1920s, Hopkins experimented with biological oxidations, finding the first clues that intermediate oxygen transportation possibly occurs in living tissues. At the time, the theory was new and queried, but today it is a well-established fundamental fact in the field of biological oxidation. In 1929, Hopkins won the Nobel Prize for Medicine and Physiology for his work in nutrition, which set the stage for those who followed him in nutritional science.

In particular, his 1932 Gluckstein Lecture on "Chemistry and Life" presented a scientific approach to the biochemistry of "living systems [that] should sometimes occupy the thought of every chemist" (Hopkins 1933: 3). This view, based on Hopkins' understanding of the complexity of nature, placed living organisms again into the realm of biochemistry, which had, by the 1930s, begun to see itself as concerned with the molecular level and as a science separate from any explanation of how actual systems work in living organisms. This return to the world of origin of biochemistry in the laboratories of Justus von Liebig (1803–73) meant a focus on processes such as metabolism in plants and animals (Hopkins 1933: 5). Liebig had begun with an understanding of how such processes were carried out, and Hopkins wished to return to this earlier model. Diet, the "intensive studies of plant and animal products," meant a return to the science that created the modern concern with diet. We now "know that the consumption of so much protein, fat and carbohydrate lead to the excretion of so much urea and so much carbon dioxide." But this tells us "nothing of that succession of complex events intervening between consumption and excretion, which it is the business of the biochemist to understand" (Hopkins 1933: 5). This, he pointed out in 1932, is the goal of biochemistry looking at the "intact and living body" (Hopkins 1933: 6).

SLG/LAURA K. GOLDSTEIN

*See also* Metabolism

### References and Further Reading

Anon. (1998) "Frederick Gowland Hopkins, Sir," in Paula K. Byers (ed.), *Encyclopedia of World Biography*, 2nd edn, seventeen volumes, Detroit, Mich.: Thompson Gale. Available online at <http://www.everything2.com/index.pl?node_id=1529200> (accessed June 23, 2007).

Hopkins, Frederick Gowland (1933) "Chemistry and Life," Gluckstein Memorial Lecture, 4, London: Institute of Chemistry.

Lerner, Lee and Lerner, Brenda Wilmoth (2002) "Frederick Gowland Hopkins," *World of Anatomy and Physiology*, two vols, Detroit, Mich.: Gale Group. Available online at <http://www.bookrags.com/browse/World%20of%20Anatomy%20and-%20Physiology> (accessed June 23, 2007).

# Hormone

A hormone is a signaling compound or molecule in the body that enables one part of the body to communicate with another part of the body. The term itself appears in the scientific literature in the opening decade of the twentieth century. In 1905, E.H. Starling, writing in the British medical journal the *Lancet* notes that "these chemical messengers [are] 'hormones' . . . as we might call them" (Starling 1905: 340). Hormones are produced by the endocrine system in organs like the thyroid and adrenal glands (Harvey 2005: 92–3). In terms of metabolism, some functions performed by hormones are to signal to the stomach when enough food has been consumed and to increase fat storage in times of calorie excess. However, hormones have many functions that go far beyond those required for metabolism.

SLG/Suzanne Judd

*See also* Calorie; Metabolism

**References and Further Reading**
Harvey, R.A. (2005) *Biochemistry*, Baltimore, Md.: Lipincott, Williams, & Wilkins.
Starling, E.H. (1904) "The Croonian Lectures on the Chemical Correlation of the Functions of the Body," *The Lancet* 166 (4275): 339–41.
Stipanuk, M.H. (2000) *Biochemical and Physiological Aspects of Human Nutrition*, Philadelphia, Pa.: Saunders.

# Hormones Used in Dieting

In 2004, *Forbes* magazine reported that the thirty-two teams in the National Football League had an operating income of 851 million dollars on revenue of 5.3 billion dollars. As a result, players on professional sports teams are making millions. In 2003, the average salary for a Major League Baseball player was 2,555,476 dollars, amazingly high but not even the highest in professional sports. Players in the National Basketball Association in 2003 brought in an *average* of 4.5 million dollars a year. This is big-time money, and the players in these leagues are big-time athletes who work hard to keep their bodies at the peak of physical performance. Many times, players do more than just eat right and exercise to stay physically competitive; they look for alternative means to enhance performance. Most often, these alternatives come in the form of supplements ranging from simple protein shakes to manufactured hormones. However, it is not just these professional athletes using hormone supplements. Rather, many "ordinary" people are using them to lose weight and increase muscle mass. Whether it's a "weekend warrior" who wants to make a big play on his company's softball team or a "soccer mom" wanting to fit into a dress for a high-school reunion (or indeed a soccer dad or a female weekend warrior), hormone manipulation has become big news and big business in dieting culture.

The most important aspect to this new method of dieting is an increase in knowledge regarding the body. The understanding of the human body and all the many ways it works has improved recently. This increased knowledge has provided people with the ability to manipulate their bodies in new and more effective ways. We now better understand how the body utilizes carbohydrates, fats, and proteins and what this means for the performance and development of the body. With scientific discoveries over the past century, we also better understand how hormones control the body, and scientists now have the ability to artificially produce hormones. As a result, the use of artificial hormones in the sporting world has become a major concern for owners, coaches, players, fans, and legislatures. In March 2005, Congress held a special hearing on the use of steroids in baseball. Their concern was about fairness in the game but also about the message that doping controversies send to young fans. According to Democratic Representative Henry A. Waxman from California,

> There is an absolute correlation between the culture of steroids in high schools and the culture of steroids in major league clubhouses. Kids get the message when it appears that it's okay for professional athletes to use steroids. If the pros do it, college athletes will, too. And if it's an edge in college, high school students will want the edge, too.
>
> (Waxman 2005)

In the human body, steroid hormones are derived from cholesterol. The most common hormones used by professional and amateur athletes today are steroidal hormones, thyroid hormones, and human growth hormones (hGHs). Understanding the way hormones work is imperative to understanding how they give athletes an edge in body shaping and athletic performance. While these hormones are commonly found in the human body at a regulated level, athletes exploit normal hormonal effects by taking artificially produced hormones and, thereby, greatly increasing the amount of hormones in the body. It is at this point that hormones begin to change the physical composition of the body.

The steroids used for performance enhancement are termed "anabolic steroids." These are converted into testosterone by the body. Steroids can be administered by mouth, injection, or in cream form. Users of steroids often administer the steroids in "cycles," which consists of taking steroids for a period of time then stopping for another period and starting again. Often users combine various types of steroids, hoping for an increased effect. The use of steroids can be dangerous with a long list of possible side effects, ranging from balding and mood swings to an increased risk of cancer, heart disease, and stroke.

There are two main steroid hormones used by athletes: cortisol, produced in the adrenal cortex, and testosterone, produced by the gonads. These two steroids have different functions and affect different parts of the body. Cortisol is produced by the body in times of stress and helps the body quickly create extra energy. In excess, cortisol stimulates glucose production, which is then converted to fat. There are products marketed to help reduce the amount of cortisol in the body, therefore, reducing the amount of glucose production, fat storage, and overeating. These products, such as Relacore and CortiSlim, are classified as herbal supplements and claim to balance cortisol in times of stress but have not been proven effective. Cortisol is used by people looking to lose weight. Testosterone, on the other hand, is carried through the blood to muscle tissue; there the steroids stimulate protein synthesis and act to increase muscle size and strength.

Steroids can produce dramatic muscle changes. For example, one study showed that

supraphysiologic doses of testosterone, especially when combined with strength training, increase fat-free mass, muscle size, and strength in normal men . . . [t]he combination of strength training and testosterone produced greater increases in muscle size and strength than were achieved with either

intervention alone. The combined regimen of testosterone and exercise led to an increase of 6.1 kg in fat-free mass over the course of 10 weeks.

(Bhasin et al. 1996: 5)

This is one of the effects athletes and bodybuilders are looking to achieve when using steroids because increased muscle size and strength leads to hitting balls farther, running faster, jumping higher, and lifting more.

A third hormonal supplement, hGH, also known as somatotropin, is synthesized and secreted by the anterior pituitary gland. hGH can directly affect cells that have a receptor specific for hGH and more importantly it has an effect on the liver, stimulating it to produce IGF-1 (insulin-like growth factor 1). IGF-1 has important effects on body mass and size; it stimulates bone growth, as well as protein synthesis in muscle cells. hGH is essential for postnatal growth and development, and its prevalence generally decreases in the human body with age. When hGH is used as a supplement, it can act to eliminate fat and increase muscle. One study found, for example, that "administration of GH alone or in combination with IGF-I caused a greater increase in fat-free mass and a greater reduction in fat mass than those achieved by diet and exercise alone" (Thompson et al. 1998: 1481). This result is the reason hGH is used by those looking to lose weight and gain muscle.

hGH is not available over the counter, but many companies offer supplements that supposedly increase the secretion of hGH. One in particular, GH+Releaser, claims to increase hGH levels by 402 percent and strengthen the immune system, reduce wrinkles, heighten sexual potency, enhance energy, improve sleep, sharpen the memory, reduce fat, increase lean body mass, and promote healing (GH+Releaser 2003). hGH has been proven to be effective in promoting weight loss and increases in muscle mass, but the long-term effects of hGH have yet to be discovered. Supplements claiming to increase hGH release have not been proven effective and may hold little or no benefit and also may be dangerous.

Finally, people may also use and abuse thyroid hormone, which has a major effect on metabolism, mainly on fat and carbohydrate metabolism. It acts within the small intestine and on fat cells to raise metabolic rate. Diet companies rely on these claims to promote products that they claim will act on the thyroid. For example, bodybuilding.com makes a claim that using thyroid supplements is great because you can regulate and optimize your thyroid so it performs at a higher level than it can on its own. And when you do this, suddenly body fat will make like the office slacker when it's time to work weekends—it'll be nowhere to be found.

(Anon. Fat Loss Help)

This is the type of statement many people use to justify the use of thyroid supplements, but the efficacy and safety of these supplements is not proven. Thyroid hormone is prescribed by doctors to treat hypothyroidism, but its use for anything other than this is not recommended.

People take a risk each time they use one of these performance-enhancing hormones or supplements. Not only are they banned by most athletic organizations, some of them are illegal without prescription, and ultimately they can be very dangerous. Those using hormones and supplements may be putting their health and life in danger to achieve a level of physical performance or physical feature. These hormones are essential at normally regulated levels, but when artificially increased they can wreak havoc on the body.

SLG/DARREN JOHNSON

*See also* Hormone; Metabolism

### References and Further Reading

Anon. "Fat Loss Help," bodybuilding.com, available online at <http://bodybuilding.com/store/fatloss.htm> (accessed November 28, 2006).

Bhasin, S., Storer, T.N., Berman, N., Callegari, C., Clevenger, B., Phillips, J., Bunnell, T.J., Tricker, R., Shirazi, A. and Casaburi, R. (1996) "The Effects of Supraphysiological Doses of Testosterone on Muscle Size and Strength in Normal Men," *New England Journal of Medicine* 335 (1): 1–7.

GH+Releaser (2003) available online at <http://www.pureghreleaser.com/index.html> (accessed November 28, 2006).

Thompson, J.L., Butterfield, G.E., Gylfadottir, U.K., Yesavage, J., Marcus, R., Hintz, R.L., Pearman, A., and Hoffman, A.R. (1998) "Effects of Human Growth Hormone, Insulin-Like Growth Factor I, and Diet and Exercise on Body Composition of Obese Postmenopausal Women," *Journal of Clinical Endocrinological Metabolism* 83 (5): 1477–84.

Waxman, Henry W. (2005) "Restoring Faith in America's Pastime: Evaluating Major League Baseball's Efforts to Eradicate Steroid Use," Committee on Government Reforms. U.S. House of Representatives, 108th Congress, March 17, available online at <http://www.businessofbaseball.com/steroidhearings/WaxmanOpeningStatement.pdf> (accessed March 11, 2007).

# Hornby, Lesley (Twiggy) (1949–)

## Model, actress, and singer

Born in London, England, her classmates called her "Sticks" because of her very slim, boyish figure, and at the age of fifteen, Hornby dropped out of school to pursue a career in modeling. She was nicknamed "Twiggy" by her boyfriend/manager, Justin De Villeneuve. In 1966, Twiggy began her modeling career in London with success following almost instantly.

England and, in fact, the world, seemed to have been searching for a change, something different, in what defined beauty and femininity. Twiggy represented that change from the 1950s curvy body type towards a modern, androgynous look. Her body appealed to men and women around the globe and influenced the general conception of femininity. The 1950s insistence that female sex symbols have curvaceous figures was destroyed by Twiggy, who became a positive celebration of androgyny. In fact, the 91-pound, saucer-eyed girl with an angelic face may have helped push standards of thinness a bit too far, leading many young women toward personal dissatisfaction with their bodies and, in some cases, chronic anorexia. For example, Gillian Bobroff, one British model of the 1960s, recalls, "It was dreadful.

... [Twiggy] started a trend, and you had to be just the same. I ... started killing myself, taking a million slimming pills. I never ate. I had bulimia. It was a nightmare, trying to keep up" (Zimmerman 1997: 22).

Twiggy modeled for only four years and became an icon and one of the most recognized models of all times. She was perhaps recognized internationally as the world's first supermodel and was named the "Face of 1966" by the London *Daily Express*. To most people's surprise, Twiggy's thin frame was far from a result of anorexia, dieting, or exercise. "She admitted to eating 'anything, absolute rubbish,' including the ice cream and chocolate sauce piece de resistance 'Bananas Twiggy' whipped up especially for her at her favorite London restaurant. Her irreverent eating habits aside, Twiggy set a standard that most models found impossible to reach" (Zimmerman 1997: 21–2).

SLG/RAKHI PATEL

*See also* Anorexia

## References and Further Reading

Gross, Michael (1996) *Model: The Ugly Business of Beautiful Women*, New York: Warner Books.

Hutton, Tim and Warner, Steven (2006) "Twiggy." Available online at <http://wwwtwiggylawson.co.uk> (accessed March 3, 2007).

Pendergast, Tom and Pendergast, Sara (eds) (2000) "Twiggy," *St. James Encyclopedia of Popular Culture*, five vols, Detroit, Mich.: St. James Press.

Zimmerman, Jill S. (1997) "An Image to Heal: Women, Supermodels, and Body Acceptance," *The Humanist* 57 (1): 20–5.

# I

## Ibn Sina, Abū 'Alī al-Husayn ibn 'Abd Allāh ibn Sīnā

### Known as Avicenna in the West (CE 980–1037)

A distinguished Persian physician and philosopher, who in his *Canon of Medicine*, also known as the *Qanun* (full title: *al-qanun fil-tibb*), Ibn Sina offered a regimen that he claimed would reduce obesity (Avicenna 1930: 441–2). This regimen resembled much later physical rather than dietary interventions but was clearly based on Galen's views of the dangers of obesity. He argued that one should have the food move quickly through the alimentary canal through the use of laxatives, eat food that is bulky but which has little nutrition, bathe before eating and follow it up with hard exercise, eat foods that attenuate the humours, and take vinegar and salt while fasting to purge the body. Still, it is Ibn Sina who provides a first major link between weight reduction and beauty. He lists those "states, which are not 'disease,' but are classed as such" (Avicenna 1930: 221). These categories in which "the beauty of the form of the body is impaired." Among his long list is to be found "great emaciation; excessive bulk; undue thinness and fatness" (Avicenna 1930: 168). Ibn Sina is the most widely known and respected of the Arab physicians to be read in the West.

SLG

*See also* Brillat-Savarin; Medieval Diets; Roman Medicine and Dieting

### References and Further Reading

Avicenna (1930) *A Treatise on the Canon of Medicine*, trans. O. Cameron Gruner, London: Luzac.
Cohen, Sheldon G. (1992) "Avicenna on Food Aversions and Dietary Prescriptions," *Allergy Proceedings* 13 (4): 199–203.

## Imes-Jackson, Mo'Nique (1967–)

### Comedienne and television and movie actress

Mo'Nique has established herself as a celebrated role model and advocate for voluptuous women. Mo'Nique has been awarded four NAACP Image awards for her performance as Nikki Parker on the television series *The Parkers*. From August 2000 until 2002 she had her own line of clothing, Mo'Nique's "Big Beautiful and Loving

It." Her *New York Times*-bestselling book *Skinny Women are Evil* also garnered much attention in 2003. The installment of the first-ever "full-figured" beauty pageant/reality television show, *Monique's F.A.T. (Fabulous and Thick)* aired on the women's television network Oxygen in August 2005. It was the most successful original program in the network's history to that date with 3.8 million viewers, attesting to the growing demand for fat-positive programming. In addition, Mo'Nique's 2006 film *Phat Girlz* highlights central themes from her book and commercial endeavors, including ideas that women can be both fat and beautiful; the valuation of skinny bodies is not universal across time and space, but rather the product of a particular fat-hating, diet-obsessed culture; the dieting industry harms women, emotionally and physically; and fat women suffer discrimination, cruelty, and lack of accessibility.

SLG/ANGELA WILLEY

*See also* Celebrities; Fat-Positive; Manheim

### References and Further Reading

Imes-Jackson, Mo'Nique (2003) *Skinny Women Are Evil*, New York: Atria Books.
—— Mo'Nique's Official Website, available online at <http://1monique.com> (accessed March 3, 2007).
Internet Movie Database (2007) "Mo'Nique Imes." Available online at <http://www.imdb.com/name/nm0594898/bio> (accessed March 3, 2007).
Yursik, Patrice Elizabeth Grell (2006) "Big-Girl Sunday: Mo'Nique's Casting Call Became a Must-See Event," *Miami New Times*, March 16.

# Infectobesity

## Fat across the Species Barrier

In 1997, researchers presented a claim at the Experimental Biology meeting in New Orleans (a city known for food) that obesity could be caused in part by an infectious agent, adenovirus-36 (Ad-36). Nikhil Dhurandhar (then at Wayne State University, Detroit, Mich. and now at the Pennington Biomedical Research Center at Louisiana State University in Baton Rouge) and Richard Atkinson (Obetech, Richmond, Virg.) undertook to show that "this increase [in obesity] is the type of pattern that might occur with a new infectious disease, as has been seen with the AIDS virus" (Anon. "Virus May Be Linked to Obesity" 1997). Both were engaged in obesity research. Indeed, Atkinson was a founder of the American Obesity Association and an editor of the association's flagship journal. They speculated that Ad-36 makes animals fat by stimulating the growth and reproduction of adipocytes (fat cells), as well as by causing immature adipocytes to mature more quickly. Thus, they claimed that animals infected with Ad-36 may have as much as three times more fat cells than uninfected animals, as well as vastly decreased metabolisms.

In a subsequent paper, Dhurandhar noted that this may well solve the mystery of the rapid spread of

obesity [which] has been called the number one public health problem in America. The etiology of obesity is considered to be multifactorial . . . While genetic and behavioral components of obesity have been the focus of intense study, an infection as an etiological factor has received little attention. Although "infectobesity," a new term to describe obesity of infectious origin, appears to be a new concept, over the past 20 years six different pathogens have been reported to cause obesity in animal models. The relative contribution of these pathogens to human obesity is unknown.

(Dhurandhar 2001: 2794S)

But, of course, no greater "magic bullet" can be imagined for human obesity than an antiviral agent that would simply "cure" obesity or even a vaccine that could prevent it. "In 10 years," Dhurandhar stated,

> people may be able to walk into a clinic and be told that their obesity is due to X cause, such as genes, the endocrine system, or pathogens. That may have a more productive outcome than a blanket treatment right now, [which] is not very successful. And because viruses are hard or impossible to treat, prevention through vaccines will be key.
>
> (Jones 2005)

These claims were based on decades of research. As early as the 1970s, Dhurandhar had observed that a chicken adenovirus, isolated in Bombay, caused chickens to accumulate as much as 50 percent more fat than healthy birds. The virus also lowered the animals' cholesterol and triglyceride levels before it killed them. "Normally, obesity in any species is associated with high levels of cholesterol and triglycerides," Dhurandhar noted (Neporent 2005). What interested him at that time though was the odd fact that infected chickens ate no more than uninfected ones. As a result, Dhurandhar and his colleagues identified the infectious agents as Ad-36. This agent was first isolated in humans in 1978 in the fecal matter of a seven-year-old diabetic girl.

Based upon the discovery of Ad-36, Dhurandhar began to theorize that it might be a contributing factor to the skyrocketing obesity epidemic in humans. He next looked for evidence of infection with the chicken virus in a group of fifty-two obese people. Ten showed signs of infection; therefore, it was an avian-spread virus that was postulated as the cause, a "bird-flu" model that might spread to human beings. This work led Steven Heymsfield of the Columbia University College of Physicians and Surgeons in New York City to observe, "Their work on obesity-related viruses has a strong experimental base in animal models and their descriptive epidemiological data appears sound. Whether or not their hypothesis holds up in appropriately designed prospective human studies remains to be answered as far as I know" (Powledge 2004).

Commentators also responded immediately to the "possibility that obesity is a viral disease." Some argued that Ad-36 had serious social consequences as "it may give people ammunition to fight for insurance coverage for weight-loss treatment because they could argue: 'I've got a reason. I'm not just a fat slob' " (Marchione 1997). The moral claim that obesity was simply a public sign of the lack of will, one of the most powerful notions driving the moral panic about obesity, could be stilled by the very notion that its cause was beyond the individual (even beyond the individual's genetic makeup) and was to be found in the ever more dangerous world of infectious diseases. "The implications are enormous," said John Foreyt, a behavioral psychologist at Baylor College of Medicine. He called the research "startling" and "potentially a real breakthrough" in explaining the swift rise of the obesity epidemic (Marchione 1997). Twenty-six percent of American adults were obese in 1980, and more than 35 percent or more are now. It also could help explain the odd demographics of the "obesity epidemic" as it moved from the coasts and then toward the midsection of the U.S.A. "People are still struggling with why this enormous increase in obesity" since "diet, sedentary lifestyles, genetic predispositions and metabolism problems don't explain the whole trend," Foreyt noted (Marchione 1997). If confirmed, these commentators argued, infectobesity would answer multiple problems and a drug that could combat it would be a worldwide blockbuster (Dobson 2004).

While clearly important, Dhurandhar's research was not the first attempt to define obesity as the symptom of an infectious disease. The noted Rockefeller University geneticist, Jules Hirsch, attempted to do so very early in his career. In a 1982 paper, he and his colleagues found "An obesity syndrome . . . in a number of mice infected as young adults with canine distemper virus, a morbillivirus antigenically related to measles" (Lyons et al. 1982: 82). These mice, according to Hirsch, had more and larger fat cells than their noninfected littermates. The researchers thought that the infections might well have altered brain pathways to encourage cell alteration and growth. No "natural" (genetic) process here but rather a response to a pathological agent (Lyons et al. 1982). This trajectory, however, was quickly abandoned for a "genetically" determined hypothesis for the existence of obesity.

Here is the perfect model to imagine how the fear that lies behind the very notion of infectious diseases can be used to focus and define a moral panic that may well have only a tangential relationship to the very notion of infection itself. What is remarkable about the notion of infectious diseases in the age of AIDS is that it couples the idea of the origin of disease in a distant foreign place with the fear of an uncontrolled spread answered almost simultaneously with the announcement of a cure, a quick fix or magic bullet. E.B.R. Desapriya warned "A 1% increase in the prevalence of obesity in such countries as India and China leads to 20 million additional cases" (Desapriya 2004). Imagine each of these cases being a potential source of infection for the West!

It is no accident that the assumption of global, evidence-based medicine is that such plagues—specifically those that deal with the transmission of disease from animals to human beings—originate in the East. "Bird 'flu" in the twentieth-first century has not crossed the "species barrier" any more than bubonic plague did, but bubonic plague had animals (rats and lice) as its vector. The relatively small number of cases of bird flu today seems to be the result of direct exposure to infected animals. Bird flu is being treated much like bubonic plague in that intimacy with animals is seen to be its cause (and more importantly) seen to pose a risk that the disease will cross the species barrier so that human beings could infect other humans without an animal vector.

The fascination with a viral cause for obesity also comes in the context of the SARS (severe acute respiratory syndrome) as well as other, more recent Asian avian influenzas of the past decade (McLean et al. 2005). The view that these diseases invade healthy spaces through an infectious process seems to be a commonplace. All of these claims about disease reflect the potential for mass death associated with an earlier disruption of the food chain: BSE (Bovine Spongiform Encephalopathy, "mad cow disease") which haunted Europe (and North America) when it entered the public's awareness in 1990 with the publication in European newspapers of the association between BSE and neurological diseases such as vCJD (Variant Creutzfeldt-Jakob disease) in human beings (Pennington 2003).

While the origin of BSE was originally not seen as the exotic reaches of the Orient or Africa, it quickly became the English disease on the continent or the Canadian disease in the U.S.A. BSE, caused evidently by the use of technology that ground animal offal (by-products) into animal feed, became the model for the notion that food kills—but only food that infiltrates from beyond our borders. Recently, the argument has been made that BSE originated in the consumption of animal feed made from bones and organic scraps imported for animal feed from Bangladesh, India, and Pakistan in the 1960s and 1970s. Rather than being an "indigenous" disease, having its source in the viral disease Scrapie among sheep in Europe, it spread from ingestion of diseased organic matter from the bodies of infected "Orientals" (Colchester and Colchester 2005). Or, as the authors of the recent study stated,

> that the route of infection was oral, through animal feed containing imported mammalian raw materials contaminated with human remains; and that the origin was the Indian subcontinent, from which large amounts of mammalian material were imported during the relevant time period. Human remains are known to be incorporated into meal made locally, and may still be entering exported material.
>
> (Colchester and Colchester 2005: 856)

Cannibalism is always a significant charge in drawing the line between acceptable and unacceptable levels of civilization and health.

Does the anxiety about barriers to disease not lie at the heart of our desire that obesity, too, can be quickly fixed, once it is recognized as "merely" an infectious disease, rather than a reflex of national or personal character? The quick fix here is not to repair the food chain or end fast food, but to change the world so that such depression is eliminated. No quick fix is promised; why not hope for a vaccine against modernity, hopelessness, and fat? Simply because such quick fixes never truly eliminate the moral panic associated with this newest epidemic.

SLG

*See also* Aboulia; Genetics; Obesity Epidemic; Metabolism

## References and Further Reading

Anon. "Virus May Be Linked to Obesity," University of Wisconsin-Madison News Service. Available online at <http://www.news.wisc.edu/4754> (accessed June 23, 2007).

Colchester, A.C. and Colchester, N.T. (2005) "The Origin of Bovine Spongiform Encephalopathy: The Human Prion Disease Hypothesis," *The Lancet* 366 (9488): 856–61.

Desapriya, E.B.R. (2004) "Letter: Obesity Epidemic," *Lancet* 364 (9444): 1488.

Dobson, Roger (2004) " 'Fat War' Scramble to Develop Wonder Pill to Fight Obesity," *Independent on Sunday* (London), May 2.

Dhurandhar, Nikhil V. (2001) "Infectobesity: Obesity of Infectious Origin," *Journal of Nutrition 131*: 2794S–2797S.

Jones, Deborah (2005) "Vaccine May Target Obesity in the Future," Agence France Presse—English, October 18.

Kolata, Gina (2007) *Rethinking Thin: The New Science of Weight Loss—and the Myths and Realities of Dieting*, New York: Farrar, Straus and Giroux.

Lyons, M., Faust, J.I.M., Hemmes, R.B., Buskirk, D.R., Hirsch, J., and Zabriskie, J.B. (1982) "A Virally Induced Obesity Syndrome in Mice," *Science* 216 (4541): 82–5.

Marchione, Marilynn (1997) "Virus Is Linked to Weight Problems in Humans," *Seattle Post-Intelligencer*, April 8.

McLean, Angela, May, Robert M., Pattison, John, and Weiss, Robert A. (eds) (2005) *SARS: A Case Study in Emerging Infections*, Oxford: Oxford University Press.

Neporent, Liz (2005) "Can a Virus Make You Fat?" *New York Daily News*, November 2.

Pennington, T. Hugh (2003) *When Food Kills: BSE, E. Coli, and Disaster Science*, Oxford, New York: Oxford University Press.

Powledge, Tabitha M. (2004) "Is Obesity an Infectious Disease?" *The Lancet Infectious Diseases* 4 (10): 599.

# Internet

The Internet has powerfully changed the world of health and nutrition so much so that the term "e-dieting" has come quickly into fashion in the beginning of the twenty-first century. By joining online communities, individuals can seek information, treatment programs, or help from experts within seconds. The World Wide Web has become a particularly popular way for people to access dieting information because of its convenience and simplicity. Whether people around the world are tracking their calories online or sharing dieting techniques, virtual communities are unique in the anonymity they prove for participants. Individuals can sit in the comfort of their homes and read about dieting plans online, tell personal stories, and even join groups focused on weight loss. As such, the powerful technology of the Internet has impacted dieting culture by making access to information fast and faceless.

The categories of health topics found on the Internet include: (1) academic resources, (2) obesity related-organizations, (3) chat groups and social support resources, and (4) commercial services and products. In each of these four areas, the Internet has become a "therapeutic tool" (Fontaine and Allison 2002). People can access innovative organizational websites that explain ways to prevent obesity and other medical problems resulting from a poor diet. Consumers can even educate themselves using these diverse resources, which may provide them a greater level of control over their weight and health in general.

The wide variety of websites and virtual tools available to the online community allow users to choose sites based on their personal preference. The Internet's 24/7 available access provides many tools including customized eating advice, plans, and information. Individuals can become members of websites, such as e-diets.com and caloriescount.com, where they can track their calories and access a diet plan with the click of a button. Some websites offer plans with specific recipes and make it convenient for dieters to keep food diaries and track their progress online (Graham 2006). Other sites have instructions for following specific popular diets, such as the Atkins diet or the South Beach diet. Cyber diet plans, however, involve a lot of time, effort, and accuracy. Users must fill out diet and activity questionnaires carefully (and truthfully) in order to effectively track their weight. In addition to these, blogs and personal websites connect dieters across the globe and create a large following of cyber social groups. These sites can play a big role in shaping people's dieting behaviors in positive and negative ways (Graham 2006). For example, while virtual weight-watchers meetings encourage people to stick to their diets, pro-anorexia websites provide those with an eating disorder dangerous weight-loss tips.

Numerous government websites also provide information on obesity, eating disorders, and nutrition. Federally funded web-based programs that promote interactive experiences for users may be some of the most helpful and safe tools available online. These sites provide education on healthy eating and exercise by outlining specific instructions that one can follow, as well as weight-management and self-monitoring systems where members can follow strict regimens to attain the optimal body weight (Fontaine and Allison 2002). For example, the Shape Up America! program, founded by U.S. Surgeon General C. Everett Koop is an important online tool in the national battle against obesity. This federally funded program is a result of collaboration between numerous health experts all focused on promoting healthy eating and physical exercise and making Americans realize that preventing obesity should be a public health priority (Fontaine and Allison 2002). The findings from Shape Up America! show the promise web-based programs have for improving the health of Americans. In addition, other sites, like the Government's mypyramidtracker.org, allow people to find out if what they are eating has the suggested amount of nutrition (Fontaine and Allison 2002). Today, federally funded health-related websites provide one way for the government to educate its citizens about how to lose weight and stay healthy; however, in order for them to work, consumers have to be invested in weight loss and healthier eating.

People's investments in dieting vary almost as much as their reasons for choosing online dieting help. While it is impossible to know exactly why consumers choose internet dieting, some may be too embarrassed to seek professional help, while others many want to feel a part of an online community where they can be held accountable for their dieting progress. Moreover, consumers may prefer the convenient and inexpensive tools on the web. Whatever a person's reason for choosing online dieting, there are several potential advantages to using cyber tools (Fontaine and Allison 2002). Primarily, the unlimited use of the Internet allows one to access thousands of individuals at an extremely low cost. In addition, the Internet can be used at any hour of the day and from any city; thus, the number of people who can access online dieting

sites is nearly limitless. Further, experts can monitor users and give quick and direct feedback on their progress. Lastly, the ability for people to participate in a treatment program tailored to their needs and yet remain anonymous is a positive aspect of Internet use.

Like any powerful technology that is convenient and for the information-savvy, there are potential drawbacks (Fontaine and Allison 2002). Many websites focusing on weight loss and health, for example, lack accurate information. Because the Internet does not require face-to-face interaction, it is also tough to know whether people are really keeping the weight off or fibbing about their smaller pant-sizes to their internet peers. In addition, though the Internet eliminates personal interactions, it allows a person to expose themselves and even sometimes overexpose themselves. Through Internet chatrooms and blogs, dieters can tell their personal stories and connect with other patrons who are experiencing similar situations; however, uncertainties about safety and truth remain a potential downside. It is ultimately the responsibility of the Internet user to ensure the accuracy of the advice that they are obtaining.

Studies have also found evidence that when compared to other treatments such as in-person therapy, internet dieting is less successful. A study conducted at the University of Vermont, for example, looked at the difference in weight maintenance programs conducted over the Internet versus in-person treatments. A record of the body weight, dietary intake, energy expended in physical activity, attendance, self-monitoring, and comfort with technology of 122 healthy, overweight adults was kept over twelve months. Results showed that the Internet group gained significantly more weight than the in-person group during the first six months of weight maintenance. These findings suggest that internet support is not as effective at facilitating the long-term maintenance of weight loss compared to in-person therapy (Harvey-Berino et al. 2002). Other studies have found that internet sites such as e-diets.com are not as effective at helping users lose weight as compared to manual in-person weight-loss programs (Womble et al. 2004).

Despite their questionable efficacy, dieting websites are becoming more and more common in the internet universe. The semi-public yet still private environment of the Internet allows dieters to feel in control of their dieting habits. In addition, if one's diet falters, it remains a behind-doors matter. While safety and oversight are problematic in cyberspace, research on the benefits of

## Popular health-related websites

| Site | What it offers | Cost | Goal |
|---|---|---|---|
| Caloriescount.com | You can pick a recipe-based plan or a convenience-based plan, or a combination of both. | $10 for the first two months; discounted rates for longer terms | Healthy weight loss (one to two pounds a week) |
| Ediets.com | Flexibility in choosing a plan; can add restaurant meals, etc. | $16 for one month; extra features are additional costs | Has plans that follow many popular plans (Mayo Clinic, Atkins, Slim Fast, etc.) |
| Weightwatchers.com | Well-balanced diet plan with support and behavior training. | $46.90 for the first month, then $16.95 a month. | Easy weighing, measuring, and counting |
| Eatright.org | Provides information on American Dietetic Association | Free | N/A |
| Something-fishy.org | Largest website for eating disorders. Includes information, conference updates, chatrooms, "treatment finder service," and help for family and friends. | Free | N/A |
| Mypyramidtracker.gov | You can fill out food-intake questionnaire and find if you're getting enough recommended nutrients. | Free | Ability to see if you follow food pyramid suggestions |

internet dieting suggests that this dieting method will continue to grow in popularity.

SLG/JESSICA SAWHNEY

*See also* Anorexia; Atkins; Food Pyramid; Nidetch

### References and Further Reading

Fontaine, Kevin R. and Allison, David B. (2002) "Obesity and the Internet," in Christopher G. Fairburn and Kelly D. Brownell (eds), *Eating Disorders and Obesity: A Comprehensive Handbook*, 2nd edn, New York: Guilford Press, pp. 609–12.

Graham, Janis (2006) "Best Sites for Staying Well and Shaping Up," *Good Housekeeping* 243 (5): 73–82.

Harvey-Berino J., Pintauro, S., Buzzell, P., DiGiulio, M., Casey Gold, B., Moldovan, C., and Ramirez, E. (2002) "Does Using the Internet Facilitate the Maintenance of Weight Loss?" *International Journal of Obesity and Related Metabolic Disorders* 26 (9): 1254–60.

Shape Up America! Healthy weight for life (2006) available online at <http://www.shapeup.org/shape/index_shape.php> (accessed December 15, 2006).

Womble, L.G., Wadden, T.A., McGuckin, B.G., Sargent, S.L., Rothman, R.A., and Krauthamer-Ewing, E.S. (2004) "A Randomized Controlled Trial of a Commercial Internet Weight Loss Program," *Obesity Research* 12 (6): 1011–18.

# Israeli, Isaac ben Salomon

## Known as Isaac Judaeus, and Abu Ya'kub ibn Sulaiman Alisr'ili (before 832–932 CE)

**A** Jewish physician, born in Egypt, Israeli had his major impact in Tunis where he died. As a student of 'Ishak ibn 'Amran al-Baghdadi, he incorporated the traditions of Greek medicine as understood by contemporary Jewish and Muslim physicians. He was court physician to the last Aghiabite prince, Ziyadat Allah, and in 909 CE became the official physician to the Fatimid caliph Ubaid Allah al-Mahdi and, as such, had enormous influence in the medical world of his day. He was the author of, among many other medical works, a treatise on disease and its cures, *Kitab al-adwiya al-mufrada wal-aghdhiya*, the last three sections of which were translated into Latin as *De diaetis particularibus*. This was the first dedicated book on dieting published in Europe. His works' initial impact on Christian Europe came with their translation into Latin in 1087 by Constantine of Carthage (the African), who claimed that he had written the works himself. His dieting book was then translated into Hebrew from the Latin as *Sefer ha-Ma'akalim* and was first published from a manuscript in Padua in 1484. This book was immediately translated into the vernacular, and a German translation by Valentin Schwendes appeared in 1498 (Nägele 2001). It was only in 1515 that these works were finally attributed to Isaac Judaeus, who was one of the most influential interpreters of Greek medical knowledge for the Muslim world. Many of his works were written in Arabic as well as Hebrew.

SLG

*See also* Greek Medicine and Dieting

## References and Further Reading

Nägele, Susanne (2001) *Valentin Schwendes "Buch von menicherhande geschlechte kornes und menicherley fruchtte."* Würzburg: Königshausen & Neumann.
Wüstenfeld, Heinrich Ferdinand (1840) *Geschichte der arabischen Ärzte und Naturforscher*, Göttingen: Vandenhoeck und Ruprecht.

# J

## Jews

### Diet and Disease

The Bible (Old Testament, Tanach) contains a long series of prohibitions concerning food. Prohibited are certain foods from any animal that does not have both cloven hooves and chew its cud (pigs) (Lev. 11:3; Deut. 14:6) or fish/seafood that does not have fins and scales (sturgeon or shrimp) (Lev. 11:9; Deut. 14:9) as well as rules concerning the combinations of foods that may be eaten. Added to these rules are specific laws concerning slaughter and the preparation of meat (Deut. 12:21). In total, these laws are called "kashrut," and food that is acceptable under these laws is called "kosher," meaning "fit" or "proper." Whatever the initial intent of such laws, and there is a long historical debate about them, they were seen as part of rituals parallel to the sacrifices of animals and food stuffs at the Temple.

The anthropologist Mary Douglas offers a compelling reading of the meaning of these dietary codes. For her, they are intended to keep order; that which is forbidden creates an awareness of where danger lies. Her reading of the "abominations" listed in Leviticus stresses the arbitrary nature of inclusion and exclusion. "The precepts and ceremonies alike are focused on the idea of the holiness of God which men must create in their own lives. So this is a universe in which men prosper by conforming to holiness and perish when they deviate from it" (Douglas 2002: 50). For Douglas, the prohibitions reflect a general rule that

defilement is never an isolated event. It cannot occur except in view of a systematic ordering of ideas [ . . . ] the only way in which pollution ideas make sense is in reference to a total structure of thought whose key-stone boundaries, margins, and internal lines are held in relation by rituals of separation.

(Douglas 2002: 41)

With the destruction of the Second Temple and the development of Rabbinic Judaism these laws became fixed as a central aspect of Jewish ritual practice.

With the reforms of the late eighteenth and nineteenth centuries, there was a long discussion about where such dietary restriction should be abandoned as a residue of earlier practices, which centered on the practice of animal slaughter. While Reform Judaism did abandon this to an extent, neo-Orthodox Jews of the nineteenth century rethought the dietary laws in term of the new understanding of hygiene. The dietary code became a means of assuring health, and Moses became "the first hygienist." As Henry Behrend observes in 1889,

The idea of parasitic and infectious maladies, which has conquered so great a position in modern pathology, appears to have greatly occupied the mind of Moses, and to have dominated all his hygienic rules. He excludes from the Hebrew diet animals particularly liable to parasites; and as it is in the blood that the germs or spores of infectious disease circulate, he orders that they must be drained of their blood before serving for food . . . What an extraordinary prescience!

(Behrend 1889: 409)

And the great Anglo-Canadian physician and essayist

William Osler stated in 1914, "we may go to Moses for instruction in some of the best methods in hygiene" (Osler 1959: 56).

The counterargument was made by animal-rights groups, which labeled Jewish ritual slaughtering procedures as signs of the innate cruelty of the Jews. In the 1883 meeting of Congress for the Protection of Animals in Vienna, the argument was made that the protection of ritual slaughter, or at least its lack of condemnation, was a sign that the Jews controlled the political process in Europe. By 1892, a law against ritual slaughter was passed in Saxony. And by 1897, there was a clear link between such attacks and the antivivisection movement, as the cruelest physicians were reputed to be Jews.

Ironically, the boom in the sale of kosher food (which only means ritually supervised) in the U.S.A. today has much the same "hygienic" rationale. Some 40 percent of foods sold in mainstream retail outlets in the U.S.A. are "kosher" (Blech 2004: xvii). Out of a market of 500 billion dollars spent on food, American food manufacturers sell more than 170 billion dollars worth of kosher-certified products each year. As one hot-dog maker's advertisement has it, kosher food answers to a higher authority, but it also carries with it the promise of better eating. Whenever a company makes a product kosher, it sees a jump in its market share. In contemporary America, kosher has become interchangeable with "organic" and is therefore deemed healthy. Ritual slaughter as a sign of Jewish cruelty disappears as a problem in this context.

Given the focus of the Jews on diet, it is surprising how little emphasis Jews placed on the representation of the overweight body. Such a body is evoked by the biblical figure of Eglon, King of Moab, who oppressed the children of Israel for eighteen years (Preuss 1978: 215). His fat (*ish bari me'od*) body was destroyed by the left-handed hero Ehud (Judges 3:17, 22). Indeed, it is even described how Eglon's fat closed about the blade when he was pierced. Ehud smuggles his sword into the presence of the King by wearing it on the "wrong-side," at least the wrong side for right-handers. He is "treacherous and sneaky; perhaps the culture of ancient Israel thought those descriptions to be synonymous, at least stereotypical" (Berquist 2002: 34–5). As for the fat king, his guards do not even notice that he has been disemboweled until they smell his feces. Is this the case of one deviant body destroying another?

The Talmudic fat body was a deviant one, but not particularly a dangerous one. Rather, there is a sort of fascination with it. The Talmud even asks whether very fat men, such as Rabbis Ishamel ben Yose and Eleazar ben Simeon (end of the second century) could ever reproduce because of their huge bellies. But Jewish attitudes toward such obesity were clearly defined by the model of the lack of self-control. Not yet a "sin," it was a sign of the lack of self-discipline appropriate for a real man, a real scholar and could be punished (Kottek 1997).

In the classic work of the twelfth-century Iberian physician-philosopher Maimonides on dietetics, *The Regimen of Health*, there is no sense that obesity was a moral or even a medical problem (at least for the rulers for whom he wrote), while he notes sexual overexertion as one (Rosner 1998: 58). However, it was still viewed as an important health issue, with repercussions upon the body of the individual; he treated the condition of "obese old men" with medication, exercise, massage, and baths (Maimonides 1992: 175–6). His work provides a synthesis of Galenic medicine and the work of the Arabic physician Ibn Sina, whose *Kitah al-Quanun* or *The Canon* includes a detailed discussion of obesity in its fourth book.

It is only in modernity that the Jew's body comes to represent all of the potential for disease and decay associated with the modern body of the fat boy. In modern medicine, there has been a preoccupation with a claimed Jewish predisposition to diabetes. The nineteenth-century practice of labeling Jews as a "diabetic" race was a means of labeling them as inferior. In the fall of 1888, the Parisian neurologist Jean Martin Charcot described to Sigmund Freud the predisposition of Jews for specific forms of illness, such as diabetes, and how "the exploration is easy" because the illness was caused by the intermarriage of the Jews. Jewish "incest" left its mark on the Jewish body in the form of diabetes as well as on the Jewish soul (indicative of his depreciatory attitude in regard to the Jews, Charcot's letter to Freud used the vulgar "juif" rather than the more polite "Israëlite" or more scientific "sémite" [Gelfand 1988: 574]). However, there are further views on why the Jews are predisposed to this illness. The British eugenicist George Pitt-Rivers attributed the increased rate of diabetes among the Jews to "the passionate nature of their temperaments." He noted that by the 1920s diabetes was commonly called a "Jewish disease" (Pitt-Rivers 1927: 82).

But over and over again it was the obesity inherent in the Jew's body (and soul) that was seen as the cause of the illness. Often the power of the racial model overwhelms any specificity of gender, even though the seemingly ungendered term "Jew" in this context is always understood to be the male Jew. The "Oriental races, enervated by climate, customs, and a superalimentation abounding in fats, sugar and pastry will inevitably progress towards the realization of fat generations, creating an extremely favourable soil for obesity" (Frumusan 1930: 9). Even in the Diaspora, the assumption is that the Jew is diabetic because of his predisposition for fat:

All observers are agreed that Jews are specially liable to become diabetic. . . . A person belonging to the richer classes in towns usually eats to much, spends a great part of his life indoors; takes too little bodily exercise, and overtakes his nervous system in the pursuit of knowledge, business, or pleasure . . . Such a description is a perfectly accurate account of the well-to-do Jew, who raises himself easily by his superior mental ability to a comfortable social position, and notoriously avoids all kinds of bodily exercise.

(Saundby 1897: 197–9)

In addition, it was claimed that Jews inherited their tendency toward fat because of their lifestyle: "Can a surfeit of food continued through many generations create a large appetite in the offspring; alternatively, can it cause a functional weakness of their weight-regulating mechanism?" asks W.F. Christie. And he answers:

Take, for instance, the Hebrews, scattered over the ends of the earth. Probably no race in the world has so apparent a tendency to become stout after puberty, or is more frequently cited as an example of racial adiposity. It is also probable that no nation is so linked in common serfdom to their racial habits and customs. [Elliot P.] Joslin says of the present generation of Jews: "Overeating begins in childhood, and lasts till old age." The inheritance of large appetites and depressed weight-regulating mechanism may exist in them, although they show no other signs of the latter; whereas the inheritance of fat-forming habits is certain.

(Christie 1937: 31)

Thus, Jews inherit the compulsive eating patterns of their ancestors and are therefore fat already as children. Their obesity and their diabetes are a reflection of their poor hygienic traditions, precisely the opposite of the claims of nineteenth-century Jewish reformers who saw Judaism as the rational religion of hygiene. Indeed, it is the "Oriental" Jew who presents the worst-case scenario for this line of argument. Max Oertel, perhaps the most quoted authority on obesity at the beginning of the twentieth century, states that "The Jewesses of Tunis, when barely ten years, old are systematically fattened by being confined in dark rooms and fed with farinaceous articles and the flesh of dogs, until in the course of a few months they resemble shapeless lumps of fat" (Oertel 1895: 647–8). Here the fantasy about the "Oriental" body in the West is heightened by the Jews feeding their daughters nonkosher food.

From the nineteenth century, diabetes had been seen as a disease of the obese and, in an odd set of associations, the Jew was implicated as obese due to an apparent increased presence of diabetes among Jews. According to a turn-of-the-century specialist, mainly rich Jewish men are fat (von Noorden 1910: 63). But rather than arguing for any inborn metabolic inheritance, he stated that it is the fault of poor diet among the rich—too much rich food and alcohol, this being yet another stereotype of the Jew. And yet, the other side of the coin is amply present. At the beginning of the twentieth century, scientists began to explore the relationship between the predisposition of the Jews for diabetes and the assumed relationship between diabetes and obesity. One physician noted that

since one in twelve obese Gentiles develops diabetes, no less than one in eight obese Jews develop it. This, it is suggested, is to be explained by the fact that a fat Hebrew is always fatter than a fat Gentile, and that it is the higher grade of obesity which determines the Semitic preponderance in diabetes.

(Williams 1926: 53)

The assumption about fat and the "Oriental" race is one that comes to haunt discussions of the meaning of fat (Leray 1931: 11–12). When W.H. Sheldon develops his "somatotypes" in the 1940s, he observes that Jews shows an exaggeration in each of his body types. Thus, fat Jews are somehow fatter than fat non-Jews (Sheldon et al. 1940: 221). More recent studies of obese Jews look at the complex behavior patterns that occur when religious demands for fasting and the psychological predisposition of the obese come in conflict.

Today, the general consensus is that diabetes is not particularly a Jewish illness. Research now follows the so-called "thrifty genotype" hypothesis that had been suggested in 1964. Simply stated, it has been observed that when mice are transferred from a harsh to a benign environment, they gain weight and are hyperglycemic. When one thus measured first generation groups of immigrants to the U.S.A. in the late nineteenth century or in Israel today, there is a substantially higher rate of diabetes. The initial groups, such as the example of the Yemenites who immigrated to Israel from a harsh environment, showed an extremely low index of diabetes when they arrived in Israel. This index, however, sky-rocketed after just a short time of living in their new environment. Thus, diabetes and obesity seem to be an index of a failure to adapt rapidly to changed surroundings (Goodman 1979: 334–41).

And yet fat still is imagined as a Jewish issue. The columnist David Margolis, writing in the *Los Angeles Jewish Journal* in 2001, observes that:

A lot of people also consider fat a Jewish issue. According to a recent survey in the New York City area, Jewish families consume "almost double" the amount of cake and donuts that non-Jewish families do and more than twice as much diet soda and cottage cheese. A professional in the eating-disorder industry claims that Jews tend to choose food over addictions to other substances. Food is just another drug, after all, the cheapest, most easily available, most socially acceptable mood-altering substance. Is it merely a coincidence that Alcoholics Anonymous was founded by two Christian men, while Overeaters Anonymous was founded by two Jewish women?

(Margolis 2001)

The image of the overfed Jew, central to the culture that needed to see the Oriental disease of diabetes as an essential aspect of the corrupt Jewish soul, now has a place in American popular culture about the Jewish body. Yet, here it is transformed into the body of the Jewish woman, as "fat" in the U.S.A. "is a feminist issue."

SLG

*See also* Ibn Sina; Religion and Dieting; Roman Medicine and Dieting

## References and Further Reading

Anon. (1994) "Talmudic Aphorisms on Diet: III. What Should We Drink?" *Israel Journal of Medical Sciences* 30 (1994): 732–3.

Behrend, Henry (1889) "Diseases Caught from Butcher's Meat," *The Nineteenth Century* 26: 409–22.

Berquist, Jon L. (2002) *Controlling Corporeality: The Body and the Household in Ancient Israel*, New Brunswick, NJ: Rutgers University Press.

Blech, Zushe Yosef (2004) *Kosher Food Production*, Oxford: Blackwell.

Christie, W.F. (1937) *Obesity: A Practical Handbook for Physicians*, London: William Heinemann.

Douglas, Mary (2002) *Purity and Danger*, London: Routledge & Kegan Paul.

Frumusan, Jean (1930) *The Cure of Obesity*, trans. Elaine A. Wood, London: John Bale.

Gelfand, Toby (1988) " 'Mon Cher Docteur Freud': Charcot's Unpublished Correspondence to Freud, 1888–93," *Bulletin of the History of Medicine* 62 (4): 563–88.

Goodman Richard M. (1979) *Genetic Disorders Among the Jewish People*, Baltimore, Md.: Johns Hopkins.

Kottek, Samuel S. (1997) "On Health and Obesity in Talmudic and Midrashic Lore," *Obesity Surgery* 7 (2): 161–2.

Lepicard, Etienne (1994) "Talmudic Aphorisms on Diet," *Israel Journal of Medical Sciences* 30 (7): 314–15.

Leray, Jean (1931) *Embonpoint et obésité*, Paris: Masson et cie.

Maimonides (1992) *Medical Writings: The Art of Cure— Extracts from Galen*, ed. and trans. Uriel S. Barzel, Haifa: Maimonides Research Institute.

Margolis, David (2001) "Fat: Remember 'Stressed' Spelled Backwards Is 'Desserts'," David Margolis Journalism, available online at <http:// www.davidmargolis.com/article.php?id=11> (accessed March 4, 2007).

Oertel, M.J. (1895) "Obesity," in Thomas J. Stedman (ed.), *Nutritive Disorders*, Vol. III of *Twentieth Century Practice*, twenty vols, London: Sampson Low, Marston and Co., pp. 626–725.

Osler, William (1959) "Israel and Medicine," in Earl F. Nation (ed.), *Men and Books*, Pasadena, Calif.: Castle Press, p. 56. Originally published in 1914 *Canadian Medical Association Journal* 4(8): 729–33.

Pitt-Rivers, George Henry Lane-Fox (1927) *The Clash of Culture and the Contact of Races*, London: Routledge.

Preuss, Julius (1978) *Biblical and Talmudic Medicine*, trans. Fred Rosner, New York: Sanhedrin Press.

Rosner, Fred (1998) *The Medical Legacy of Moses Maimonides*, Hoboken, NJ: KTAV.

Saundby, Robert (1897) "Diabetes mellitus," in Thomas Clifford Allbutt (ed.) (1990) *A System of Medicine*, London: Macmillan, Vol. III, pp. 197–9.

Schwarz, D. (1990) "Jüdische Speisegeetze und Gesundheitserziehung," *Zeitschrift für die gesamte Hygiene und ihre Grenzgebiete* 36 (12): 641–4.

Sheldon, W.H., Stevens, S.S. and Tucker, W.B. (1940) *The Varieties of Human Physique*, New York: Harper.

von Noorden, Carl (1910) *Die Fettsucht*, Vienna: Alfred Hölder.

Williams, Leonard (1926) *Obesity*, London: Humphrey Milford/Oxford University Press.

# Johnson, Samuel (1709–84)

## English wit and raconteur

Compiler of what is seen as the first English dictionary, Johnson suffered from chronic illness from his childhood in Lichfield. When he was two and a half, he contracted scrofula and was taken by his mother in March 1712 to be "touched" by Queen Anne for what was then called the King's Evil (Keynes 1995). This "cure" had as little impact on his future life as did his later recourse to dieting. As Johnson aged, he became corpulent. At this time, some of the older traditions of weight loss, such as the use of the flower "Thrift" (*Armeria maritima*), were still in use, but it was diet that was the newest fad (Jacquin 1770: I, Table 42).

In his *Dictionary of the English Language*, Johnson defined diet both in the older sense of "food, provisions for the mouth; victuals" as well as the more modern sense of "food regulated by the rules of medicine, for the prevention or cure of any disease" (Johnson 1819). Johnson, whose odd-looking body was then wracked by innumerable ailments, both inherited and acquired, undertook such a "cure" in September of 1780: "I am now beginning the seventy-second year of my life, with more strength of body and greater vigour of mind than, I think, is common at that age . . . I have been attentive to my diet, and have diminished the bulk of my body" (Johnson 1958: 301).

Johnson's fat was an ailment of his middle age, but according to James Boswell's (1740–95) biography *The Life of Samuel Johnson LL.D.* (1791), he viewed obesity as purely a product of bad diet: "whatever be the quantity that a man eats, it is plain that if he is too fat, he has eaten more that he should have done" (Boswell 1980: 958). Boswell, however, disagreed with Johnson, stating "you will see one man fat who eats moderately, and another lean who eats a great deal" (1980: 958). This was in response to Johnson who said that he "fasted from the Sunday's dinner to the Tuesday's dinner, without any inconvenience" (Boswell 1980: 958). Boswell noted that this may well have been true, but he also explained that Johnson could "practise abstinence, but not temperance" (Boswell 1980: 1121). Nevertheless, Johnson's recourse to the "cure" of dieting was a typical approach of the first great age of public dieting, the Enlightenment (Rogers 1993).

SLG

*See also* Enlightenment Dietetics

## References and Further Reading

Boswell, James (1980) *Life of Johnson*, ed. R.W. Chapman, Oxford: Oxford University Press.

Jacquin, Nicholaus Joseph von (1770) *Hortus Botanicus Vindobonensis*, Vienna: Leopold Johann Kaliwoda.

Johnson, Samuel (1819) *Johnson's Dictionary: Volume 1 A-K*, Philadelphia, Pa.: James Maxwell.

—— (1958) "Diaries, Prayers, and Annals," in E.L.

McAdam, Jr., D. Hyde, and M. Hyde (eds) *The Yale Edition of the Works of Samuel Johnson*, New Haven, Conn.: Yale University Press.

Keynes, Milo (1995) "The Miserable Health of Dr. Samuel Johnson," *Journal of Medical Biography* 3 (3): 161–9.

Rogers, Pat (1993) "Fat Is a Fictional Issue: The Novel and the Rise of Weight-Watching," in Marie Mulvey Roberts and Roy Porter (eds), *Literature and Medicine during the Eighteenth Century*, London: Routledge, pp. 168–87.

# K

## Kellogg, John Harvey, MD (1852–1943)

**B**est known for his invention of flaked breakfast cereals, Kellogg was also one of the most outspoken health reformers in the late nineteenth century. Raised as a Seventh-Day Adventist, he was inspired by founder Ellen G. White's writings on health reform that stressed healthy living as a religious duty. Kellogg began to write and lecture prolifically, becoming a powerful advocate for healthy diet, exercise, sexual repression, and natural remedies for health problems. Kellogg's published works range from a monthly Adventist magazine called Health Reformer to an anti-tobacco book, *Tobaccoism or How Tobacco Kills* (1922), to *Plain Facts about Sexual Life* (1877). The linking of all types of reform, including sexual reform, was part of the moralizing tendency in which diet and dieting played a large role in nineteenth- and twentieth-century America.

In his *The Stomach: Its Disorders, and How to Cure Them* (1896), Kellogg presents a cure for the new "American malady," dyspepsia. For him "Americans enjoyed the unenviable, but nevertheless deserved, reputation of being a nation of dyspeptics" (Kellogg 1896: 17). It is dyspepsia, rather than George Miller Beard's "American Disease" of "neurasthenia" (1869) that defined the pathology of modernity for Kellogg. Indeed, he lumps such nervous disorders under "gastric neurasthenia" and argues that they can be cured through diet, rather than through electrotherapy. To prove this, Kellogg presented his theory of diet and dieting in light of the newest science of bacteriology. It is a new science for a new reformed America.

Quoting Pasteur, David, and others who showed that the digestive tract is full of "a vast number of microbes capable of producing various acids, poisonous ptomains and toxins," Kellogg argued that only correct dieting can prevent disease (Kellogg 1896: 19). It is the "modern stomach" that demands a modern cure for this "formidable disease" (Kellogg 1896: 55). He provides a detailed list of what to do, including slow and regular chewing (Kellogg 1896: 58) and the avoidance of substances like vinegar (because it is "an alcoholic liquor" [1896: 112]), too much sugar (1896: 105), uncooked food (1896: 96), and abundant use of fat. But, most importantly, Kellogg provides a detailed diet regimen for all people to follow to prevent or to cure dyspepsia. He begins with an "aseptic dietry" which advocates sterilized food prepared without milk or eggs, whole grains, fresh fruits raw, or cooked without sugar or with grains (Kellogg 1896: 227ff). Page upon page of proscriptive diets follow, all of which are intended to cure and prevent various forms of disease. In addition, all of Kellogg's diets focus on vegetarian diets, with the preparation or manufacture of the foods being part of the diet.

His dietary beliefs may have been influenced by his professional training but were also the result of a general interest in health reform at the time. Kellogg was trained as a surgeon at Bellevue Hospital Medical College in New York. Shortly after receiving his medical degree, he became superintendent of the Western Health Reform Institute in Michigan, which he renamed Battle Creek Sanitarium (also known as "The San"). The health retreat became the most popular health sanatorium of its time, boasting patients like Henry Ford (1863–1947), John D. Rockefeller (1839–1947), and J.C. Penney (1875–1971). Patients at "the San" closely followed Kellogg's "Battle Creek Idea," a diet that excluded meat and recommended sparing use of eggs, refined sugar, milk, and cheese. This demanded a "lifestyle change," which advocated abstaining from alcohol, tea, coffee, tobacco, and chocolate. The diet also prescribed daily enemas, drinking large quantities of water, and participating in regular exercise and outdoor activity.

"The San" was originally affiliated with the Adventist Church but had moved away from religious practice to a more medical and scientific focus by 1907. Kellogg now appealed to "rational medicine" as "nature alone possesses the power to heal." As in "The San," "patients, and not disease are to be treated" (Kellogg 1907: 593). As such, "The San" included a "Laboratory of Hygiene" that aimed to create new nutritious food products by undertaking the "preliminary digestive work" of the body by "kettle cooking, oven cooking, and toasting" (Kellogg 1907: 1561).

Kellogg's brother, William Keith Kellogg (1860–1951), joined him in his research, and they began experimenting with new kinds of grain products, imitation meats, coffee substitutes, and soy-milk. At this time, manufactured and processed foods were believed to be healthier than "natural" foods. In 1895, they accidentally left a batch of boiled grain (dough) out for several days, allowing it to dry out and become crisp. When they rolled out the dried dough, it formed flakes and a new kind of cereal was born. The flakes, originally named Granose and later known as Toasted Wheat Flakes, immediately became popular, and they sold over 100,000 pounds of the cereal in the first year. The Kellogg brothers established Sanitas Food Company for their new products but experienced major ideological differences relating to both health reform and business. The company split into John's Battle Creek Food Company and William's W.K. Kellogg Company. The latter went on to become one of the most popular food companies, ironically abandoning the "health food" label of its origins. Many have argued today that it was the advent of convenience food that led to many of the problems with obesity, currently considered a major public-health problem in the U.S.A.

SLG/Sarah Gardiner

*See also* Electrotherapy; Fat Camp; Fletcher; Graham; Medieval Diets; Post; Sex; White

## References and Further Reading
Anon. (1943) "J.H. Kellogg Dies; Health Expert, 91," *New York Times*, December 16: Obituaries.

Anon. (1973) "John Harvey Kellogg," *Dictionary of American Biography, Supplement 3: 1941–1945*. American Council of Learned Societies.

Anon. (2001) "John Harvey Kellogg," *Encyclopedia of World Biography Supplement*, Vol. XXI, Detroit, Mich.: Gale Group.

Anon. (2002) "John Harvey Kellogg, Dr.," *Gale Encyclopedia of Medicine*, 2nd edn, five vols, Detroit, Mich.: Gale Group.

Kellogg, J.H. (1896) *The Stomach: Its Disorders, and How to Cure Them*, London: International Tract Society.

—— (1907) *The Home Book of Modern Medicine*, London: C.D. Cazenove & Sons.

Schwarz, Richard, W. (1970) *John Harvey Kellogg, MD*, Nashville, Tenn.: Southern Pub Association.

# Kneipp, Sebastian (1821–97)

One of the major advocates of the use of water to cure disease, Kneipp was born in Stephansried, Germany and died in Wörishofen. He was a Bavarian priest and one of the founders of the nineteenth-century naturopathic ("Naturheilkunde") movement. He is most commonly associated with the "Kneipp Cure" form of hydrotherapy, a system of healing involving the application of water through various methods, temperatures, and pressures. Such cures were commonplace for disorders of metabolism and formed a part of most therapies for overweight until the mid-twentieth century. His Austrian contemporary Vincenz Priessnitz also treated his overweight patients with baths, packs, and showers of cold water. Such approaches are still standard models of therapy in Spain and India. Though today he is mostly known in Norway for his bread recipe (Kneipp Bread), Kneipp was an advocate of a strict "naturopathic" diet including whole grains, fruits, and vegetables with very limited amounts of meat of all kinds. He also advocated the use of regular exercise. His system is spelled out in a series of widely popular books translated into all major languages, many of which are still in print: *My Water Cure*, *Thus Shalt Thou Live*, and *My Will*. In 1997 the German Government printed a stamp in his honor.

SLG

*See also* Fat Camp

## References and Further Reading

Kneipp, Sebastian (1894) *Thus Shalt Thou Live: Hints and Advice for the Healthy and the Sick on a Simple and Rational Mode of Life and a Natural Method of Cure*, London: H. Grevel & Son.
—— (1896) *My Will: A Legacy to the Healthy and the Sick*, London: H. Grevel.
—— (1898) *My Water-Cure: Tested for More Than 35 Years and Published for the Cure of Diseases and the Preservation of Health*, London: H. Grevel.
—— (1996) *Healing and Treatment of Diseases through Water*, Delhi: Sri Satguru Publications.
Richter, Thomas and Caesar, Wolfgang (1998) "Von Kneipp bis zur Phytotherapie: Geschichte der Naturheilverfahren," *Deutsche Apotheker Zeitung* 138: 2848–9.
Schomburg, Eberhard (1963) *Sebastian Kneipp, 1821–1897: Bildnis eines dienenden Lebens*, Bad Wörishofen: Sanitas Verlag KG.

# L

## LaLanne, Jack (1914–)

Also known as Francois Henri LaLanne, the "God-father of fitness." His career in the field spans more than seventy years. At the time of writing ninety-two, LaLanne claims to have begun exercising and eating a healthy diet at the age of fifteen, at which time he considered himself to be a weak, sugarholic junk-food junkie. Suffering from bulimia and headaches, LaLanne decided to get healthy after his father's early death, which was caused in part by poor nutrition (Gentle 2000). LaLanne claims that he was inspired by Paul Bragg, a pioneer nutritionist, who promised him that if he exercised and ate a proper diet, he could regain his health. Highly impressed by Bragg's advice and theories, he cut out sweets and began to exercise. This strict regime helped make him, as he claims, into one of the world's healthiest and finest built men. His muscular development at 5 foot 7 inches, 175 pounds was symmetrical, making him look good from any angle, with especially well-developed abdominals. After seven years of vegetarianism, he slowly reintroduced meat protein to his diet but continued to stay low on carbohydrates, making sure his meals contained all the required vitamins and minerals, through plenty of fruits and vegetables (Gentle 2000).

In 1936, LaLanne became part of a new movement of exercise and diet as part of body reform. He opened the nation's first modern health studio, the Jack LaLanne Physical Culture Studio in Oakland, in 1936. This studio prefigured modern health clubs in many ways, combining a gym, juice bar, and health-food store. At a time when doctors claimed weight-lifting would cause heart attacks and coaches predicted their athletes would become muscle-bound and banned the activity, LaLanne gave athletes keys to his facility so they could work out at night (Gentle 2000). He has since claimed, "Time has proven that what I was doing was scientifically correct—starting with a healthy diet followed by systematic exercise, and today everyone knows it. All world class athletes now work out with weights, as do many members of the general public, both male and female" (LaLanne 1997).

LaLanne also developed many of the first prototypes of exercise equipment used in most modern-day gyms, including the first leg-extension machine, the first pulley machines using cables, and the first weight selectors (Gentle 2000). He eventually opened a chain of gyms (later licensed to Bally) and, in 1951, launched his fitness show. From a sparse set with only a handful of props, LaLanne showed the folks at home how he got—and stayed—strong. "Viewers could see I knew what I was talking about," says LaLanne. *The Jack LaLanne Show* enjoyed immense popularity with viewers and aired for thirty-four years.

As fitness moved into the mainstream during the 1980s, a new generation of instructors promised dramatic results fast, and LaLanne's show, which focused on the fundamentals, was canceled. He became an infomercial staple, hawking high-powered juicers—so far, he's sold more than a million of the 150-dollar machines (Gentle 2000). However, LaLanne continues to extol the virtues of diet and, most importantly, exercise to his fans and followers. He explains,

You can eat perfectly but if you don't exercise, you cannot get by. There are so many health food nuts out there that eat nothing but natural foods but they don't exercise and they look terrible. Then there are other people who exercise like a son-of-a-gun but eat a lot of junk. They look pretty good because the exercise is king. Nutrition is queen. Put them together and you've got a kingdom!

(LaLanne 1997)

Some of LaLanne's most public feats of stamina include 1,033 pushups in twenty-three minutes in 1956, setting a world record at the age of forty-two on *You Asked for It*, a television show with Art Baker. In 1959, he also completed 1,000 pushups and 1,000 chinups in one hour and twenty-two minutes at the age of forty-five (Gentle 2000). At the age of ninety-two, LaLanne continues to exercise routinely and encourages people of all ages to do the same. He has made recent appearances on talk shows such as the *Tonight Show* with Jay Leno on NBC, and he was also commemorated on his ninety-second birthday on *Pardon the Interruption*, a sports commentary/talk show on ESPN.

SLG/JASON WEINSTEIN

*See also* Anorexia; Macfadden; Vegetarianism

## References and Further Reading

Anon. (1994) "Jack LaLanne," *Current Biography* 55 (10): 26–30.

Anon. (2000) "LaLanne, Jack," in Tom Pendergast and Sara Pendergast (eds), *St. James Encyclopedia of Popular Culture*, five vols, Detroit, Mich.: St. James Press.

Gentle, David (2000) "King of Fitness, Jack Lalanne," NaturalStrength.com, June 30, available online at <http://www.naturalstrength.com/history/detail.asp?ArticleID=316> (accessed March 7, 2006).

Katz, Donald (1995) "Jack Lalanne Is Still an Animal," *Outside Magazine*, November, available online at <http://outside.away.com/magazine/1195/11f_jack-.html> (accessed March 7, 2007).

Kolata, Gina (2002) "Ageless Apostle of Muscle," *New York Times*, November 19.

LaLanne, Jack (1997) The Official Jack LaLanne World Wide Web Site, available online at <http://www.jacklalanne.com> (accessed March 7, 2007).

Ottum, Bob (1981) "Look, Mom, I'm an Institution (Jack Lalanne)," *Sports Illustrated* 55 (November 23): 64–9.

# Lambert, Daniel (1770–1809)

## The exemplary fat man of the nineteenth century

By profession a jailer, Lambert came to represent the freakish nature of fat. The novelist George Meredith described London as the Daniel Lambert of cities, and the sociologist Herbert Spencer used the phrase a Daniel Lambert of learning. A wax model of Lambert found its way to America and was shown in the Mix Museum in New Haven in 1813 and later in P.T. Barnum's famous American Museum. Lambert had been displayed as a wonder of nature along with giants and dwarfs much against his own desires (Ritvo 1997: 148–9). He was huge, and yet the contemporary literature stressed that he neither drank nor ate "more than one dish at a meal," and after his death he was remember as a man of great "temperance" (Clarke 1981: 3). Other than his size, he was deemed to be of "perfect health: his

breathing was free, his sleep undisturbed, and all of the functions of his body in excellent order" (Bondeson 2000: 243). In other words, he was huge but healthy and happy.

His early death (at the time he measured 5 feet, 1 inch in height and weighed 739 pounds) was bemoaned by fashionable London that had made him one of the sights that had to be visited when you were on the town. When he died, his body had to be removed from the room in which he was staying by demolishing a wall! As his body weight increased, he went on a perpetual diet, without any decrease in his rate of weight gain. Lambert functions here as an exemplar of great size but also of a social status that is attributable to his "freakish" character. Lambert was one of the "case studies" of obesity of the time and created much interest in obesity as part of the world of medical freakishness.

Indeed, Dr. T. Coe's earlier 1751 letter to the Royal Society about Mr. Edward Bright, the "fat man at Malden in Essex," has a certain breathless quality about it. Bright was "so extremely fat, and of such an uncommon bulk and weight, that I believe there to be very few, if any, such instances to be found in any country, or upon record in any books" (Coe 1751–2: 188). According to Coe, Bright was descended from a lineage of "remarkably fat" people. Extremely fat as a child, he grew in size and weight over the years until at his death at thirty when he weighted more than 616 pounds at 5 feet 9 inches. He was "the gazing-stock and admiration of all people" (Coe 1751–2: 189). He ate "remarkably" and drank much beer, a gallon a day (Coe 1751–2: 191). Those about him saw his "life as a burthen, and death as a happy release" (Coe 1751–2: 192). No respite could have been had by diet or therapy.

William Harvey, one of the noted British obesity specialists turned to the study of obesity in 1872, spurred on, he wrote, by William Banting's success (Harvey 1872: vi). Harvey stressed that the new scientific advances in "physiology and animal chemistry" have meant that one could treat obesity as a disease. To that point, he cited the case of Daniel Lambert, the fattest man on record to that time, who died in 1809 at the age of forty weighing 739 pounds. It was suggested there seemed to have been no attempt to "arrest the progress of the disease" in Lambert's case (Harvey 1872: viii). More insights, Harvey opined, could now have "cured" Lambert.

SLG

*See also* Banting

### References and Further Reading

Bondeson, Jan (2000) *The Two-Headed Boy and Other Medical Marvels*, Ithaca, NY: Cornell University Press.

Clarke, David T.D. (1981) *Daniel Lambert*, Leicester: Leicestershire Museums, Art Galleries and Records Service.

Coe, T. (1751–2) "A Letter . . . Concerning Mr. Bright, the Fat Man at Malden in Essex," *The Royal Society: Philosophical Transactions* 47: 188–9.

Harvey, William (1872) *On Corpulence in Relation to Disease: with Some Remarks on Diet*, London: Henry Renshaw.

Ritvo, Harriet (1997) *The Platypus and the Mermaid and Other Figments of the Classifying Imagination*, Cambridge, Mass.: Harvard University Press.

---

# Leibel, Rudolph, MD (1942–)

## American physician, professor of medicine and pediatrics, Director of the Division of Molecular Genetics, and Co-Director of the Naomi Berrie Diabetes Center, Columbia University

Leibel was known in his younger years, practicing at Harvard and Cambridge City Hospital, as an outstanding pediatric endocrinologist who specialized in hormone disorders. When one of his young patients' frustrated parents made him realize how little he really knew about obesity, he took up a position in Jules Hirsch's laboratory at Rockefeller University in 1978.

Leibel was particularly interested in finding out how the body controlled its weight: altering the "set point". Sometimes thought of as the "Holy Grail" of obesity research, the idea of the set point comes from Jean Mayer (Harvard psychologist), who hypothesized that the body contains a "lipostat" that keeps the amount of fat in the body constant. If researchers learned how to adjust the set point, they could literally control the amount of fat in the body. Leibel threw himself into this work, examining the records of severely obese patients and normal controls at Rockefeller who had lost weight by consuming a special liquid formula as part of clinical studies. Leibel found that the important variable in comparing energy requirements was fat-free body mass—no matter the amount of fat, people with a similar fat-free body mass would require a similar amount of calories. What this meant in practice was that after patients had lost fat below their standard homeostatic point, they would literally require fewer calories to maintain their weight than people who had weighed the same amount as they now weighed and not dieted. Otherwise, they would gain weight.

Leibel realized that some of this body-weight regulation must be genetic, so in 1986 he turned his attention with his collaborator Jeff Friedman (then an assistant professor at Rockefeller) to cloning the ob gene, which was thought to be the cause of obesity in rodents. Graduate student Nathan Bahary, lab technician Ricardo Proenca, and postdoctoral fellows Yiying Zhang and Margherita Maffei did painstaking work over the course of six years in the lab to find the mutation, which resulted in the rodent's fat cells producing a nonfunctional version of a protein that would ordinarily function as a hormone that signaled satiety, a hormone called leptin. Their work was published in *Nature* in 1994, but Bahari and Leibel were left off the author list by Friedman (Shell 2001: 77–104). When the gene was sold by Rockefeller to Amgen for a staggering 20 million dollars up front (the

largest sum at the time a patent had ever been sold for) plus promised future payments as the drug based on leptin got closer to market, Leibel was not eligible for a cut of this money because he was not on the author list. As a result, he left Rockefeller for Columbia University with Zhang to set up his own laboratory.

According to Leibel's website, the lab's current research in the Genetics of Complex Disorders training program at Columbia includes identifying genes in both rodents and humans related to obesity and Type 2 diabetes, particularly those that regulate homeostasis, leptin, and the glucose/insulin cycle at the molecular level.

SLG/KATHARINE MANCUSO

*See also* Friedman; Genetics; Homeostasis; Hormone; Metabolism

### References and Further Reading
Anon. "Rudy Leibel, MD," Genetics of Complex Disorders Training Program, available online at <http://cpmcnet.columbia.edu/dept/sph/epi/gcd/ Preceptors/Leibel.html> (accessed April 20, 2006).

Kolata, Gina (2007) *Rethinking Thin: The New Science of Weight Loss—and the Myths and Realities of Dieting*, New York: Farrar, Straus and Giroux.

Shell, Ellen Ruppel (2001) *The Hungry Gene: The Science of Fat and the Future of Thin*, New York: Atlantic Monthly Press.

# Lessius, Leonard (1554–1623)

## Flemish Jesuit and theologian

In 1613, Lessius wrote his account of his struggles with dieting, the *Hygiasticon*. This text simply repeated much of the diet reformer Cornaro's life as his own; nevertheless, it was widely translated from the Latin and often cited by those arguing for a sober lifestyle, which would assure longevity. It is still in print today.

Rescued from a world of dissipation and fat after his physicians had given him up as lost, he found the simple

pleasures of sobriety and self-limitations, which enabled him to become manlier in his deeds and actions. Lessius not only mirrors the autobiography of Cornaro but also cites St. Augustine's struggle with the pleasures of gluttony as one of his main witnesses (Lessius 1742: 20–1). Lessius paraphrases him, stating that "Lust knows not where Necessitie ends," which is, for Lessius, why one may grow fat (Lessius 1742: 21). He stresses, like

Augustine, that we must all control our desire to "feast and banquet" (Lessius 1742: 85). We can do this is by imagining food as disgusting and bad smelling, for if we do not we shall certainly die, as almost all diseases come from taking more food into the body than "nature requires" (Lessius 1742: 103). Lessius continues by amplifying the arguments of Cornaro about longevity and diet, as well as echoing the theological and moral underpinnings of his text.

SLG

*See also* Christianity; Cornaro

## References and Further Reading

Bailey, John Burn (1888) *Modern Methuselahs: or, Short Biographical Sketches of a Few Advanced Nonagenarians or Actual Centenarians Who Were Distinguished in Art, Science, Literature, or Philanthropy. Also, Brief Notices of Some Individuals Remarkable Chiefly for Their Longevity*, London: Chapman & Hall.
Boia, Lucian (2004) *Forever Young: A Cultural History of Longevity from Antiquity to the Present*, London: Reaktion Books.
Lessius, Leonard (1742) *Hygiasticon*, trans. Timothy Smith, London: Charles Hitch.

# Lindlahr, Henry (1862–1924)

Lindlahr first achieved success in politics and was appointed Mayor of Kalispell, Montana in 1893. At the height of his political success, he began to suffer from diabetes, which he believed was due to his excessive weight. Because insulin was yet to be discovered, his condition was thought to be incurable. Leaving the U.S.A. to search for a cure, Lindlahr sought out Father Sebastian Kneipp's hydrotherapy center at Woerishoffen, Bavaria. There he underwent water therapy and began a new vegetarian diet. His weight quickly dropped, and he regained his health.

Thereafter, Lindlahr returned to the U.S.A. and became very interested in natural healing methods. He read Russell Trall and J.H. Kellogg's works and began to study osteopathy, at that point an alternative approach to medical care (today it is a complementary one). After receiving his license to practice medicine and opening up his own office, he continued his studies on "natural" cures. In 1906, he opened the Lindlahr Sanitarium, which stressed the importance of hydrotherapy, a natural diet that restricted meat, and sunbathing. Lindlahr became one of the chief proponents of iridology, a system of diagnosing disease from study of the iris, the circular colored portion of the eye. As the sanitarium had great success, Lindlahr opened up the Lindlahr College of Nature Cure and Osteopathy.

Lindlahr's system is delineated in his *Nature Cure* (1913). For him, this, and not allopathic medicine, is the exact science because the "underlying laws which correlate and unify its scattered facts and theories have been discovered" (Lindlahr 1921: 17). Thus, the "Nature Cure" "is a system of man-building in harmony with the constructive principle in Nature on the physical, mental, moral, and spiritual planes" (Lindlahr 1921: 17). It is thus so simple that it is difficult to accept, a standard argument against the new complexity of modern medicine (Lindlahr 1921: 10). It treats the entire body and all of its systems. This holistic approach incorporates the moral aspects of human beings in its treatment, and dieting becomes both prevention and cure. If you are ill, a diet of "easily digestible foods as white of egg, milk, buttermilk, whole grain bread with butter in combination with raw and stewed fruits, and with vegetable salad with lemon juice and olive oil" is prescribed (Lindlahr 1921: 130). This diet is one aspect of treatment in addition to fasting, cold packs, and the water cure. To become or remain healthy, Lindlahr provides a detailed account of "natural dietetics" (Lindlahr 1921: 271ff). At its core stands "MILK, which is the only perfect natural food combination in existence" (Lindlahr 1921: 271). Clearly, Lindlahr's notion of cure is aimed against the innovations of allopathic medicine of his day. He condemns "the terrible after effects of X-ray treatment, of extirpation of the ovaries, the womb, and of other vital organs" so common at the time that he wrote (Lindlahr 1921: 271). Natural cure is the opposite of such technological innovations.

In addition, Lindlahr wrote and self-published widely on his theory. His works include: *Acute Diseases Their Uniform Treatment by Natural Methods: Mental, Emotional and Psychic Disorders* (1918); *The Lindlahr Vegetarian Cook Book and ABC of Natural Dietetics* (with his wife Anna in 1918); *Iridiagnosis and other Diagnostic Methods* (1919); and *Philosophy of Natural Therapeutics* (1918).

SLG

*See also* Alternative Medicine; Fat Camp; Kellogg; Kneipp; Milk; Trall; Vegetarianism

## References and Further Reading

Lindlahr, H. (1921) *Nature Cure: Philosophy and Practice Based on the Unity of Disease and Cure*, 17th edn, Chicago, Ill.: Nature Cure Publishing House.

Melton, J. Gordon (1990) *New Age Encyclopedia: A Guide to the Beliefs, Concepts, Terms, People, and Organizations That Make Up the New Global Movement Toward Spiritual Development, Health and Healing, Higher Consciousness, and Related Subjects*, Detroit, Mich.: Gale Research, pp. 164–5.

# Linn, Robert (1933–)

## Creator of a 1970s fad diet that entailed fasting and consuming a drink called Prolinn

Robert Linn is a doctor of osteopathy, and his diet was known as "The Last Chance Diet." Prolinn was a drink, consisting of animal hooves, hides, tendons, horns, bones, and other animal products, which people on the diet drank numerous times a day. In a day, this drink provided 400 calories. The Prolinn diet created a lot of controversy, and there were warnings issued about the drink and its lack of nutrients. At the time, many people thought that it could harm the kidneys due to the protein content. It has been estimated that 2 to 4 million people have tried the diet. While some people claimed to lose weight, at least fifty-eight people reportedly had heart attacks while on the diet. However, it is now thought that the drink itself was not dangerous; it was the fasting that caused health complications.

Linn also co-authored a book called *The Last Chance Diet: A Revolutionary Approach to Weight Loss* in which he presented his diet to the general public. There was, again, legal trouble when, in 1989, a lawsuit was filed against his publisher because someone had allegedly died while on the diet. The judge dismissed the suit on the basis of the First Amendment right of free speech. The court claimed that there was no warranty made through the publication of the book that the diet would work or, indeed, would not be hazardous to a person's health (*Smith* v. *Linn*; Anon. First Amendment Protects). Diet books are thus sheltered from any measure of the efficacy of their suggested methods, and subsequent authors have been free to promote ineffective and even dangerous dietary advice.

SLG/MARY STANDEN

*See also* McGraw; Very-Low-Calorie Diets

**References and Further Reading**

Anon. (1989) "First Amendment Protects Deadly Diet Books:—Smith v. Linn, 386 Pa.Super. 392, 563 A.2d 123 (Pa.Super. 1989)," LSU Law Center's Medical and Public Health Law Site, available online at <http://biotech.law.lsu.edu/obesity/cases/last_chance_diet.htm> (accessed March 12, 2007).

Burros, Marian (2004) "Dieter Sues Atkins Estate and Company." Available online at <http://www.newsmine.org/archive/nature-health/health/obesity/atkins-diet-clogged> (accessed March 12, 2007).

CBC News Online (2004) "Diets: A Primer." Available online at <http://www.cbc.ca/news/background/food/diets.html> (accessed April 5, 2006).

Linn, Robert (1976) *The Last Chance Diet—When Everything Else Has Failed: Dr. Linn's Protein-Sparing Fast Program*, Secaucus, NJ: Lyle Stuart.

*Smith* v. *Linn*, 386 Pa.Super. 392, 563 A.2d 123 (Pa.Super. 1989).

Stahl, Linda (2005) "A Who's Who of American Dieting History." Available online at <http://www.courierjournal.com/apps/pbcs.dll/article?AID=/20051103/FEATURES03/511030322> (accessed April 10, 2006).

# Literature and Fat Bodies

The image of the female body and questions of ideal beauty and its relationship to size have been central to many works of modern fiction. For example, in British author Fay Weldon's *The Life and Loves of a She Devil* (1983) (made into a movie starring Meryl Streep and Roseanne Barr in 1989), the protagonist, Ruth, described on the book's flap copy as a "lumbering, clumsy woman, over six feet tall, with a jutting jaw topped by spouting moles," revenges herself on her petite (and beautiful) rival by destroying her life and then having cosmetic surgery so that she can literally assume her physical presence. Weldon's novel and the film based on it provide a caustically humorous look at society's expectations of women—especially of women who become mothers and wives. More recently, author Jennifer Weiner, herself a plus-size Jewish-American woman, has come out with romantic comedies, such as *In Her Shoes* (2002) (made into a film in 2005 and starring Cameron Diaz and Toni Collette) and *Good in Bed* (2001), in which the heroines are also plus-size. They don't, however, lose weight at the end of the tale. Instead, they have healthy and very active sex lives and also find Mr. Right without transforming into delicate beauties.

Helen Fielding's wildly successful *Bridget Jones's Diary* (1996) (filmed in 2001 with a "zaftig" Renée Zellweger) is also a candid look at the various demons that plague single, almost middle-aged, white-collar women in a late-capitalist world. The eponymous Ms. Jones is forever on a diet because she sees herself as too large, but she is just as forever reneging on them. Indeed, each of the entries in her fictional diary is prefaced by weight measurements and food or alcohol intake. In a bit of irony toward the end of the novel, Bridget reaches her goal weight, and people tell her she does not look well. Popular literary representations of dieting tend to focus on middle- to upper-middle-class white women trying to fit a hegemonic body ideal. Success is often in spite of one's body not because of it. The proof is heterosexual love.

The focus of literary representations of obesity and bodily difference has not, however, been exclusively on women. At the beginning of the twentieth century, Edna Ferber's "The Gay Old Dog" (1917) condemns Jo Hertz, an old bachelor, to a single life with his demanding sisters and mother. At fifty, he is fat, and his body rebels in "his fat-encased muscles" when he tries to look youthful (Ferber 1947: 12). After a love affair destroyed by the demands of his family, he falls into a bachelor's life as his sisters move on to their own married or professional lives. He becomes "a rather frumpy old bachelor, with thinning hair and a thickening neck" (Ferber 1947: 19). During the beginning of the Great War, he watches the troops march down Michigan Avenue as they go off to war when a voice in back of him shouts "Let me by! I can't see! . . . You big fat man! My boy's going by—to war—and I can't see!" It is his former lover who has married and whose son is marching. He sees the boy and "picked him assuredly as his own father might have" (Ferber 1947: 26). He returns to his home and his sisters confront him about his social life, at which time he turns on them: "You two murderers! You didn't consider me, twenty years ago. . . . Where's my boy! You killed him, you two, twenty years ago. And now he belongs to somebody else. Where's my son that should have gone marching by today?" (Ferber 1947: 27). Rendered impotent by his family, Jo's body is the public sign of his thwarted reproductive drive.

The quintessential fat boy's novel in American literature is John Kennedy Toole's *A Confederacy of Dunces* (1980). His protagonist, Ignatius J. Reilly, is depicted as "waves of flesh rippling beneath the tweed and flannel, waves that broke upon buttons and seams" (Toole 1980: 13–14). His external appearance reflects his own asexuality. Reilly's New York-born, Jewish college girlfriend Myrna Minkoff has failed in her many attempts to seduce him because "my stringent attitude toward sex intrigued her; in a sense I became another project of sorts" (Toole 1980: 137). Are fat men asexual, or are they perceived as asexual, or are they made asexual by marriage, or is their sexuality damaged by their fat?

The protagonist of Kingsley Amis's *One Fat Englishman* (1963), Roger Micheldene, is concerned with "keeping hidden the full enormity of his fatness" when he is off to seduce women. "Recent experience suggested that that belly, exposed in a moment of inattention or abandon, could cause total withdrawal of favours previously granted" (Amis 1963: 18). In Salman Rushdie's first novel, *Grimus* (1977), a fantasy work centering on a quartet of misfits, one of them, Virgil Jones, "gross of body" (Rushdie 1977: 12), is in love with the hunchbacked Dolores O'Toole: "they loved each other and found it impossible to declare their love. It was no beautiful love, for they were extremely ugly" (Rushdie 1977: 12). When they finally do make love, their "disfiguration [is] transformed into sexuality" (Rushdie 1977: 50). "Her hands grasping great folds of his flesh . . . It's like making bread, she giggled, pretending to work his belly into a loaf" (Rushdie 1977: 50). Only the disfigured may love the disfigured, and in the rhetoric of the novel the fat boy is as disfigured as the hunchbacked woman. The power of literary representations can allow characters to use their weight as a protection against the world or as a

sign of their own impotence. In the end, no one loves a fat man.

There is also a body of literature for young adults, which deals with issues of body image and dieting. There is one particular subgenre called the young adult (YA) romance whose themes often revolve around young women and body politics. As Brenda O. Daly remarks, this fiction is an exploration of "the quest for thinness, which sometimes, leads to eating disorders, [and] is most common among white girls in the middle and upper-middle classes, the exact readership of YA romances" (Daly 1989: 52). Daly argues that the belly/viscera, which is the site for both sexual urges as well as hunger pangs, has become a site of conflict for the upper-class woman, who must suppress both kinds of appetites.

This phenomenon is reflected in YA fiction: The heroines of these books tend to be "saintly" and constrained, neither admitting to a desire for their lovers, nor to a desire for food. Daly also notes that psychological as much as physical nourishment is at the heart of this genre and suggests that the young women in these books experience a continued and often frustrated need for the mother's nurturing influence (which is typically terminated at the oedipal turn). This lack expresses itself in how the heroine's conflicted relationship with food is also connected to her strained, unfulfilling relationship with her mother. As an example, Daly refers to a book written as part of the *Starfire* series, created in the 1980s by the author/creator of the Sweet Valley High franchise, Francine Pascal (and written by a wide range of ghostwriters). *True Love* is about Caitlyn Ryan, a student at the upper crust HighGate academy. She is madly in love with Jed Michaels but pretends when she sees him that she doesn't want to, because, "ladies (and only ladies are allowed in HighGate Academy) do not admit to such desires" (Campbell and Pascal 1986: 52). Most popular literature that engages dieting as a theme, then, is raced, classed, and gendered.

The YA fiction for adolescent boys that deals with weight, weight reduction, and the social stigma of obesity aims for the most part to ameliorate the difficulty of such a social position rather than to encourage weight loss. Certainly, the most appalling model for the fat male child is in William Golding's *Lord of the Flies* (1954), where the character of Piggy is described as a "bag of fat." He is introduced to us as a fat boy defined by his pathologies: " 'I was the only boy in our school what had asthma,' said the fat boy with a touch of pride. 'And I've been wearing specs since I was three' " (Golding 1954: 8). Suffering from asthma, he becomes the representative of the rational trapped in the body of the fat boy. Thus, he is eventually the human sacrifice that signals the final breakdown of all civilization among the children on the island:

> Piggy fell forty feet and landed on his back across the square red rock in the sea. His head opened and stuff came out and turned red. Piggy's arms and legs twitched a bit, like a pig's after it has been killed. Then the sea breathed again in a long, slow sigh, the water boiled white and pink over the rock; and when it went, sucking back again, the body of Piggy was gone.
>
> (Golding 1954: 181)

He is the most degenerate of the children in terms of his dependence on civilization (his glasses as an example) and, at the same time, the most civilized. Once his tenuous ties to civilization are destroyed, he is unable to function in the "natural" world of childhood thinness and cruelty. His "asthma" marks his body as much as does his corpulence.

Golding's novel, popular with young readers, does not offer the "moral" lessons of confronting one's own difference that is demanded by YA literature dealing with obese males. By 1971, Robert Lipsyte's autobiographical novel *One Fat Summer*, recounts how his alter ego, Bobby Marks, struggles through a summer at Rumson Lake, where he learns both moral and physical self-control. Likewise, the Australian author Ian Bone's *Fat Boy Saves the World* (1998) shows how the fat but graceful "Neat" can change others while being true to his own "fat" self. Catharine Forde's *Fat Boy Swim* (2000) shows how morbidly obese fifteen-year-old Jimmie learns to swim and shows the athlete hidden under the layers of fat. Chris Crutcher's *Staying Fat for Sarah Byrnes* (1993) pairs the obese narrator Eric Calhoune with Sarah Byrnes, whose face and hands were hideously disfigured in a childhood accident. Outsiders show great moral courage to aid one another. There is no Piggy here.

In dealing with dieting, certain genres also validate, albeit implicitly, the extreme consumerist ethic that informs dieting culture. Jan Cohn analyses the centrality of the market and themes of ownership and exchange in the romance novel genre. She cites research by feminist journalist and thinker Barbara Ehrenreich, who found in her review of magazines like *Playboy* in the late 1970s/ early 1980s that the image of the ideal American man had changed over the years. In popular representations, the model American male went from being frugal, hardworking, and family-oriented to being an individualist who worked hard but played harder, when it came to money and women (Cohn 1988). The women who figure in popular fiction as a whole and in the romance novel in particular are configured to be the handsome, well-built, successful hero's perfect counterpart. They often have bodies and consumption patterns that conform to and perpetuate the dominant social ideal. Many of these women eat conscientiously, with an eye on their weight.

SLG/SHRUTHI VISSA

*See also* Southern Fat

## References and Further Reading

Amis, Kingsley (1963) *One Fat Englishman*, New York: Summit.

Bone, Ian (1998) *Fat Boy Saves the World*, New York: Pocket Pulse.

Campbell, Joanna and Pascal, Francine (1986) *True Love*, Toronto: Bantam.

Cohn, J. (1988) *Romance and the Erotics of Property: Mass Market Fiction for Women*, Durham, NC: Duke University Press.

Crutcher, Chris (1993) *Staying Fat for Sarah Byrnes*, New York, N.Y: Greenwillow Books.

Daly, Brenda O. (1989) "Laughing WITH, or AT, the Young Adult Romance," *The English Journal* 78 (6): 50–60.

Ferber, Edna (1947) "The Gay Old Dog," in *One Basket*, Chicago, Ill.: Peoples Book Club, pp. 11–28.

Fielding, Helen (1996) *Bridget Jones's Diary*, New York: Penguin Books.

Forde, Catharine (2000) *Fat Boy Swim*, Harlow, Essex: Pearson/Longman.

Golding, William (1954) *Lord of the Flies*, New York: Berkley.

Lipsyte, Robert (1971) *One Fat Summer*, New York: Harper & Row.

Rushdie, Salman (1977) *Grimus*, London: Granada.

Toole, John Kennedy (1980) *A Confederacy of Dunces*, New York: Grove Press.

Weiner, Jennifer (2001) *Good in Bed*, New York:
   Washington Square Press.
—— (2002) *In Her Shoes*, New York: Pocket Star Books.

Weldon, Faye (1983) *The Life and Loves of She-Devil*,
   New York: Pantheon Books.

# Low-Fat and Fat-Free Foods

For years, people have debated the efficacy of diets that promise to help one lose weight and keep it off. The subjects of these debates include low-carbohydrate, no-carbohydrate, low-fat, fat-free, and high-fiber diets, among others. As dieting has become an integral part of American culture, specific foods and diets have been created and marketed to appeal to the desires of the public. In recent years, supermarkets have continuously been filled with new food products created and labeled as "low-fat," or "fat-free," making them more alluring to those who are seeking weight loss or a healthy lifestyle. Fad diets have proliferated in the U.S.A. since the nineteenth century; however, they just as often fall out of favor. Within the span of only a year or two, a diet can go from being endorsed by nutritional sponsors to being shunned. In comparison to extreme diets, such as the Atkins Diet, which were rejected by nutritionists soon after they become popular, a diet low in fat has been popular for decades.

According to the U.S. Food and Drug Administration, in order for a food to be considered fat-free, it must have less than 0.5 grams per reference amount and per labeled serving, (for meals less than 0.5 grams per labeled serving). A low-fat food has 3 grams or less per reference amount (and per 50 grams if reference amount is small and for meals, less than 3 grams per serving). During the past twenty years, however, the amount and type of dietary fat that one should consume in order to maintain a healthy diet has become the source of great controversy. While fat is often portrayed as a dietary scoundrel, it ironically has many health benefits. According to the *Nutrition and Health Encyclopedia*, fats should take up 30 percent of caloric intake, functioning to supply the majority of food energy (Tver and Russel 1989: 375). While the consumption of fat is essential for one to live and maintain a healthy diet and body, the right types of fats must be consumed. Modern societies generally eat a diet high in saturated fat, sugar, refined foods, and low in fiber—often termed the "Western Diet." Many believe that this diet is the reason for the prevalence of obesity as well as high levels of chronic and degenerative diseases (Popkin 1993: 138). Ironically, as the prevalence of obesity in America and most Western cultures is climbing by the year, more low-fat and fat-free foods are appearing and being endorsed on the market.

There may, however, be a cause-and-effect relationship between the popularity of low-fat and fat-free foods and the rising levels of obesity. Nutritionist Barry M. Popkin has observed that the rise in diseases related to high fat intake and obesity has caused a health-conscious behavioral change. During the 1980s and 1990s, the U.S. population started increasingly to eat low-fat foods and reject high-fat foods (Popkin 1993: 145). As the variety of low-fat and fat-free foods continues to increase, it becomes easier to attain and eat these types of foods.

In the U.S.A., dietary patterns often differ by income. People who earn higher incomes and are generally more educated are more likely to follow a low-fat diet than those who earn low incomes. Fat and sugar provide dietary energy at a very low cost and are, therefore, all the more appealing to low-income people. Low-fat products are also more expensive in comparison to similar foods with higher fat contents. For example, at the online grocery store, www.netgrocer.com, Baked Lays, which are low-fat, cost 61 cents per ounce, while Regular Lays, which are not low-fat, cost 35 cents per ounce.

Food consumption is very much based on price, explaining the recent studies, which have applied economic theories to changing dietary behavior. For example, two community-based intervention studies completed by the University of Minnesota School of Public Health revealed that price reductions are an effective strategy to increase the purchase of more healthful foods in community-based settings, such as work sites and schools

(French 2003: 841S). In twelve Minnesota work sites and twelve secondary schools, when the prices of low-fat foods in vending machines were reduced by 10, 25, and 50 percent, the percentage of sales of the low-fat foods increased by 9, 39, and 93 percent respectively (French 2003: 842S). Based on this study, which demonstrates the importance of price in relation to food consumption, the high acquisition of fast food and "supersize portions" makes sense because they are large quantity/low price foods.

While a portion of the population in recent years has been consuming a lower-fat diet, consisting of many low-fat and fat-free foods, a great number of people in the Western world have been consuming high-fat foods. This has resulted in the rise of obesity rates and high health risks for more and more people. Being overweight or obese increases the risk of many health conditions, including hypertension, dyslipidemia, Type 2 diabetes, coronary heart disease, stroke, gallbladder disease, osteoarthritis, sleep apnea, respiratory problems, and specific cancers (Centers for Disease Control). Due to rising obesity rates and obesity-related health problems, the promotion of low-fat and fat-free foods and healthy fats (i.e., Omega 3 Fatty Acids) have become ever more important. The U.S. Department of Health and Human Services recommends that total fat intake should not exceed more than 30 percent of total caloric intake and that saturated fat should account for no more than 10 percent of daily caloric intake. Increased consumption of low-fat and fat-free foods aids in weight loss and benefits an individual's health, possibly preventing certain diseases as well as lowering cholesterol and blood pressure. Considering that 1 gram of fat has 9 calories in it, while 1 gram of protein or carbohydrate contains only 4 calories, it is clear why diets lower in fat often lead to weight loss.

However, while it would make sense for people who consume many low-fat and fat-free foods to lose weight, this is not always the case. For some people, consuming a low-fat diet does lead to a lower calorie diet and weight loss, but for others, low-fat diets do not correlate with lower-calorie diet. Often, when a food is labeled low-fat or fat-free, people eat more in quantity, canceling out the weight-loss effect of the food. This particular phenomenon would explain the increasing rates of obesity as more low-fat and fat-free foods are available, and more people consume a smaller percentage of calories from total fat (Kennedy et al. 1999: 207).

In 1998, the U.S. Department of Agriculture performed a study, which focused on the patterns of dietary fat intake of the U.S. population. The study concluded that while the general fat and saturated-fat intakes as a percentage of total calories have been declining over the past thirty years, a majority of individuals do not consume a diet which meets the levels of fat and saturated fat recommended by the Dietary Guidelines for Americans (Kennedy et al. 1999, 211). In essence, individuals are generally consuming more calories while simultaneously reducing fat intake as a percentage of total calories.

Often people who eat low-fat and fat-free foods, reducing their overall fat intake, also suffer from an energy loss and, therefore, start to eat higher-fat foods. The energy loss is usually a result of eating the wrong foods. In order to keep energy levels high on a low-fat diet, it is important to consume foods which are low in fat but also nutrient-dense. For example, an individual could switch from a high-fat snack to a piece of fruit or from full-fat cottage cheese to low-fat cottage cheese. These tradeoffs allow the dieter to consume needed nutrients while lowering the fat and calorie content of their food.

The obesity epidemic has become a global concern. In recent years, society has facilitated an environment where palatability rather than health is most salient, which explains the rise in obesity (Roefs et al. 2005: 733). As the importance of a healthy diet is continually and publicly stressed, the general population, be it a result of taste, cost, lack of education, or apathy, continues to consume a diet too high in fat. While fat is essential to living, consuming the right amount and types of fat are necessary to maintain a healthy diet. Though low-fat and fat-free foods will aid weight loss, it is also important keep caloric intake equal to caloric expenditure and lead an active lifestyle.

SLG/Laura Goldstein

*See also* Atkins; Obesity Epidemic; Ornish; Socioeconomic Status

## References and Further Reading
Centers for Disease Control and Prevention "Overweight and Obesity: Home," Department of Health and Human Services, available online at <http://www.cdc.gov/nccdphp/dnpa/obesity> (accessed March 12, 2007).
Center for Food Safety and Applied Nutrition (2004)

"Definitions of Nutrient Content Claims," U.S. Food and Drug Administration food labeling guide, available online at <http://www.cfsan.fda.gov/~dms/flg-6a.html> (accessed March 12, 2007).

French, Simone A. (2003) "Symposium: Sugar and Fat—from Genes to Culture-Pricing Effects on Food Choices," *American Society for Nutritional Sciences* (March): 841S–843S.

Kennedy, Eileen T., Bowman, Shanthy A., and Powell, Renee (1999) "Dietary-Fat Intake in the U.S. Population," *Journal of the American College of Nutrition* 18 (3): 207–12.

Popkin, Barry M. (1993) "Nutritional Patterns and Transitions," *Population and Development Review* 19 (1): 138–54.

Roefs, A., Quaedackers, L., Werrij, M.Q., Wolters, G., Havermans, R., Nederkoorn, C., Breukelen, G. van, and Jansen, A. (2005) "The Environment Influences Whether High-Fat Foods Are Associated with Palatable or with Unhealthy," *Behavior Research and Therapy* 44 (5): 715–34.

Tver, David F. and Russel, Percy (eds) (1989) *The Nutrition and Health Encyclopedia*, New York: Van Nostrand Reinhold.

U.S. Department of Agriculture "Choose a Diet Low in Fat, Saturated Fat, and Cholesterol," the United States Department of Agriculture, available online at <http://www.health.gov/dietaryguidelines/dga95/lowfat.htm> (accessed March 12, 2007).

# Luther, Martin (1483–1546)

## German reformer, polemicist, and theologian

An advocate of the abandonment of celibacy for the clergy, and creator of the Protestant distinction between the merely huge and the obese, Luther's is the central theological statement of a distinction that remained in place until at least the mid-twentieth century, which sees a difference between a "healthy" and a "pathologically" fat body. Luther condemned the excesses of Catholic fasts, yet he advocated moderate fasting to make the body able to care for others' needs. There is a none-too-subtle view that religious fasting must have consequences in this world. For Luther, the distinction is always between the healthy and the diseased body, rather than between the fat and thin body.

This distinction is found in Martin Luther's commentary on 1 Cor. 15, the text that set the modern image of the bloated body (Luther 1973: 28 and 196). Man must bear his earthly body as a confinement for the soul. He drags his heavy paunch about with him, and the mortal body is symbolized by the paunch, the sack of stench, which man must endure. He stuffs himself, evacuates, discharges mucus, and suppurates, as a consequence of his mortality (Luther 1973: 172). The ailments that plague fat bodies are sickness, misfortune, frailty, filth, blemishes, and stench, which are always attributed to the influence of Satan (Luther 1973: 203). This heavy existence contrasts with the heavenly body that will move though all the heavens as swiftly and lightly as lightning and soar over the clouds among the dear angels (Luther 1973: 143, 188, 196). Above all, it will be devoid of all infirmities and wants (Luther 1973: 172). The contrast between heavy and light bodies, which Luther occasionally employs, is common among the Greek and Latin fathers. Luther's text depicts only fat bodies this side of heaven (Cornfield 1996). Indeed, any of the Commentary's descriptions of life on earth are bound to mention the paunch and the gut that extends out in front of us, a perpetual reminder of our fleshiness. This paunch eclipses the genitalia as the most salient image of carnality.

However, Luther also differentiates good fat from bad fat and Christian bodies from diabolical bodies in describing distinct types of fat bodies: the bloated and solid. Each of these bodies corresponds to a mode of being in the world. The bloated body relies on the image of the puffed up body from Paul. When Luther observes that the opponents of Paul in Corinth claimed that they knew better than he about God, Luther compares them to Isaiah's audience whom he describes as "arrogant and miserly paunches" and "vexatious windbags" (Luther 1973: 158). Their proud bellies are expansive but only because they are filled with air. These bodies are fat but certainly not solid. In keeping with this image, Luther continually invokes the image of the pig which, although bulky, has a reputation as perhaps the least solid of all animals. It waddles on stubby legs, fat jiggling, and resembles a curious balloon more than a mass of solid flesh. Invoking this fat flimsiness, Luther makes an explicit connection between the pig and the arrogant, bloated body (Luther 1973: 148). "Swinish" becomes his preferred adjective for this type of existence. For Luther the swinish man stuffs his paunch until it covers his penis, thereby eliminating his sexuality.

The opposite of this puffy, bloated figure of false belief is the fat but solid body. These are healthy bodies. Every human being, without exception, gains weight for the slaughter (i.e., death) when Satan will devour us. The difference is that the swinish herd actively fatten themselves, while true Christians passively endure being stuffed by Satan. Luther writes of the bloated ones: "Let those people go their way with their mocking, their carousing and swilling and living like swine that wallow around among the husks and fatten themselves until they are slaughtered" (Luther 1973: 164). But regarding the Christians he writes: "Satan dispenses no other food than pestilence and every other sickness and pours no other wine of drink than pure poison. Therefore we can expect nothing else than that he will fill us with this and then butcher and flay us" (Luther 1973: 111–12). The bloated body and the solid body acquire their fat differently and mean something quite different. True Christians possess a remedy for Satan's poisonous edibles, and that is nourishment from God's Word. Unlike the bloated glutton who is always looking for food to consume, the Christian (again passively) receives sustenance from God. Luther writes: "See to it that you remain in the Word. By it God wants to bear you up and sustain you, so that you will not be lost" (1973: 75). The Christian has access to God's nourishment through the Word and is, thereby, given a healthy supplement to his or her diabolical diet.

For Erik Erikson, this passivity is a return to the mother who "taught him to touch the world with his searching mouth and his probing senses." He writes that "I think that in the Bible Luther at last found a mother whom he could acknowledge: he could attribute to the Bible a generosity to which he could open himself, and which he could pass on to others, at last a mother's son" (Erikson 1993: 208). A mother with her suckling child (Mary and Jesus) is Luther's crucial image for establishing a healthy relation to the Word. Above all, the solid constitution is characterized by its passive relation to external powers, both to Satan who inflicts disease and to God whence flows the maternal milk of the Word. Thus, the moral order of Pauline Christianity and its image of the fat body are converted into a diet culture rooted in belief and sustenance.

SLG

*See also* Christianity; Religion and Dieting

## References

Cornfield, Thomas (1996) "Luther, Paracelsus, and the Spirit," Ph.D. diss., University of Chicago.

Erikson, Erik H. (1993) *Young Man Luther: A Study in Psychoanalysis and History*, New York: W.W. Norton & Company Inc.

Luther, Martin (1973) "Commentary on 1 Corinthians 15," in Hilton C. Oswald (ed.), *Luther's Works*, Vol. XXVIII, Saint Louis, Mo.: Concordia Publishing House.

# M

## Macfadden, Bernarr (1868–1955)

### Known as the "Father of Physical Culture" and was nicknamed "Body Love" Macfadden by *Time* magazine

**B**orn Bernard Macfadden, he was a weak and sickly child. Orphaned at a young age, Macfadden seldom had time for exercise. At age sixteen, disgusted by his physical form, which he referred to as "a complete wreck" and mistrusting of the medical profession, Macfadden bought a pair of dumbbells and created a daily exercise schedule for himself. He was inspired after reading William Blaikie's *How to Get Strong and How to Stay So* (1879), which was also a weight-loss system. Blaikie advocated exercise and diet for those with "considerable superfluous flesh" (Blaikie 1879: 155). Macfadden quickly added long walks outside, cold baths, minimal clothing, and mostly vegetarian eating habits to this regimen. In 1887, he opened his first studio in St. Louis under the name "Bernard Macfadden—Kinestherapist—Teacher of Higher Physical Culture." Having coined the new "scientific" label of "kinestherapist," he also created the slogan that he would use all his life: "Weakness is a crime; don't be a criminal!"

Macfadden first advertised this health regimen, which he dubbed "physical culture" at the Chicago World's Fair in 1893, which is also where he saw Eugene Sandow, the first great celebrity bodybuilder. Knowing the value of publicity, such as that which propelled Sandow's career, in 1898 Macfadden began publishing a monthly magazine called *Physical Culture*. It was at this time that he changed his name to Bernarr, which he believed was a stronger version of his given name. By 1900, the magazine, which featured scantily clad but physically fit individuals, was selling thousands of copies at 15 cents per issue. The link between bodybuilding culture and the erotic, especially the male erotic, was clear. This was a surprising antidote to the early link between "unnatural sexuality" and the diet culture. Macfadden went on to start Macfadden Publications and the Bernarr Macfadden Foundation, as well as "healthatoriums" and vegetarian restaurants where he promoted his philosophies on health and fitness. His most grandiose plan was "Physical Culture City," which was to have 30,000 inhabitants whose "alert minds would be sheltered in healthy bodies" on 1,900 acres in New Jersey. However, the cult of bodybuilding and nudism made the project scandalous. It floundered when, in 1907, *Physical Culture* was accused of obscenity and Macfadden was sentenced to two years of hard labor and a 2,000-dollar fine. While William Howard Taft pardoned him, the stigma of pornography remained associated with Macfadden's "health culture."

In 1919, Macfadden achieved huge success with the young working-class audience when he published *True Story*, a magazine focusing on first-hand confessions of sex and other sins. By 1930, Macfadden was worth 30 million dollars, but the Great Depression hurt him severely. He died in 1955 trying to cure himself of jaundice by fasting.

SLG/Sarah Gardiner

*See also* Bodybuilding; Graham; Taft; Vegetarianism

**References and Further Reading**

Bennett, Jim (2007) "Bernarr Macfadden (1868–1955), the "Father of Physical Culture." Available online at <http://www.bernarrmacfadden.com> (accessed March 11, 2007).

Blaikie, William (1879) *How to Get Strong and How to Stay So*, New York: Harper Brothers.

Ernst, Robert (1991) *Weakness Is a Crime: The Life of Bernarr Macfadden*, Syracuse, NY: Syracuse University Press.

Hunt, William R. (1989) *Body Love: The Amazing Career of Bernarr Macfadden*. Bowling Green, Ohio: Bowling Green State University Popular Press.

Todd, J. (1987) "Bernarr Macfadden: Reformer of Feminine Form," *Journal of Sport History* 14 (1): 61–75.

# McGraw, Phil, Ph.D. (1950–)

## Psychologist and former American collegiate football player, who became a television talkshow host by providing quasi-therapeutic approaches to personal problems

McGraw's show is the middle-brow answer to the American reveal-all, confrontational shows created by Sally Jessy Raphaël (beginning in 1983) and then honed by Jerry Springer. Like his predecessors, *The Dr. Phil Show* features programs dedicated to weight issues, including obesity and eating disorders. For example, Raphaël dealt critically with the dieting culture on a show aired on August 17, 1990. McGraw, however, seems to accept the body norms of the society in which he works and advocates weight reduction through altering what he calls the "personal truth ... whatever you, at the absolute core of your being, believe to be true about yourself" (McGraw 2003: 49).

McGraw was born in Wichita Falls, Texas, and he developed his interest in psychology after his father returned to college at the age of forty to pursue a degree in psychology. He began his career as a television psychologist as a regular guest on *The Oprah Winfrey Show* in 1988. In 2002, he was given his own self-help television show on CBS and became widely recognized in the U.S.A. as "Dr. Phil."

In September of 2003, he published *The Ultimate Weight Loss Solution* in which he details a dieting program based on his psychology of dieting. His selling point, as with such self-help books since William Banting, rested on autobiography as proof of the efficacy of his method. In addition to his dieting book, he has written a stream of other books on relationships and coping with difficult personal situations through psychological counseling and therapy. His promise at the beginning of his dieting book is that through this approach one will not only lose weight but have a new (and happy) life: "When you follow my instructions and take decisive and effective action ... you will begin to live with such a high level of health, energy, vitality, and control that your life will seem like new" (McGraw 2003: 5). His approach is a variant on the behavior modification method.

McGraw advocates "managing" rather than losing weight by creating "right thinking, emotional control, a no-fail environment, habit control, food control, body control, social control." The mantra of "control" means that older notions of "willpower" are done away with: "You don't need willpower.... You have been lied to by the diet industry that you require willpower ... You believed that you failed because ... you were weak and inadequate" (McGraw 2003: 17). His claim, as with other advocates of behavior modification, is that dieters must change their self-image and their pattern of relating to food and eating in all possible circumstances. As is evident from the work done evaluating behavior modification this approach has a high level of immediate effectiveness (as most diets do) but does not actually maintain weight loss over time. McGraw also advocates "high-response, high-yield" (food-group balancing of protein, fats, and carbohydrates) as opposed to "low-response cost, low-yield foods" (McGraw 2003: 302).

The latter consists of high-carbohydrate and high-fat foods from carbonated, sugar-sweetener drinks to ice cream. He thus supplies nutritional as well as psychological approaches to weight loss.

The tie-in with his television show and his connection with American television's favorite dieter, Oprah Winfrey, has made him the most visible public advocate for psychological interventions for weight loss at the beginning of the twenty-first century. Yet his function as a paid spokesman for Texas-based CSA Nutraceuticals, which makes the "Shape Up" shakes, bars, and multivitamins, as dieting aids has led to a lawsuit by those who tried these products with no appreciable weight loss. The company settled the lawsuit for 10.5 million dollars.

By 2005, McGraw had abandoned his advocacy of the "Shape Up!" diet plan, and dieting advocacy seems to have become much less important on his television show. Nevertheless, his books have been a commercial success, published in thirty-seven languages with more than 23 million copies in print.

SLG/Suzanne Judd

*See also* Aboulia; Banting; Professionalization of Dieting; Psychotherapy and Weight Change; Self-help

### References and Further Reading

Anon. "About Dr. Phil, Biography," Dr. Phil's Official Website, available online at <http://www.drphil.com/shows/page/bio> (accessed March 18, 2006).

Anon. "Dr. Phil," The Biography Channel, available online at <http://www.thebiographychannel.co.uk/biography_story/1111:242/1/Dr_Phil.htm> (accessed March 18, 2006).

McGraw, Phil (2003) *The Ultimate Weight Solution: The 7 Keys to Weight Loss Freedom*, New York: Free Press.

# Manheim, Camryn (1961–)

## Jewish American actress

**B**orn Debra Francis Manheim. No one, she writes, "understood what it was like to grow up as a fat, Jewish girl in America" (Manheim 1999: 161). Ethnicity and body size still play a major role in her self-representation. She is considered overweight by the American public because she is 5 foot 10 inches tall and weighs over 200 pounds; however, she is also a highly visible celebrity and icon of the fat-positive movement. In 1998, she won an Emmy Award for Best Supporting Actress for her performance as Ellenor Frutt on the television series *The Practice* (1997–2004) and, during her acceptance speech, she jovially exclaimed, "This is for all the fat girls!"

As evidenced by her speech, Manheim is an active feminist and a self-proclaimed champion of curvy, voluptuous bodies; she is against the existence of a weight standard. In essence, she is an activist of fat-acceptance. In her autobiography, she explains how she came to realize her potential as a spokesperson for fat acceptance when, "a friend of mine told me about the size-acceptance movement. She told me there was a whole subculture in which fat was not only accepted but celebrated. I was told to check out Dimensions magazine" (Manheim 1999: 118). This investigation paid off, and Manheim has now turned fat acceptance into a productive part of her work.

In her autobiographical one-woman off-Broadway show, *Wake Up, I'm Fat!* (1995), Manheim candidly reveals how American culture fosters eating disorders and dangerous behavior in its insistence that people lose weight. She recounts her own experiences with addiction to speed pills, which she took in order to increase her metabolism. Her role as the celebrity representative of the fat-acceptance movement seems to have surprised her: "I never intended to become the spokesperson for the fat-acceptance movement. But I did want to provide an alternative role model to young girls so they wouldn't feel such pressure" (Manheim 1999: 217).

Manheim later rewrote her play into a bestselling

book of the same name. The book, like the play, has been well received by critics and members of the public who are looking for alternatives to the stick-thin role models who dominate fashion and media. According to the *Village Voice*, Manheim is regarded as a "supersize role model, especially for women struggling with body issues, dieting, eating disorders, and low self-esteem" (Taormino 2000). She is active in the civil-rights world at large, which she sees as a legacy of her Jewish, academic parents (Manheim 1999: 74).

SLG

*See also* Celebrities; Fat-Positive

**References and Further Reading**

Heyamoto, Lisa (1999) "Camryn Manheim Delivers Wake-Up Call to Kane Hall," *University of Washington Student Newspaper: The Daily*, March 25.

Manheim, Camryn (1999) *Wake Up I'm Fat!* New York: Broadway Books.

Taormino, Tristan (2000) "Pucker up: XXL," *Village Voice*, February 16–22, available online at <http://www.villagevoice.com/people/0007,taormino,12533,24.html> (accessed April 19, 2006).

# Marcé, Louis-Victor (1828–64)

## French physician best known for his work regarding psychiatric disorders in postpartum women

In 1858, Marcé wrote *Traité de la folie des femmes enceintes*, a treatise about emotional disorders during pregnancy and after delivery. Equally important was his role in understanding anorexia nervosa in the nineteenth century. In a paper delivered to the Medical Psychological Society in Paris on October 31, 1859, Marcé described "young girls, who at the period of puberty and a precocious physical development, become subject to 'inappetency' carried to the utmost limits. Whatever the duration of their abstinence they experience a distaste for food" (1860: 833). Publishing in French and in English more than a decade before William Gull (who cites him), Marcé is regarded as "anorexia nervosa's forgotten man" because his commentary and evaluation of the disorder was generally ignored (Silverman 1989: 833). Yet, Marcé's descriptions of anorexia nervosa and the "inflexible, rigid, and stubborn characteristics of the personalities of anorexia nervosa patients" (Halmi 1999: 1673) are the first of their kind in modern medicine. The researchers and physicians of the twentieth century went on to follow Marcé's diagnostic criteria.

Marcé believed that the first physicians who addressed this "obstinate refusal of food" misunderstood its true significance (Marcé 1860: 264). He advocated the change of habitat in order to remedy the "sufferings of the stomach" because he believed that the family surroundings perpetuated the disorder (Silverman 1989: 833). Marcé ascribed the symptoms to a "hypochondrial delirium." He also argued that what such sufferers eat helps define the syndrome: "the majority of hysterical and nervous sufferers make themselves remarkable for the slenderness of their diet, for their liking for indigestible food, and their antipathy for bread, meat, and strengthening dishes" (Marcé 1860: 264). Here, the ghost of Marcé's contemporary Brillat-Savarin and the question of taste and cure reveals the symptoms of anorexia to be very much in line with the notion of "healthy" and "unhealthy" foods of mid-nineteenth-century Paris. The cure is not, however, in the kitchen; rather, it is "a sustained effort of the will" that leads to recuperation (Marcé 1860: 834).

SLG/JESSICA RISSMAN

*See also* Anorexia; Brillat-Savarin; Gull

## References and Further Reading

Blewett, Andrew and Bottéro, Alain (1995) "L.-V. Marcé and the Psychopathology of Eating Disorders," *History of Psychiatry* 6 (21): 69–85.

Halmi, Kathrine (1999) "Eating Disorders: Defining the Phenotype and Reinventing the Treatment," *American Journal of Psychiatry* 156 (11): 1673–5.

Marcé, Louis-Victor (1860) "On a Form of Hypochondrial Delirium Occurring Consecutive to Dyspepsia and Characterized by Refusal of Food," *Journal of Psychological Medicine and Mental Pathology* 13: 264–6.

Silverman, Jason (1989) "Louis-Victor Marcé, 1828–64: Anorexia Nervosa's Forgotten Man," *Psychological Medicine* 19 (4): 833–5.

---

# Mazel, Judy

## Creator of the Beverly Hills Diet (1981)

The Beverly Hills Diet is a fad diet that focuses on a lifestyle of "conscious combining," a technique, which involves eating specific mixtures of food in a specific order for optimum digestion. Mazel asserts, "It isn't *what* you eat or *how much* you eat that makes you fat; it is *when* you eat and *what you eat together*" (Mazel and Shultz 1981: vi). The diet relies heavily on fruit (especially pineapple) and recommends never eating protein with carbohydrates, eating carbohydrates with fats and other carbohydrates, eating fruit alone, as well as a variety of other rules regarding the order in which foods maybe eaten. The key to her system is her reliance on "enzymes," both in the foods consumed and in the process of digestion, to break down foods without gaining weight. She also advocates avoiding the "perfect food," milk and most dairy products as difficult to digest. In addition, she stresses over and over again, though this is not part of her "combination" theory, that portion size is also vital.

Mazel was the youngest of three daughters and "began life as a skinny" (Mazel and Schultz 1981: 10). She began to gain weight in puberty: "When I graduated from grammar school, my mother was shocked because I was too fat to fit into children's clothes" (Mazel and Shultz 1981: 11). Her autobiography is the keystone to her argument about successful weight loss. This claim (if I could do it, so can you) was first developed in the mid-nineteenth century by William Banting as a layperson's answer to the medicalization of dieting. Mazel struggled with her weight for many years, trying everything from diet pills to thyroid medication, smoking, and laxatives. But she found success in none of these. She was riddled with guilt, hiding pizza boxes under the bed and dumping them in the neighbor's trash.

It took a skiing accident in the mid-1970s that left her bedridden to make her rethink her perceptions of food and metabolism. After researching the literature, she began dieting and experimenting with food combining based on her understanding of food's enzymatic content. The modern origins of this approach lie in the food faddism of the nineteenth century. Within the next few years, she lost 78 pounds, which she kept off for twenty-two years. Based on her success, Mazel, together with the ghostwriter, Susan Schultz, published the first edition of *The Beverly Hills Diet*. It became a *New York Times* bestseller that year, selling more in a shorter period of time than any other book in history up to that point.

In the twenty-five years since the original publication, Mazel has published *The Beverly Hills Diet Born Again Skinny Trilogy*, which includes *The New Beverly Hills Diet* (1996), *The New Beverly Hills Diet Little Skinny Companion* (1996), and *The New Beverly Hills Diet Recipes to Forever* (1996), as well as books like *The Beverly Hills Style: How to Be a Star in Your Own Life* (1986), and the *Beverly Hills Diet Lifetime Plan* (1983). The diet, which promises at least 15–20 pounds of weight loss in the first thirty-five days, boasts support from celebrities such as Jack Nicholson, Jodie Foster, and

Maria Shriver. As with her first book, all of her subsequent volumes rely heavily on testimonials. Most recently, Mazel branched into the world of children's diets, coauthoring *Slim and Fat Kids: Raising Healthy Children in a Fast-Food World* (1999).

SLG/Sarah Gardiner

*See also* Banting; Celebrities; Graham; Hay; Milk; Self-help

**References and Further Reading**
Anon. (2006) "About the Author," New Beverly Hills

Diet, Inc., available online at <http://www.newbeverlyhillsdiet.com/about/aboutthe author.html> (accessed April 18, 2006).
Anon. (2006) "Cell Tech Celebrity—Judy Mazel, a Woman Ahead of Her Time," Cell Tech International, available online at <http://www.celltech.com/resources/judymazel.html> (accessed April 18, 2006).
Anon. "Judy Mazel, 1996–2004," HCI: The Life Issues Publisher, available online at <http://www.hci-online.com/jmazel> (accessed March 11, 2007).
Mazel, Judy and Schultz, Susan (1981) *The Beverly Hills Diet*, New York: Macmillan.

# Media

The media (loosely defined here as mass market films, television, popular magazines and music) is an oft-beaten scapegoat, taking the blame for everything from violent children to casual sex. It has also been accused in recent decades of causing negative body-image perceptions (specifically in young women) by promoting unrealistically thin bodies. Young men, it has been reported, read only 10 percent of the articles and advertisements about dieting as young women (Andersen 2002: 189). One scholar notes that a full quarter of all of the female models in some fashion magazines fulfill the clinical description of anorexia nervosa, while few "overweight" individuals appear in a culture in which approximate a quarter of the population is overweight (Stice 2002: 104). Viewers and readers, in this argument, believe that they must have this "ideal" body, become depressed, start dieting, or develop an eating disorder. Besides representing a slender, fit body ideal that may encourage dieting, the media also reflects and perpetuates our dieting obsession, normalizing and thereby promoting the practice. The media is thus seen as presenting impossible body types for emulation and perpetuating a dieting culture to achieve such ends.

The media has often been noted as the cause of disordered eating and body-image issues because it promotes thinness as our culture's idea of beauty. Research has shown that interest in weight loss increases after exposure to television across the globe. Adolescent girls

in Fiji were studied, and they were interested in dieting to look like television characters from *Beverly Hills, 90210* (1990–2000) and *Xena, Warrior Princess* (1995–2001) (Becker et al. 2002: 509). The influence of Western mass media was further shown in a study of women in Ukraine. For these women, exposure to Western media was correlated with internalization of the thin ideal, and those women were also more likely to diet (Bilukha and Utermohlen 2001: 120).

Aside from the ubiquity of magazines more or less devoted to helping readers shape their bodies, there has been an obvious increase in the number of stories relating to dieting in other magazines as well. While the presence of stories about fad diets can be expected in news magazines, the fact that they are cover stories reflects the nation's growing obsession. For example *Time* magazine's November 1, 1999 cover featured the story "Low-Carb Diets." Is this what it takes to lure readers? Or is it simply an acknowledgment of dieting's growing relevance? Magazines also show that dieting has now expanded its horizons. Teen magazines regularly include diet and fitness tips for their young readers although very self-consciously, often with a disclaimer about the seriousness of eating disorders. *Seventeen* magazine's website even includes a BMI calculator along with sample menus to gain or lose weight. In addition, *Parade* magazine included an article titled "Help Your Pet Shed

Pounds." Just like human diets, the magazine suggests reducing caloric intake and increasing exercise for obese pets (Wilson and Kilcommons 2006).

Dieting has become such a regular part of modern life that media producers can allow their characters to remain "average" while still dieting. In "The Real Me" (Episode 50 of the wildly popular television series *Sex and the City*), Samantha Jones (played by Kim Catrall) went on a hot water and lemon diet to lose weight. All of this to take a few good photos—it was a moment to which the primarily female audience could relate. In the film *Mean Girls* (2004), new girl Cady Heron (played by Lindsay Lohan) seeks revenge on the popular Regina George (Rachel McAdams) by telling her that protein bars would help her lose weight, when in fact they do the opposite. The underlying truth is this: We are appalled that anyone would be mean enough to trick another girl into getting fat, yet fat jokes are hilarious. The ubiquity of dieting is also a constant theme in the animated sitcom *The Simpsons* (1989–): After eating too much junk food, Bart gains weight, has a heart attack, and is forced to go on a diet that he can't keep; Lisa is teased for having a "big butt" so she reads "Thin by Third Grade" and goes to the mall where a store employee makes a pre-teen mannequin even thinner; Homer orders a "Lose Weight in Your Sleep" audio cassette.

Perhaps because of widespread accusations of media culpability, the media has become increasing self-aware (to the point of shamelessness) of its role in promoting dieting. For example, some television programs have straddled the line between blatantly promoting thin body types and the exhibition of dieting as a normal societal practice. For example, NBC's reality show *The Biggest Loser* (2004–), which also has U.K. and Australia editions, featured fitness trainers and health experts who helped contestants competitively lose a large amount of weight. One segment included a food temptation; contestants would win a prize if they chose to eat it and would gain nothing, including extra pounds, if they didn't. Such a challenge promotes the importance of self-control but also ironically underlines the unimportance of it all: Eating a cupcake doesn't really make any difference. VH1 had a similar show called *Celebrity Fit Club* (2002, 2005) where B-list celebrities tried to lose weight with the help of a U.S. Marine drill coach and were weighed publicly at the end of every show. Besides using the celebrity as a hook, viewers gain the satisfaction of knowing that dieting is the great equalizer: Famous

people have to work just as hard as anyone else to lose weight. The subtle promotion of diets, dieting tips, or the "need" to go on a diet can also be seen in the casual conversation or monologues of other reality programs, talk shows, and, ironically enough, cooking shows.

Research has also shown that the amount of time one watches music videos is a fairly good predictor of the desire to be thin (Tiggemann and Pickering 1996: 199). The role of music, unlike music videos, in body-shaping behaviors is seldom addressed, largely because of its lack of visual images of bodies. Grammy Award winning hip-hop artist Kanye West managed to use both visual and textual cues in his song, "The New Workout Plan" (2004). The lyrics include exercise advice to do Pilates and food tips, like eating salad instead of dessert. Meanwhile, the satirical but catchy music video featured fit women at the gym, testimonials with before and after pictures, and an image of Kanye scolding one girl who wanted to eat a doughnut. The song and its video, which included the disclaimer "Call your plastic surgeon before beginning this workout," rapidly became a hit. Meanwhile, the satirist Weird Al Yankovic more bluntly sings about a specific fad diet in his song "Grapefruit Diet" (1999), using his lyrics to poke fun at our diet-crazed society. More recently, female pop artist P!nk's song and video "Stupid Girls" (2006) mock super-skinny Hollywood celebrities such as Lindsey Lohan and Nicole Richie while creating a powerful critique of the dieting and plastic surgery industries.

Aside from being commentary, the music industry has also squeezed its way into the multibillion-dollar dieting industry. In 1997, new-age musician Steven Halpern released a CD with the not-so-subtle title "Achieving Your Ideal Weight." His website advertises to "play this program during mealtimes or whenever hungry to help you attain and maintain your desired weight." *Cduniverse.com* explains that the album was "designed with meal times in mind" and "under a layer of relaxing music . . . are subliminal affirmations like, 'You chew your food slowly. You love and accept your body fully.' " This technique is far more direct than the other link between music and dieting: the suggestion that music, any music, might be helpful when dieting. The Women's Centre for Health Matters' "Exercises for Very Large Women" suggests using music to lose weight, whether it is playing an instrument or listening to music while exercising (Anon. "Exercises for Very Large Women": 3).

Some studies support the idea that media affects

people's dieting behavior, while others refute it. Still others believe that while media influence is a factor, it is by no means the only one involved (Field et al. 2001: 54). Regardless, our popular perception of media influence on body-shaping has affected the media industry's manipulation of the subject, from promotion to awareness and even criticism. It is clear that our obsession with dieting has entered all aspects of popular media magazines, films, television, and music.

SLG/DOROTHY CHYUNG

*See also* Celebrities; Children; Fashion; Internet; Men; Pets

## References and Further Reading

Andersen, Arnold (2002) "Eating Disorders in Males," in Christopher G. Fairburn and Kelly D. Brownell (eds), *Eating Disorders and Obesity: A Comprehensive Handbook*, 2nd edn, New York: Guilford Press, pp. 188–92.

Anon. "BMI Calculator: Calculate Your Body Mass Index," *Seventeen* magazine online, available online at <http://www.seventeen.com/health/bmi/spc/0,665141_665142,00.html> (accessed May 4, 2006).

Anon. (2004) "Exercises for Very Large Women," *Women's Centre for Health Matters HEAL fact sheet* (August): 1–4, available online at <http://www.wchm.org.au/pdf/LL%20exercises.pdf> (accessed May 10, 2006).

Becker, Anne E. (1995) *Body, Self and Society: The View from Fiji*, Philadelphia, Pa.: University of Pennsylvania Press.

Becker, Anne E., Burwell, Rebecca A., Herzog, David B., Hamburg, Paul, and Gilman, Stephen E. (2002) "Eating Behaviours and Attitudes Following Prolonged Exposure to Television Among Ethnic Fijian Adolescent Girls," *British Journal of Psychiatry* 180: 509–14.

Bilukha, Oleg O. and Utermohlen, Virginia (2001) "Internalization of Western Standards of Appearance, Body Dissatisfaction and Dieting in Urban Educated Ukrainian Females," *European Eating Disorders Review* 10 (2): 120–37.

Field, Alison E., Camargo, Carlos A., Taylor, C. Barr, Berkey, Catherine S., Roberts, Susan B., and Colditz, Graham A. (2001) "Peer, Parent, and Media Influences on the Development of Weight Concerns and Frequent Dieting Among Preadolescent and Adolescent Girls and Boys," *Pediatrics* 107 (1): 54–60.

Stice, Eric (2002) "Sociocultural Influence on Body Image and Eating Disturbance," in Christopher G. Fairburn and Kelly D. Brownell (eds), *Eating Disorders and Obesity: A Comprehensive Handbook*, 2nd edn, New York: Guilford Press, pp. 103–7.

Tiggemann, M. and Pickering, A.S. (1996) "Role of Television in Adolescent Women's Body Dissatisfaction and Drive for Thinness," *International Journal of Eating Disorders* 20 (2): 199–203.

Wilson, Sarah and Kilcommons, Brian (2006) "Help Your Pet Shed Pounds," *PARADE*, January 29.

Wykes, Maggie and Gunter, Barrie (2005) *The Media and Body Image: If Looks Could Kill*, Thousand Oaks, California: Sage.

# Medical Use of Dieting

According to the cliché, "You are what you eat." More recently, in the medical field, the phrase has become praxis, and dieting is used to cure and prevent various illnesses. The use of diet has gone much further than the proverbial "an apple a day keeps the doctor away," "eating carrots will improve your vision," or "have some chicken soup to cure . . . everything." In our seemingly rational, enlightened era, science and medicine are generally accepted as unquestionable truths. With the backing of these fields, the dieting industry has gained power, legitimacy, and sustainability. Viewed as a cure for diabetes, heart disease, sleep apnea, and obesity, the medical support of dieting has provided justification for dieters who are seeking health and longevity.

The connection between medicine and dieting has a long history, extending back into the ancient world. The primary focus of the Hippocratic School of Medicine was an emphasis on lifestyle, including diet, nutrition, exercise, and a reliance on calm, moderate living. Plato believed that excessive eating led to illness and that disease should be cured not by drugs, but by food. *Samuel Johnson's Dictionary* (1799) claimed that "to diet" meant "to feed by the rules of medicine (to eat by the rules of physick); to give food to." In addition, Hillel Schwartz traces the history of dietary regulation of salt intake:

> Athletes were the first to be hostile to salt, since it causes water retention and may add pounds to body weight. From this came the association with obesity, Bright's disease and diabetes in the early part of this century and the first suggestions that dieters should watch salt intake. Then came stronger associations with heart disease and high blood pressure, until in 1973 Cosmopolitan's Super Diets & Exercise Guide would claim that most Americans consumed ten to twenty times as much salt as they should.
>
> (Schwartz 1986: 259)

Some of the earliest diets, too, sought to cure ailments through dieting. John Wesley wrote *Primitive Physick* (1747) with the aim of bringing practical medical advice to those who could not afford to see physicians, and Gaylord Hauser used lemons to fight tuberculosis. The trend has continued with contemporary diets like the DASH diet (Dietary Approaches to Stop Hypertension) and the creation of "nutraceuticals," chemically engineered foods that cure diseases.

In addition, diabetes has been treated through diet since antiquity. In ancient India, the classical medical author Susruta described a diabetes-like disease which was understood as the result of the gluttonous overindulgence in rice, flour, and sugar (Papaspyros 1964). In 1796, Dr. John Rollo devised a treatment for diabetics: a low-carbohydrate diet high in fat and protein. In contrast, in the late 1850s, French Dr. Priorry prescribed eating large amounts of sugar to treat diabetes. The French Dr. Bouchardat also had the idea in the 1870s of personalizing diets for his diabetic patients after the glucose levels in their urine decreased following the rationing of food during the Franco-Prussian War. In the late nineteenth century, Catoni, an Italian diabetes specialist, used a lock and key to force his patients to follow their diets. From 1900 to 1915, diets for diabetes included the "oat(meal)-cure," the milk diet, the rice cure, and "potato therapy." In 1914, American Dr. Frederick Allen prescribed low-calorie diets of as little as 450 calories a day to his diabetic patients, believing that less food would reduce the strain on the body since it was believed that a diabetic's body was unable to process food. Again, in 1921, Dr. Elliot P. Joslin linked diabetes to obesity and thought that thin people might be immune to the disease. In contrast, another diet to treat diabetes was based on overfeeding and the belief that excess food could make up for the diabetic body's loss of weight and fluids. Even following the discovery of insulin, treatment was administered along with a reducing diet that "required the weighing of foods" (Schwartz 1986: 173).

Medicalization, or the identification of nonmedical problems as medical ones, is also evidence of medicine's authority. Specific attention to body size increased after a space for weight was introduced to standard forms in 1866, and life-insurance companies eventually began connecting weight with lifespan. Many fad diets, sometimes created by "doctors" with the title yielding legitimacy, also supported the idea that weight loss through a reducing diet would lead to health. However, medical concern about weight emerged only after public anxiety regarding excess weight had already begun. In addition, the growing attention toward degenerative diseases and studies on nutrition contributed to the growing medical attention on weight (Stearns 2002).

The use of diet as a cure was also supported by *The China Study*, which was able to show the link between nutrition and heart disease, diabetes, and cancer. This 1983 study surveyed the diet, lifestyle, and disease mortality data of 130 villages in sixty-five counties of rural China in hope of finding the causes of some diseases. Their results found that "the richer the diet is in native nutrients provided by plant matter, the greater are the reductions of degenerative diseases and the more beneficial are their biochemical indicators" (Campbell and Chen 1994: 103). This implies that a diet with proper nutrition can reduce or eliminate these diseases, as well as obesity. Yet the problem with such a bold assertion is the nature in which the belief was proven. That is, the collection of such statistics neglects many other factors that may contribute to a decreased prevalence of disease. Other clinical studies that have supported dieting for health are also limited by their methodology; it is impossible to make the control group and dieting group exactly the same.

The promotion of dieting as a medical cure has also been criticized for reinforcing the stigma against fat and for emphasizing weight loss over healthy eating and exercise (Germov and Williams 1996: 103; Campos 2004). In addition, the target audience is unclear such that many people who are encouraged to diet don't need to. The possible negative consequences of dieting, such as nutritional deficiencies and anxiety, are often overlooked, as are the problems associated with being underweight. Paul Campos pointedly asks, "If we were to employ the logic of the anti-fat warriors, does this latter fact mean that Americans should be encouraged to *gain* weight so as to protect themselves from, among other things, cancer, osteoporosis, and most of the major pulmonary diseases?" (Campos 2004: 25). It has also been suggested that the use of dieting as a cure caused the Food and Drug Administration (FDA) to be more lenient in the regulation of dieting drugs with dangerous side effects, such as "fenphen" and Redux (Klein 1997). The FDA believed that the effects of obesity outweighed the consequences of taking these drugs. On the other hand, some just do not believe that dieting is a sufficient cure. In a statement by the American Obesity Association (2004), the organization claims that dietary interventions may not be enough, and direct surgical intervention, such as gastric bypass surgery, is sometimes necessary to improve health.

The medical industry's use of dieting as a cure can be seen throughout history, generally for diseases associated with obesity. Although many still claim that they diet for overall health and not necessarily to cure a particular ailment, the evidence backing the health claims of diets is not irrefutable. In addition, society's influence on the medical field, in particular its aversion towards fat, should not be overlooked.

SLG/DOROTHY CHYUNG

*See also* Bariatric Surgery; China Today; Greek Medicine and Dieting; Hauser; Milk; Noorden; Wesley

## References and Further Reading

American Obesity Association (2004) "Statement of the American Obesity Association before the Medicare Coverage Advisory Committee Review of Bariatric Surgery," November 4, available online at <http://

## "You are what you eat"

This sentiment is ancient, appearing in one form or the other from the Greeks on. Martin Luther, in his conversations collected in *Table Talk*, states that: "When it comes to eating, we are the ilk of every tyrannical sort of animal. The wolf eats sheep, so do we; the fox chickens and geese, just like us; hawks and vultures eat birds as we do; pike eat fish, like us. We eat grass as do oxen, horses, and cows. And like pigs we eat dung and filth. But internally everything becomes shit." This phrase was first recorded in modern writing about diet by Jean-Anthelme Brillat-Savarin in 1826 and repeated in a different context by the German philosopher Ludwig Andreas Feuerbach in his essay of 1863 on "Spiritualism and Materialism." Friedrich Nietzsche employs the same formulation in an ironic comment on the studying of German philosophy in his cryptic autobiography of 1888, *Ecce Homo* (first published in 1908):

But as to German cookery in general—what has it not got on its conscience! Soup before the meal (still called *alla tedesca* in the sixteenth-century Venetian cook-books); meat cooked till the flavor is gone, vegetables cooked with fat and flour; the degeneration of pastries into paper-weights! Add to this the utterly bestial post-prandial habits of the ancients, not merely of the ancient Germans, and you will begin to understand where German intellect had its origin—in a disordered intestinal tract. . . . German intellect is indigestion; it can assimilate nothing.

Such a view is very much in line with his own failure at dieting. If you study bad philosophy because you are a German you are, of course, what you eat! Such a metaphoric use came into practical application with its introduction in English by nutritionist Victor Lindlahr in the 1920s, with a meat market slogan reading "Ninety per cent of the diseases known to man are caused by cheap foodstuffs. You are what you eat." He later published a book entitled *You Are What You Eat: How to Win and Keep Health with Diet*. In the 1960s, the meaning of this phrase became much more specific. It was used to mean that you would be healthy from eating "healthy food," here defined as macrobiotic whole foods. Some also trace the roots of this phrase to the Christian communion, where bread and wine represent the body and blood of Jesus Christ.

*See also* Brillat-Savarin; Cornaro; Lindlahr; Luther

www.obesity.org/subs/advocacy/MCAC2004.shtml> (accessed March 11, 2007).

Anon. "The History of Diabetes," Canadian Diabetes Association, available online at <http://www.diabetes.ca/Section_About/timeline.asp> (accessed March 11, 2007).

Anon. (1992) "History of Diabetes: From Raw Quinces & Gruel to Insulin," *Diabetes Health Magazine* (November), available online at <http://www.diabeteshealth.com/read,1012,25.html> (accessed May 8, 2006).

Campos, Paul (2004) *The Obesity Myth: Why America's Obsession with Weight Is Hazardous to Your Health*, New York: Gotham.

Campbell, T. Colin and Chen, Junshi (1994) "Diet and Chronic Degenerative Diseases: A Summary of Results from an Ecologic Study in Rural China," in Norman J. Temple and Denis P. Burkitt (eds), *Western Diseases: Their Dietary Prevention and Reversibility*, Totowa, NJ: Humana Press, pp. 67–118.

Germov, John and Williams, Lauren (1996) "The Epidemic of Dieting Women: The Need for a Sociological Approach to Food and Nutrition," *Appetite* 27 (2): 97–108.

Klein, Richard (1997) "Dieting Dangerously," *The New York Times on the Web: Women's Health* (July 14), available online at <http://www.nytimes.com/specials/women/warchive/970714_613.html> (accessed April 9, 2006).

MacCracken, Joan and Donna Hoel (1997) "From Ants to Analogues: Puzzles and Promises in Diabetes Management," *Postgraduate Medicine* 101 (4), available online at <http://www.postgradmed.com/issues/1997/04_97/diabetes.htm> (accessed March 11, 2007).

Papaspyros, Nikos S. (1964). *The History of Diabetes Mellitus*. Stuttgart : G. Thieme.

Sattley, Melissa (1996) "The History of Diabetes," *Diabetes Health Magazine* (November), available online at <http://www.diabeteshealth.com/read,1012,715.html> (accessed May 8, 2006).

Schwartz, Hillel (1986) *Never Satisfied: A Cultural History of Diets, Fantasies, and Fat, New York*: The Free Press.

Skiadas, P.K. and Lascaratos, J.G. (2001) "Original Communication Dietetics in Ancient Greek Philosophy: Plato's Concepts of Healthy Diet," *European Journal of Clinical Nutrition* 55 (7): 532–7.

Stearns, Peter (2002) *Fat History: Bodies and Beauty in the Modern West*, 2nd edn, New York: New York University Press.

# Medieval Diets

In the medical school at Salerno in the thirteenth century, the standard textbook of medicine, the *Regimen sanitatis salernitanum*—the *Salernitan Regime of Health*—was composed. A book of verses attributed to Arnald of Villanova (1240–1311), it provided practical guidelines for good living, but also definitions of the healthy and pathological bodies. Extraordinarily popular, it summarized and informed much of the later views of obesity. In a seventeenth-century English translation, it provided a snapshot of the humoral obese body in the light of the medieval reception of Greek medicine:

Men that be flegmatik, are weak of nature,
  Most commonly of thick and stubbed stature.
And fatnesse overtaketh them amain,
For they are slothfull, and can take no pain.
Their sences are but dull, shallow and slow,
Much given to sleep, whence can no goodnesse grow,
They often spet: yet natures kind direction,
Hath blest them with a competent complexion.
                              (Holland 1806: 35)

Thus phlegmatic fat persons cannot stand pain; they suffer from character flaws and are lazy, and nonproductive. But there is also a healthy fat that dines on "sweet wine, delicious meats, eggs that are rare / Over ripe figs and raisins, these appear. / To make the body fat, and nourish nature, / Procuring corpulence, and growth of stature" (Holland 1806: 7). This fat can itself become diseased but is of a different nature than the inherent obesity of the phlegmatic body because it comes from a different source. Food can cause illness, as Galen states, but there is also a "healthy" fat that is the result of eating without overindulgence. The cure for overindulgence is to eat foods with the antithetical humoral traits as the fat person. Thus, drinking vinegar (which is dry and cool) as therapy for the obese body (wet and cool), "unto fat folks, greatly doth no good" (Holland 1806: 19).

The sixteenth-century Italian physician Gerolamo Mercuriale also stressed that obesity is the result of internal and external factors, paraphrasing Galen. Yet, he also understands that the obese are not all stupid; indeed, they can be as intellectual as the thin person. Any given person can be born with the tendency towards *obesitas*. But *adventitia*, the acquired fat of a dissolute life, makes the mind crude. It is the result of an oily blood that turns to fat. Mercuriale's contemporary Tommaso Minadoi follows Galen's theory of the temperaments seeing damp and cold as the origin of fat. Such people are born not made; they are soft, hairless, pale and cold. Those who become fat are quite different. They are of a reddish complexion, hairy, have hard rather than soft flesh. They suffer from a constant hunger that drives them to become fat. Such theories build on the notion of a "natural" and an "unnatural" obesity, which demand different types of diets.

SLG

*See also* Brillat-Savarin; Ibn Sina; Roman Medicine and Dieting

## References and Further Reading

Bondio, Mariacarla Gadebusch (2005) *Medizinische Ästhetik: Kosmetik und plastische Chirugie zwischen Antike und früher Neuzeit*. Munich: Fink.

Cohen, Sheldon G. and Saavedra-Delgado, A.M. (1990) "Through the Centuries with Food and Drink, for Better or Worse. VIII: The School of Salerno," *Allergy Proceedings* 11 (6): 313–17.

Holland, P. (trans.) (1806) *Regimen sanitatis salernitanum*, in John Sinclair (ed.), *The Code of Health and Longevity*, 4 vols, Edinburgh: Arch. Constable & Co., pp. 5–46.

# Men

## Dieting and Eating Disorders

It is easy for anyone who has been exposed to mass and popular culture in the U.S.A. in the past twenty years to believe that dieting is an exclusively female activity and that eating disorders only affect woman. Advertisements for weight-loss companies such as Weight Watchers and Jenny Craig primarily feature women, and young women have also been, until recently, the primary focus of discussions about anorexia and bulimia. Since the 1990s, however, diet companies, doctors, and the media have "discovered" that men deal with body-image problems and struggle with overweight and disordered eating as well. While men have actually been dieting and struggling with eating disorders for centuries, an increasing number of popular and professional publications in the past fifteen years have focused on the unique problems of obesity in men, male dieting, and men with eating disorders.

In twentieth-century Western culture, overweight and eating disorders have largely been perceived as a female problem because of social and ideological gender constructs (Gilman 2004: 4). In the past thirty years, feminist writers, like Susan Orbach, have declared fat a "feminist issue" and sought to understand why women are particularly vulnerable to the "tyranny of slenderness" (Orbach 1978; Chernin 1981). However, this discourse, while essential to understanding the complex relationship between gender, the body, and social power, has neglected and almost effaced a very long history of anxieties about men's bodies and eating behaviors.

Until the end of the nineteenth century, concerns about obesity centered on men's bodies, and men generated the bulk of dietary advice literature (Gilman 2004: 4–5). Even in the early twentieth century when women received "the most biting commentary" on their weight, attention to male standards continued, and both men's and women's magazines featured slim male models (Sterns 1997: 98–9). In fact, during World War I, there was widespread cultural anxiety about the fitness of men's bodies as emblematic of the health of the nation overall. In the first two decades of the century, scientists and physicians sought to create a powerful, "gutsy" nation through transforming men's physical bodies (Carden-Coyne 2005). In the 1950s, diet books written particularly for men began to emerge, and they developed an "immediate and huge" following. This literature, however, rejected the aesthetic concerns most often associated with women and promoted weight loss, instead, as a means of improving one's masculinity and competitive edge (Sterns 1997: 101).

Similarly, the early contemporary literature on men and dieting tended to reinforce the idea that men diet for objective reasons, like health and performance, have more realistic body images, and are not vulnerable to the same aesthetic social pressures that women are. For example, sources on men and weight consciousness in the 1980s generally concluded that men do not worry that being fat will make them less attractive or socially acceptable. Instead, they think about fat and losing weight, "mainly in terms of their concerns about health" (Millman 1981: 235–6). Even studies of male eating disorders in the 1980s concluded that men "set more realistic weight goals for themselves, and have a less distorted image of themselves, than do females" (Schneider and Agras 1987: 239). These early discussions placed men in a privileged position in dieting culture by suggesting that their inherent rationality made them less susceptible to vain (pun intended) quests for slenderness. At the same time, however, these writings did a disservice to men by relegating their problems with weight and food to the margins because they included chapters on men and dieting merely as "a concession" to men who claim that it's "just as bad for them" (Ogden 1992: 74).

More recently, scholars have treated the topic of men and dieting much more seriously in an increasing number of book-length projects. This new material also shows more awareness of and sensitivity to the struggles that men have with their bodies and the role that culture and gender expectations play in those struggles (Andersen 2000: 70; Bordo 1999; Grogan 1999: 58–67). In general, research has shown that men desire larger, more muscular (mesomorphic) bodies because greater physicality is associated with desirable masculine traits like strength, power, and aggression (Bederman 1995: 42; Grogan 1999: 58). According to silhouette studies, questionnaires, and interviews conducted between 1985 and 1997, men aspire to muscular physiques, and their self-esteem is influenced by the ways in which they measure their own bodies in relationship to the mesomorphic ideal (Grogan 1999: 59–67).

This measurable body dissatisfaction in men and boys is referred to by some as "the Adonis complex," "a widespread crisis among today's boys and men" (Pope et al. 2000: iii). In this argument, men and boys are preoccupied with the appearance of their bodies but have no outlet for discussing this preoccupation in a society that has taught them not to be "hung up about how they look" (Pope et al. 2000: xiii). The "secret crisis of male body obsession" afflicts adults, as well as teenagers and young boys, who as early as elementary school indicate dissatisfaction with their bodies and who may even grow to develop eating disorders, use steroids, or suffer from depression (Pope et al. 2000: xiii–xiv). While this "crisis" in male bodies is not new, the "Adonis complex" is an important recognition that in contemporary diet culture; men too are concerned about their weight; and they also diet to improve their appearance and self-esteem, as well as their health.

Nevertheless, dieting can be very different for men than it is for women. There is physical evidence that men's bodies respond differently to diet and exercise than women's do. Men are, on average, taller than women and predisposed to have a higher percentage of body weight as lean muscle (Andersen 2000: 69). This advantage in height and lean muscle mass, which contributes to a higher resting metabolic rate in men, may make it easier for men to lose weight and sculpt their bodies (De Souza and Ciclitira 2005: 795). For example, a moderately active 125-pound woman needs, on average, only 2,000 calories a day, while a 175-pound man with a similar exercise pattern needs 2,800 calories ("Good Nutrition"). There may also be even more subtle differences that we have yet to uncover in the ways that men's bodies respond to particular diets. One small study conducted by Tufts University in 2004, for example, found that men responded more effectively to a diet low in saturated fat that was intended to lower total cholesterol (Li et al. 2003: 3431–2).

In addition, while men's health has been receiving more attention in recent years and the percentage of obese males is on the rise, men may be reluctant to diet or seek medical treatment (De Souza and Ciclitira 2005: 794–5; Drewnowski and Yee 1987: 632–3). According to a 1988 study, only 25 percent of men diet at some time in their lives, compared with about 95 percent of women (Grogan 1999: 67). The 1994–6 Survey of Food Intakes by Individuals similarly found that between 24 and 29 percent of men survey reported trying to lose weight. The reluctance of men to diet or report dieting can be attributed to the cultural constraints of masculinity, which construct men as strong and resistant to disease and dieting as a female activity (De Souza and Ciclitira 2005: 794).

Even when men do diet, they appear to approach and understand weight loss in very gendered ways. Men more often than not employ weight-lifting as a method for improving their body image because of the mesomorphic body ideal (Grogan 1999: 69), and, overall, men report exercising rather than counting calories to change their body shapes (Grogan 1999: 79; Drewnowski and Yee 1987: 626). Men may also purchase diet books and engage in activities like dieting groups and weight-loss classes that have traditionally been associated with women (De Souza and Ciclitira 2005). However, these dieters still frame their weight loss in masculinist terms. Echoing the "gutsy" rhetoric of early twentieth-century physical culture, contemporary diet books for men promise "you'll be in control and it will show," and "you'll have more vigor and stamina" physically and sexually (Goor and Goor 2000: 5–6). In addition, British men who joined a slimming class to lose weight asserted that they dieted to improve health rather than appearance. These men clearly viewed dieting for aesthetic reasons as a less legitimate, female activity and tried to distance themselves from it even though behavioral evidence suggested that they were concerned about their appearances (De Souza and Ciclitira 2005: 800).

Despite gendered differences in their reasons for and methods of dieting, men seem to share with women a susceptibility to the eating pathologies that plague consumer culture. Some of these extreme dieting practices, such as the abuse of steroids or human growth hormone, are generally associated with men (Grogan 1999: 76). However, men also fall victim to eating dis-

orders like anorexia, bulimia, and compulsive exercise, which have traditionally been associated with young women (Andersen 1990, 2000: 205, 2002: 188). While early sources on eating disorders focused primarily on white, middle-class adolescents (Bruch 1978; Brumberg 1988; Chernin 1981), medical professionals have since realized that eating disorders affect members of all ages, races, classes, and genders (Muise et al. 2003: 427). As a result, a growing body of literature on the subject of male eating disorders has emerged since the 1990s, and its authors are concerned with identifying, understanding, and treating pathological eating patterns in men (Muise et al. 2003: 433–4).

Much of this new material employs the rhetoric of "discovering" pressures on men to conform to unrealistic body types and suggests that these pressures are increasing, resulting in "as many as a million men" with eating disorders (Bordo 1999: 168; Langley 2005; Pope et al. 2000: 29; Pappano 2004; Stafford 2006). Still, it is not clear that eating disorders in males have actually increased; it is possible that greater awareness that eating pathologies can afflict multiple populations has merely allowed doctors to better recognize disordered eating in men. One of the first two reported cases of anorexia in 1689 was, in fact, found in a sixteen-year-old male (Andersen 1990: 3), and men appeared prominently in the earliest literature on eating disorders (Silverman 1987). Yet, only 0–5 percent of men reportedly suffer from bulimia (Andersen 1990: 10), and males only account for 10–20 percent of cases of anorexia today (Andersen 2002: 189).

It is difficult, however, to accurately measure the prevalence or increase of eating disorders in men because male anorexics and bulimics have been frequently misdiagnosed or overlooked by doctors who were culturally and scientifically conditioned to recognize pathological eating primarily in women (Andersen 2002: 188–9). Males with eating disorders may also be underrepresented in medical literature because they have been unlikely to seek treatment or reveal their problems to a doctor for fear that their masculinity would be undermined by a "feminized illness" like anorexia or bulimia (Laws and Drummond 2001: 29). Increases in self-reporting of anorexia and bulimia by men and boys may reflect a new comfort with "coming out" as professional discourse, popular literature (Krasnow 1996), and male celebrities like Billy Bob Thornton validate the experiences of men with eating disorders.

While popular media may help men and boys with

eating disorders to recognize and come forward with their disorders, it is also implicated in their etiology. Theorists and eating disorder researchers argue that advertising and entertainment media increasingly objectify men's bodies, promote ideals of slenderness, and represent men in unrealistic and damaging ways. Magazines, such as *Men's Health* and *GQ*, which give dieting and exercise advice and contain images of hyper-fit male models are frequently mentioned as contributing to unrealistic body ideals and increased body dissatisfaction among men (Bordo 1999: 218–19; Grogan 1999: 67–8; Pope et al. 2000: 32–33 and 45–6). Clinicians, too, see the media as an important causal factor in male body dissatisfaction. One eating disorders program director explains, "With more men's fashion magazines on the market, more emphasis being put on the way men look. Now they're subjected to the same concerns about body image that plagued women for years" (Sterns 1997: 99). Research has shown that magazine exposure increases psychosocial stress and may lead to unhealthy dieting behaviors among male and female adolescents (Utter et al. 2003).

Participation in certain sports, like swimming and wrestling, also seem to contribute to increased risk for developing eating disorders in men and boys (Dale and Landers 1999, 1382; Drewnowski and Yee 1987: 627; Langley 2005: 5). Pressures to "make weight," improve performance, or "bulk up" may lead athletes to engage in unhealthy behaviors, including excessive food restriction, over-exercise, purging, intentional dehydration, or steroid abuse. Men and boys in sports that emphasize muscular development, like bodybuilding, football, and competitive weight-lifting, are particularly vulnerable to a lesser-known disorder known alternately as "reverse anorexia nervosa" and "muscular dysmorphia." Males suffering from this disorder believe that they are overly thin even when they are highly muscular and may use anabolic steroids in an attempt to increase their muscle mass even further (Andersen 2002: 188).

Finally, researchers have also identified other factors, which might place specific groups of men at greater risk of developing eating disorders. For example, several studies in the 1980s and 1990s suggested that gay and bisexual men are more likely to be dissatisfied with their bodies and develop eating disorders than are homosexual or bisexual women or heterosexual men (Siever 1994; Williamson and Hartley 1994; Yager et al. 1988). However, these findings may be complicated by the possibility that gay men are more willing to divulge their problems with eating disorders because they feel less constrained by traditional masculine ideals (Kaminski et al. 2005: 180). It is likely that sexual orientation and homophobia are factors in men's willingness or unwillingness to admit to having an eating disorder or to seek treatment for it; however, scholars agree that more research is needed in this area.

Dieting and eating disorders are not solely the purview of women in contemporary culture despite their over-representation in popular and professional discourse. Like pressures on the female body, body dissatisfaction and dieting in men are powerfully framed by gender imperatives, which demand that men be strong, fit, and muscular but not "hung up about their appearance." This paradox has contributed to what some call a "crisis" for men, who suffer from anxiety about their bodies but cannot express their suffering because it would be considered weak or feminine. As a result, men are less likely than their female counterparts to seek help or to be correctly diagnosed when they do so. It appears hopeful, however, that these barriers to diagnosis and treatment will erode in the future as more and more people come to realize that, in a consumer culture, fat and the fear of it are men's issues too.

SLG/C. MELISSA ANDERSON

*See also* Anorexia; Banting; Brillat-Savarin; Celebrities; Children; Craig; Hormones; Morton; Nidetch; Self-help; Sexual Orientation; Sports

## References and Further Reading
Andersen, Arnold (1990) *Males with Eating Disorders*, New York: Brunner/Mazel.
—— (2000) *Making Weight: Healing Men's Conflicts with Food, Weight, and Shape*, Carlsbad, Calif.: Gurze Books.
—— (2002) "Eating Disorders in Males," in Kelly Brownell and Christopher G. Fairburn (eds), *Eating Disorders and Obesity: A Comprehensive Handbook*, 2nd edn, New York: Guilford Press, pp. 188–92.
Anon. (2006) "Good Nutrition: Should Guidelines Differ for Men and Women?" *Harvard Men's Health* (September): 4–6.
Bederman, Gail (1995) *Manliness and Civilization: A Cultural History of Gender and Race in the United States, 1880–1917*, Chicago, Ill.: The University of Chicago Press.

Bordo, Susan (1999) *The Male Body: A New Look at Men in Public and in Private*, New York: Farrar, Strauss and Giroux.

Bruch, Hilde (1978) *The Golden Cage: The Enigma of Anorexia Nervosa*, Cambridge, Mass.: Harvard University Press.

Brumberg, Joan Jacobs (1988) *Fasting Girls: The History of Anorexia Nervosa*, New York: Vintage Books.

Carden-Coyne, Ana (2005) "American Guts and Military Manhood," in Christopher E. Forth and Ana Carden-Coyne (eds) *Cultures of the Abdomen: Diet, Digestion, and Fat in the Modern World*, New York: Palgrave Macmillian, pp. 71–83.

Chernin, Kim (1981) *The Obsession: Reflections on the Tyranny of Slenderness*, New York: Harper & Row.

Dale, K.S. and Landers, D.M. (1999) "Weight Control in Wrestling: Eating Disorders or Disordered Eating?" *Medicine and Science in Sports and Exercise* 31 (10): 1382–9.

De Souza, Paula and Ciclitira, Karen E. (2005) "Men and Dieting: A Qualitative Analysis," *Journal of Health Psychology* 10 (6): 793–804.

Drewnowski, A. and Yee, D.K. (1987) "Men and Body Image: Are Males Satisfied with Their Body Weight?" *Psychosomatic Medicine* 49 (6): 626–34.

Gilman, Sander L. (2004) *Fat Boys: A Slim Book*, Lincoln, Nebr.: University of Nebraska Press.

Goor, Ron and Goor, Nancy (2000) *Choose to Lose Weight-Loss Plan for Men: A Take-Control Program for Men with the Guts to Lose*, Boston, Mass.: Houghton Mifflin Company.

Grogan, Sarah (1999) *Understanding Body Dissatisfaction in Men, Women, and Children*, New York: Routledge.

Kaminski, P.L., Chapman, B.P., Haynes, S.D., and Own, L. (2005) "Body Image, Eating Behaviors, and Attitudes Toward Exercise Among Gay and Straight Men," *Eating Behaviors* 6 (33): 179–87.

Krasnow, Michael (1996) *My Life as a Male Anorexic*, Binghamton, NY: Haworth Press.

Langley, Jenny (2005) *Boys Get Anorexia Too: Coping with Male Eating Disorders in the Family*, London: Lucky Duck Publishers.

Laws, Tom A. and Drummond, Murray (2001) "A Proactive Approach to Assessing Men for Eating Disorders," *Contemporary Nurse* 11 (1): 28–39.

Li, Zhengling, Otvos, James D., Lamon-Fava, Stefania, Carrasco, Wanda V., Lichtenstein, Alice H.,

McNamara, Judith R., Ordovas, Jose M. and Schaefer, Ernst J. (2003) "Men and Women Differ in Lipoprotein Response to Dietary Saturated Fat and Cholesterol Restriction," *Journal of Nutrition* 133 (11): 3428–33.

Millman, Marcia (1981) *Such a Pretty Face: Being Fat in America*, New York: Norton.

Muise, Alexio, Stein, Debra G. and Arbess, Gordon (2003) "Eating Disorders in Adolescent Boys: A Review of the Adolescent and Young Adult Literature," *Journal of Adolescent Health* 33 (66): 427–35.

Ogden, Jane (1992) *Fat Chance!: The Myth of Dieting Explained*, New York: Routledge.

Orbach, Susie (1978) *Fat Is a Feminist Issue: How to Lose Weight Permanently Without Dieting*, New York Paddington Press.

Pappano, Laura (2004) "Not for Girls Only: Boys with Eating Disorders," in Shasta Gaughen (ed.) *Eating Disorders*, San Diego, Calif.: Greenhaven Press, pp. 39–44.

Pope, Harrison G., Phillips, Katharine A. and Olivarda, Roberto (2000) *The Adonis Complex: The Secret Crisis of Male Body Obsession*, New York: The Free Press.

Schneider, John A. and Agras, W. Stewart (1987) "Bulimia in Males: A Matched Comparison with Females," *International Journal of Eating Disorders* 6 (2): 235–42.

Siever, M.D. (1994) "Sexual Orientation and Gender As Factors in Socioculturally Acquired Vulnerability to Body Dissatisfaction and Eating Disorders," *Journal of Consulting and Clinical Psychology* 62 (2): 252–60.

Silverman, J.A. (1987) "Robert Whytt, 1714–66, Eighteenth-Century Limner of Anorexia Nervosa and Bulimia: An Essay," *International Journal of Eating Disorders* 6 (1): 431–3.

Stafford, Duncan E. (2006) "Fat: A Male Issue Too," *Therapy Today* 17 (5): 27–9.

Sterns, Peter (1997) *Fat History*, New York: New York University Press.

Utter, J., Neumark-Sztainer, D., Wall, M. and Story, M. (2003) "Reading Magazine Articles About Dieting and Associated Weight Control Behaviors Among Adolescents," *Journal of Adolescent Health* 32 (1): 78–82.

Williamson, I. and Hartley, P. (1994) "British Research into the Increased Vulnerability of Young Gay Men to

Eating Disturbance and Body Dissatisfaction,"
*European Eating Disorders Review* 6 (3): 160–70.
Yager, J., Landsverk Kurzman, J., and Wiesmeier, E.

(1988) "Behaviors and Attitudes Related to Eating
Disorders in Homosexual Male College Students,"
*American Journal of Psychiatry* 145 (4): 495–7.

# Metabolism

People eat a variety of foods, which are broken down by the body and used to build muscle, keep the body warm, and provide energy throughout the day. Metabolism is a term used to describe this breakdown of food into energy in the body. Each person has a different metabolic set point based on a variety of factors, including hormones, which are the main communication tool within the body. Examples of hormones include: insulin, glucagon, thyroid hormone, cortisol, estrogen, and testosterone. Each of these hormones plays a role in the regulation of metabolic rate, which ultimately controls hunger and weight gain or loss. The breakdown of food is the primary manner by which the body produces energy; the energy gained from the food is determined by the number of calories contained in each meal.

The thyroid gland is one of the key organs that regulates metabolic rate through the release of thyroid hormone. People who produce too much thyroid hormone will often be hot, hungry, and unable to gain weight. When someone produces too much thyroid hormone, the body is unable to store any of the energy from the food and, therefore, converts it all to heat. This is what makes the person hot all the time. The opposite of producing too much thyroid hormone is not producing enough. The thyroid gland was one of the first inborn errors of metabolism noted in individuals who were unable to lose weight even after dieting. An individual who does not produce enough thyroid hormone will be cold all the time and will gain weight. This condition is treatable by placing the person on oral thyroid hormones. People attempting to diet have, at times, even resorted to taking oral thyroid hormone to increase metabolic rate and, thereby, lose weight.

When a person limits the amount of food eaten by dieting, the metabolic rate can be affected in a number of ways. Basal or resting metabolic rate (RMR) is a term that describes the lowest number of calories a particular person needs to eat in order to fuel basic life functions. If a person consumes fewer calories than are needed for survival (fewer calories than the RMR), the body will go into starvation mode. In starvation mode, the body begins to shut down processes which are not essential for life. For example, the body will tear down muscle tissue in order to get protein and energy to maintain heart and kidney function, which provides an additional challenge for weight management because muscle uses more energy than fat. A person who has lost muscle after dieting, therefore, has the potential to gain fat after going back to eating regularly. This happens because the reduction in muscle leads to a reduction in RMR, which ultimately means the person needs less food to maintain body weight now than was needed before the diet began.

Severe reduction in the amount of food that a person consumes, as happens when a person is dieting, can also lead to feelings of anxiety, sluggishness, and irritability. These and other side effects have led to the development of dieting drugs that combat the slowing metabolism that sometimes occurs in dieting. Drugs like ephedrine and caffeine stimulate the metabolism, which helps to maintain higher energy levels. These drugs do not prevent the loss of muscle tissue that occurs if a person consumes fewer calories than are required by that person's RMR. For this reason, dieticians and doctors have recommended that people never consume less than 1,200 calories per day. Although 1,200 calories per day is a good estimate for the average person, many people have a higher RMR. In order to better determine RMR, many gyms and health clubs have purchased machines that measure personal RMR. Knowing this information helps dieticians and trainers to develop a dieting strategy that will produce more effective results for a person trying to lose weight.

SLG/Suzanne Judd

*See also* Calorie; Homeostasis; Hormones Used in Dieting; Very-Low-Calorie Diets

**References and Further Reading**

Black, A.E., Coward, W.A., Cole, T.J., and Prentice, A.M. (1996) "Human Energy Expenditure in Affluent Societies: An Analysis of 574 Doubly-Labeled Water Measurement," *European Journal of Clinical Nutrition* 50 (2): 72–92.

Flatt, J.P. (1993) "Dietary Fat, Carbohydrate Balance and Weight Measurement," *Annals of the New York Academy of Sciences* 683 (1): 122–40.

Jebb, Susan A. (2002) "Energy Intake and Body Weight," in Christopher G. Fairburn and Kelly D. Brownell (eds), *Eating Disorders and Obesity: A Comprehensive Handbook*, 2nd edn, New York: Guilford Press, pp. 37–42.

Ravussin, Eric (2002) "Energy Expenditure and Body Weight," in Christopher G. Fairburn and Kelly D. Brownell (eds), *Eating Disorders and Obesity: A Comprehensive Handbook*, 2nd edn, New York: Guilford Press, pp. 55–61.

# Metcalfe, William (1788–1862)

## The first public advocate of vegetarianism in the U.S.A.

Born in England, Metcalfe immigrated to America to preach the gospel of temperance, vegetarianism, and health. He was a member of the "New Church," which, following the Swedish mystic Emanuel Swedenborg (1688–1772), advocated abstinence based on his theological views. Likewise, Metcalfe "gave up, at once and entirely, fish, flesh and fowl as food, and every kind of intoxicating liquor as drink" in 1809 (Metcalfe 1872: 12).

His dietary choices, however, met with some resistance. Metcalfe explained that,

> friends laughed at me, and entreated me to lay aside my foolish notions of a vegetable diet. They assured me I was rapidly sinking into a consumption, and tried various other methods to induce me to return to the customary dietetic habits of society; but their efforts proved ineffectual.
>
> (Metcalfe 1872: 13)

Nevertheless, Metcalfe did not renounce his vegetarianism, which became central to his preaching in the "Bible-Christian Church" that he helped to found. Like the New Church, Metcalfe's sect advocated temperance and vegetarianism. The Bible-Christian Church resulted, in part, from Metcalfe's break with the New Church over the question of revelation. He argued that only the Bible was a "divinely inspired record of the word of God" (Metcalfe 1872: 16). In 1816, forty-one followers of Metcalfe and the Bible-Christian Church departed Liverpool for Philadelphia. Their numbers actually decreased on the trip over as "the strong sea breeze of the Atlantic" made them "give way to indulgences in eating and drinking those things which their principles had forbidden" (Metcalfe 1872: 19). However, once in Philadelphia, Metcalfe preached the new doctrine of temperance and vegetarianism to ever-greater audiences.

His periodical *The Rural Magazine and Literary Evening Fireside* also promulgated his views. From 1820, he began to publish a series of widely read and quoted tracts against alcohol and the eating of flesh. His argument here was moral: When men and women gather together for whatever purpose, and alcohol is served, the potential for immorality is present (Metcalfe 1872: 31). The temperance movement grew much more quickly than "dietetic reform," yet it too was "as criminal, as debasing, and as barbarous as that or any other known evil" (Metcalfe 1872: 32). In 1821, Metcalfe published the tract *Abstinence from the Flesh of Animals*, and, in 1839, he met Sylvester Graham, who was then preaching temperance and, through Metcalfe, later added vegetarianism to his cause. In addition, Metcalfe's tracts had a major influence on William Alcott, whose work emphasized the moral basis of health and education. As such, Metcalfe continued to be a major feature of the growing diet-reform movement until his death in 1862.

Metcalfe based his ideas about diet on strict biblical interpretations, which were always combined with notions of health and hygiene: "The system of temperance which we thus religiously practice, furnishes us with strength and activity sufficient to support the most laborious occupations, secures one of the all-important blessings of life,—the possession of health—and qualifies us for the enjoyment of a more perfect mode of being" (Metcalfe 1872: 153). This combination is fundamental to his notion of biblical revelation, which assures not only salvation but health: "It is clear from the nature of the Law, as recorded in the text before us, that man was originally intended to live upon vegetables only" (Metcalfe 1872: 156). Thus the commandment "Thou shall not kill" applies to any living thing (Metcalfe 1872: 163). Metcalfe sees in Paul's break with Jewish law, especially with the law of sacrifices, his opening (Metcalfe 1872: 190). Christ was an advocate of temperance and of vegetarianism. Even Christ's miracle of the loaves and fishes, is reread to stress the bread and to deny the fishes (Metcalfe 1872: 180). Never mind turning water into wine! It is the "hardness of their hearts" that makes the Jews continue to sacrifice after Christ's preaching (Metcalfe 1872: 191). The Jews are "so carnal as to be incapable of understanding the nature of spiritual worship, they were mere performers of external rites and ceremonies" (Metcalfe 1872: 193). Here Metcalfe is not very far from the German atheist philosopher Ludwig Feuerbach's (1804–72) dismissal of Judaism, in his *Essence of Christianity* (1841) as not a religion at all, but a gastronomic cult, as "the Israelites opened to Nature only the gastric sense; their taste for Nature lay only in the palate; their consciousness of God in eating manna" (Feuerbach 1841).

SLG/ANGELA WILLEY

*See also* Christianity; Graham; Jews; Vegetarianism

### References and Further Reading

Feuerbach, Ludwig (1841) *Essence of Christianity*, trans. Zawar Hanfi and George Eliot, available online at <http://www.marxists.org/reference/archive/feuerbach/works/essence/ec11.htm> (accessed March 12, 2007).

Metcalfe, William (1872) *Out of the Clouds: into the Light. With a Memoir of the Author by His Son, Rev Joseph Metcalfe*, Philadelphia, Pa.: J.B. Lippincott.

Nissenbaum, Stephen (1980) *Sex, Diet, and Debility in Jacksonian America: Sylvester Graham and Health Reform*, Westport, Conn.: Greenwood Press.

Wharton, James C. (1981) "Muscular Vegetarianism: The Debate over Diet and Athletic Performance in the Progressive Era," *Journal of Sport History* 8 (2): 58–75.

# Milk

Milk and dairy products (from cows) are prevalent in the American diet. A healthy diet is supposed to include school lunches with pints of milk and is further promoted through the commercial association of athletes and milk. Recently, milk cooperatives started an advertising campaign, claiming that if dieters drink 24 ounces of low-fat or fat-free milk every day, they will lose weight. This is surprising because milk is designed to help young mammals gain weight. Nevertheless, milk has historically played a central role in dieting and continues to do so today.

All mammals produce milk for their young (which is why they are called "mammals" from *mammae*, the Latin word for breast), but this milk varies greatly in terms of proteins and fat content (Schiebinger 1993). Humans, however, are the only mammals that drink milk into adulthood (but not human milk), and not all humans can even do this. Most Americans are of European descent, and this means that they continue to produce the enzyme lactase throughout their lives, but because this enzyme was never meant to be used to digest large quantities of milk, their bodies do not produce very much lactase (Kottak 2008). This is why it is impossible for a normal person to drink an entire gallon of milk without becoming very ill. However, members of the American population who are not of European descent are, to a greater or lesser degree, lactose intolerant.

Cow's milk consists basically of all the proteins and fats that baby cows need to grow, but these proteins, most especially lactose, are difficult for humans to digest once they reach the age of five. This is with the exception of two African tribes and most northern Europeans, who have a genetic trait that allows them to digest milk proteins (Kottak 2008). Lactose is found in all milks, though in varying amounts. Milk thus varies greatly in nutritional quality. Goat's milk, for example, is much closer to human milk in terms of lactose content and so is easier for us to digest, but it is almost universally more expensive than cow's milk in stores. For many people it also has an odd taste, perhaps because they are not used to consuming it or perhaps because it is so similar to human milk that we have a natural aversion to it after the age of five.

Cow's milk did not really become part of the human diet until well after the agricultural revolution and the subsequent domestication of animals (Eaton et al. 1988). In the beginning of the nineteenth century, Cow's milk started to be called the "perfect food" because it was believed to be the only natural food to have the right balance of proteins, carbohydrates, fats, and other nutrients. As such, many diets called for people to drink more milk, though some of these diets were encouraging weight gain in neuresthenics. Even in the twenty-first century, the USDA recommends three servings (24 oz) of dairy per day.

In many ways, milk is the perfect food, for baby cows, but there is little evidence that milk is a balanced food for humans. One 8-ounce serving of skim milk contains about 8 grams of protein, 12 grams of carbohydrates, a small amount of fat (about 0.4 grams), and 80 calories. Some people cannot digest any of the proteins or sugars (carbohydrates) in milk and so receive none of its purported benefits. There are also people who cannot fully digest milk and, therefore, do not receive the full amount of protein that the food contains.

SLG/Joe Bauer

*See also* Food Pyramid; Lindlahr; Mitchell

## References and Further Reading

Anon. "Mypyramid.gov," United States Department of Agriculture, available online at <http://www.mypyramid.gov> (accessed March 12, 2007).

Eaton, S.B., Shostak, Majorie, and Konner, Melvin (1988) *The Paleolithic Prescription*, New York: Harper & Row.

Kottak, C.P. (2008) *Anthropology: The Exploration of Human Diversity*, 12th edn, New York: McGraw-Hill.

Reuters (2007) "Tea's Benefits Ruined by Milk." Available online at <http://www.msnbc.msn.com/id/16540633/print/1/displaymode/1098> (accessed January 1, 2007).

Schiebinger, Londa (1993) *Nature's Body: Gender in the Making of Modern Science*, Boston, Mass.: Beacon.

# Mitchell, Silas Weir (1829–1914)

## American neurologist and novelist

Mitchell trained at the Jefferson Medical College in Philadelphia where he received his MD. In 1850, Mitchell was in charge of nervous and mental diseases at Turners Lane Hospital in Philadelphia. His experience during the American Civil War led him to develop the "rest cure," which is associated with his name.

As the author of *Injuries of Nerves and Their Consequences* (1872) and *Fat and Blood* (1877) he was a powerful advocate for the use of diet to treat both mental and physical illnesses. He advocated using diet specifically to treat "neurasthenia," a weakness of the nervous system "discovered" by the electrotherapist George

Miller Beard (1839–83) and described as early as 1869 as "The American Disease." This is the disease of urban, stressful life, the suffering of those unable to keep up with the speed of modernity, whose nervous system collapses under the strain. In order to cure this disease, rest and a fat-rich diet were necessary. As Beard noted:

> Indigestion may excite and maintain neurasthenia and may result from it . . . in the body, though there may be much force in the nerve centers, yet if digestion be clogged and the waste matters are suffered to accumulate in the digestive apparatus . . . the amount of force generated and usable will be very much diminished.
>
> (Beard 1881: 42)

Diet would cure this, and Beard advocated eating "no fruits, no vegetables, [and] no cereals except wheat" (Beard 1881: 42). Instead, he prescribed a diet of beef, mutton, lamb, fowl, eggs, and milk.

In Mitchell's America, thinness rather than obesity is the problem. In 1877, he noted in *Fat and Blood and How to Make Them* that " 'Banting' is with us Americans a rarely needed process, and, as a rule, we have much more frequent occasion to fatten than to thin our patients" (Mitchell 1877: 16). Fat, in his opinion, is necessary for good health:

> The exact relations of fatty tissue to the states of health are not as yet well understood; but, since on great exertion or prolonged mental or moral strain or in low fevers we lose fat rapidly, it may be taken for granted that each individual should possess a certain surplus of this readily-lost material. It is the one portion of our body which comes and goes in large amount. Even thin people have it in some quantity always ready, and, despite the fluctuations, every one has a standard share, which varies at different times of life.
>
> (Mitchell 1877: 15)

Mitchell tied the lack of "visible" body fat to the notion of an insufficiency of the nerves. It is mental illnesses, such as neurasthenia, that can result when the body becomes too thin: "I think the first thing which strikes an American in England is the number of inordinately fat people, and especially fat women . . . this excess of flesh we usually associate in idea with slothfulness" (Mitchell

1877: 15). In fact, he claims that such fat is a prophylaxis against disease: "This must make . . . some difference in their relative liability to certain forms of disease" (Mitchell 1877: 15).

It is primarily women who suffer from this loss of fat and the resulting nervousness: "a large group of women, especially said to have nervous exhaustion, or who are described as having spinal irritation . . . They have a tender spine, and soon or later enact the whole varied drama of hysteria" (Mitchell 1877: 25–6). They are, he claims, "lacking in color and which had not lost flesh" (Mitchell 1877: 27). However, men too can suffer from such a debility of the nerves, specifically through traumatic experiences: "Nor is this less true of men, and I have many a time seen soldiers who had ridden boldly with Sheridan or fought gallantly with Grant, become, under the influence of painful nerve wounds, as irritable and hysterically emotional as the veriest girl," undergoing "moral degradation" (Mitchell 1877: 28). Fat men and women are mentally healthy; thin men and women suffer.

The exemplary case of treating neurasthenia though enforced inactivity and a diet of fat-rich foods is documented in Charlotte Perkins Gilman's (1860–1935) autobiographical short story "The Yellow Wallpaper" (1892). She writes of her character's malady as "but temporary nervous depression—a slight hysterical tendency" to be treated with diet, "phosphates or phosphites—whichever it is, and tonics, and journeys, and air, and exercise, and am absolutely forbidden to 'work' until I am well again" (Gilman 1997). Her husband who is also her physician suggests that " 'Your exercise depends on your strength, my dear,' said he, 'and your food somewhat on your appetite; but air you can absorb all the time' " (Gilman 1997). Gilman recounts how the boredom of inactivity and diet drives her character to the brink of true madness.

This treatment is, of course, the "rest cure." For S. Weir Mitchell, a certain amount of fat was necessary to protect the nervous system and thus the psyche from distress. He argued that "blood thins with the decrease of tissues and enriches as they increase" (Mitchell 1877: 15). And the more blood, the more psychic energy. It is a sign of "nutritive prosperity" (Mitchell 1877: 16). Such prosperity is signaled by the social station of the individual. Thus, he proposes that the "upper classes gain weight in the summer" (Mitchell 1877: 16) (and intelligence) while the working classes lose it. But it is also determined by the individual's gender. Fat men are, all in all, healthier than fat women.

Yet there is also a fat which is itself diseased. This is a fat fatter than fat. Such fat is bad; just look at the street scene in London through his eyes:

> This excess of flesh we usually associate in idea with slothfulness, but English women exercise more than ours, and live in a land where few days forbid it, so that probably such a tendency to obesity is due chiefly to climatic causes. To these latter also we may no doubt ascribe the habits of the English as to food. They are larger feeders than we, and both sexes consume strong beer in a manner which would in this country be destructive of health. These habits aid, I suspect, in producing the more general fatness in middle and later life, and those enormous occasional growths which so amaze an American when first he sets foot in London. But, whatever be the cause, it is probable that members of the prosperous classes of English, over forty, would outweigh the average American of equal height of that period, and this must make, I should think, some difference in their relative liability to certain forms of disease, because the overweight of our trans-Atlantic cousins is plainly due to excess of fat.
>
> (Mitchell 1877: 15)

The British are too fat, unlike the healthily corpulent Americans. It is a fat of excess not of health. But it too can be cured with diet, especially the consumption of large amounts of "milk is the best and most easily managed addition to a general diet" (Mitchell 1899: 119).

Mitchell was part of the growing milk cult in the nineteenth century, which saw in cow's milk the "perfect food." He presents a number of case studies such as the forty-five-year-old Mrs. P. "weight one hundred and ninety pounds, height five feet four and a half inches, had for some years been feeble, unable to walk without panting, or to move rapidly even a few steps." She is self-treating, which physicians of the nineteenth century see as dangerous: "Two years before I saw her she had been made very ill owing to an attempt to reduce her flesh by too rapid Banting, and since then, although not a gross or large eater, she had steadily gained in weight, and as steadily in discomfort" (Mitchell 1899: 231). She needs the ministrations of a physician who keeps her

in bed for five weeks. Massage was used at first once daily, and after a fortnight twice a day, while milk was given, and in a week made the exclusive diet. Her average of loss for thirty days was a pound a day, and the diet was varied by the addition of broths after the third week, so as to keep the reduction within safe limits. . . . At the seventh week her pulse was 70 to 80, her temperature natural, and her blood-globules much increased in number. Her weight had now fallen to one hundred and forty-five pounds, and her appearance had decidedly improved. She left me after three and a half months, able to walk with comfort three miles. She has lived, of course, with care ever since, but writes me now, after two years, that she is a well and vigorous woman. Her periodical flow came back five months after her treatment began, and she has since had a child.

> (Mitchell 1899: 231)

Thus, Mitchell's medicalization of diet can treat the nervous and the obese—and make veterans whole and women fecund.

SLG

*See also* Banting; Electrotherapy; Medical Use of Dieting; Milk

## References and Further Reading

Beard, George Miller (1881) "American Nervousness: Its Causes and Consequences," New York: G.P. Putnam's Sons.

Cervetti, Nancy (2003) "S. Weir Mitchell Representing 'a Hell of Pain': From Civil War to Rest Cure," *Arizona Quarterly* 59 (3): 69–96.

Gilman, Charlotte Perkins (1997) *The Yellow Wallpaper*, Electronic Text Center, University of Virginia Library. Available online at <http://etext.lib.virginia.edu/modeng/modeng0.browse.html> (accessed June 23, 2007).

Lovering, Joseph P. (1971) *S. Weir Mitchell*, New York: Twayne Publishers.

Mitchell, S. Weir (1877) *Fat and Blood and How to Make Them*, Philadelphia, Pa.: Lippincott.

—— (1899) *Fat and Blood and How to Make Them*, 8th edn, Philadelphia, Pa.: Lippincott.

Ryals, Kay Ferguson (2002) "Bedside Manners and the

Social Body: S. Weir Mitchell and the Virtues of Medical Practice," Ph.D. diss., University of California, Irvine.

Walter, Richard D. (1970) *S. Weir Mitchell, Neurologist:* *A Medical Biography*, Springfield, Ill.: Thomas.

Will, Barbara (1996) "Nervous Systems, 1880–1915," in Tim Armstrong (ed.), *American Bodies*, New York: New York University Press, pp. 86–100.

# Monroe, Marilyn (1926–1962)

## Iconic American screen actress

Born Norma Jeane Mortenson, Monroe starred in such celluloid hits as *Gentlemen Prefer Blondes* (1953), *The Seven Year Itch* (1955), and *The Prince and the Showgirl* (1957). She played the role of Sugar Kane Kowalczyk, which encapsulated her public image, in *Some Like it Hot* in 1959. Immortalized in print and on canvas by the likes of Norman Mailer and Andy Warhol, Monroe's voluptuous physique and girlish vulnerability embodied a mid-twentieth-century Western ideal of femininity.

She was one among a group of mid-century American and European stars famed for their "pin-up girl" figures. Others included American contemporary Jayne Mansfield and French star Brigitte Bardot. The popularity of these actresses signaled resurgence of an ideal of female beauty that had peaked in the late nineteenth century with the Gibson Girl look but waned in the 1920s during the jazz age.

Monroe's one-time assistant, Lenia Pepitone, states in a memoir she later wrote about her relationship with Monroe that when she met the actress on her job interview, she didn't look "voluptuous" to her but, instead, appeared "overweight" (Pepitone and Stadiem 1979). Monroe herself was alive to the extremely thin line between the two terms and was deeply self-critical of her body. Yet, on what would have been her eightieth birthday, a columnist imagined what she would be like had she lived to that date:

if Marilyn Monroe were alive today she'd be a militant feminist. She would have had an awakening in the 1970s after reading "Our Bodies, Ourselves," and realizing that she had been a mere pawn in Hollywood's insatiable quest for actresses with sex appeal. Monroe would have been close to 50 at that point, and sick of dieting in order to keep the tabloids and their cellulite-seeking cameras off her back. She would have admired Elizabeth Taylor's doffing of the sex goddess yolk, and would do the same—adding perhaps 40 pounds as she learned how to relax and enjoy life off the Hollywood grid.

(Ganahl 2006)

As Monroe's iconic status shows, body size and beauty are very much in the eye (and the memory) of the beholder.

SLG/Shruthi Vissa

*See also* Russell

## References and Further Reading

Ganahl, Jane (2006) "Happy 80th Birthday, Ms. Monroe. What Paths Might Your Life Have Taken?" *San Francisco Chronicle*, June 1: E1.

Leaming, Barbara (1998) *Marilyn Monroe*, New York: Crown Publishers.

Pepitone, L. and Stadiem, William (1979) *Marilyn Monroe Confidential: An Intimate Personal Account*, New York: Simon & Schuster.

# Morton, Richard (1637–98)

Morton was raised in Suffolk, England and eventually attended medical school at Oxford before earning his fellowship in London in 1678. Morton was credited with writing the first medical description of "nervous consumption" in 1689, which is known today as anorexia nervosa (Pearce 2004: 191). It is with Morton that the clinical history of anorexia nervosa begins; prior to that, the distinction between "fasting" and pathologies of eating was not clearly differentiated (Gutierrez 2003).

In his written account of his patients, published in *Phthisiologia*, translated to English in 1694, subtitled *A Treatise of Consumptions*, Morton characterized the illness as a wasting condition due to emotional turmoil. For Morton, this was seldom seen in England; it seemed to be an "American" disease, "most frequently amongst those that have lived in Virginia, after they have come over hither" (Morton 1694: 4). Moreover, he claimed that the disease was the result of "violent Passions of the Mind, the intemperant drinking of Spirituous Liquors, and an unwholsom Air, by which it is no wonder if the Tone of the Nerves, and the Temper of the Spirits are destroy'd" (Morton 1694: 5). The cure for this disease that "does almost always proceed from Sadness, and anxious cares" is "very good Air" but "because the Stomack in this Distemper is principally affected, a delicious diet will be convenient, and the Stomack ought not to be too long accustomed to one sort of Food" (Morton 1694: 8). Fasting diseases are disease of the spirit and the stomach, cured by healthy living and a better diet.

In order to illustrate his argument, Morton described two case histories. He saw them in the light of his understanding of consumption (tuberculosis), noting that "I do not remember that I did ever in all my Practice see one, that was conversant with the Living so much wasted with the greatest degree of consumption (like a Skeleton only clad with skin)" (Morton 1694: 9). He makes a differential diagnosis, noting that there is neither cough nor fever in these patients. Nevertheless, they demonstrate self-starvation, emaciation, a refusal to gain weight, body image distortion, and a denial of illness—the symptoms that, centuries later, would define anorexia nervosa.

Mr. Duke's daughter, the first documented patient, was a twenty-year-old woman who presented a two-year history of weight loss and amenorrhea ("suppression of her Monthly Courses" [Morton 1694: 9]). One contributing factor, according to Morton, was that "she was wont by her studying at Night, and continual poring upon Books" to be exposed to unhealthy night air. She died a few months after consulting Morton, having been "taken with a Fainting Fit" (Morton 1694: 9). The second patient, the sixteen-year-old son of Reverend Minister Richard Steele, "fell gradually into a total want of appetite, occasioned by his studying too hard, and the Passions of his Mind" (Morton 1694: 10). Morton advised him to give up his studies, go to the country, ride, and drink milk. The patient recovered his health to a certain degree. According to Morton, both Miss Duke and young Mr. Steele were documented to have severe weight loss resulting from emotional causes. Morton was the first to record observations regarding eating disorders not tied to physical illness and to argue their intractability.

SLG/JESSICA ELYSE RISSMAN

*See also* Anorexia

## References and Further Reading

Gutierrez, Nancy A. (2003) *"Shall She Famish Then?" Female Food Refusal in Early Modern England*, Aldershot: Ashgate.

Morton, Richard (1694) *Phthisiologia or, a Treatise of Consumptions*, London: Smith and Walford.

Ove, Marcia K. (2002) "The Evolution of Self-Starvation Behaviors into the Present-Day Diagnosis of Anorexia Nervosa: A Critical Literature Review," Ph.D. diss., California School of Professional Psychology.

Pearce, J.M.S. (2004) "Richard Morton: Origins of Anorexia Nervosa," *European Neurology* 54 (4): 191–2.

Silverman, Joseph A. (1988) "Richard Morton's Second Case of Anorexia Nervosa: Reverend Minister Steele and His Son—a Historical Vignette," *International Journal of Eating Disorders* 7 (3): 439–41.

# Murray, George R., MD (1865–1939)

## Physician and endocrinologist, who discovered the effect of thyroid extract

Educated at Cambridge (MD, 1896), Murray studied in Paris and Berlin and returned to the United Kingdom in 1890 to take an appointment as a pathologist at the University of Durham. He was engaged as part of a larger committee to investigate the cause of myxedema, a widespread disease with prominent signs and symptoms: Bulging eyes, increased body weight, mental confusion, and, often, goiter. This disease, found also in sheep, was variously labeled Grave's or Basedow's Disease. In 1873, Sir William Withey Gull (1816–90), one of the early promoters of anorexia nervosa as a diagnosis, had postulated that the disease was the result of the atrophy of the thyroid gland. Earlier, in 1855, the great Parisian researcher Claude Bernard (1813–78) had developed the notion that there was internal secretion from the thyroid (and other glands) that had a regulating effect on bodily systems. Gull had, in fact, diagnosed one of his patients who had shown "general increase of bulk ... Her face altering from oval to round" as suffering from some type of thyroid insufficiency (Gull 1874: 315).

Murray also hypothesized that the disease was the result of an insufficiency of thyroid production, but he sought to treat this disease through the replacement of the thyroid secretion. He ordered sheep thyroids from a slaughterhouse, had them removed in an antiseptic manner, strained them through a handkerchief, and prepared emulsions of dried sheep thyroid in glycerin. Despite being scoffed at by his colleagues, who claimed that it would be as likely to treat locomotor ataxia with an emulsion of spinal cord, he injected the thyroid extract into a patient with myxedema and was completely successful on his first such attempt with the treatment.

Murray published his results in 1891 and thus began the field of therapeutic endocrinology. With the successful reduction of symptoms in myxedema, including weight loss, thyroid extract quickly became part of the therapy for obesity. Indeed, the claim of endocrinologists after the beginning of the twentieth century was that all obesity was the result of such pathological states. In 1924, the editors of the *Journal of the American Medical Association* published an editorial entitled "What Causes Obesity?" In it, they argue, following a powerful antipsychological strand in obesity research that began in the late nineteenth century, that obesity is the result of a malfunction of normal metabolic processes. When obesity is viewed as a "scientific problem," they write, the "fat woman" will be freed from the stigma that she "has the remedy in her own hands—or rather between her own teeth" (Anonymous 1924: 1003). The subsequent use of thyroid extract and then "synthroid" (artificial thyroid extract) as a therapy for obesity is often successful as it creates a state of hyperthyroidism, a pathology, which is noted by extreme weight loss (and many other symptoms). Thus, ironically enough, one pathology is treated through the creation of another.

SLG

*See also* Gull

## References and Further Reading

Anon. (1924) "What Causes Obesity?" *Journal of the American Medical Association*, September 27: 1003.

Anon. (1967) "George R. Murray (1865–1939): Clinical Endocrinologist," *Journal of the American Medical Association* 201 (5): 321–2.

Armstrong, C.M. (1993) "George Redmayne Murray 1865–1939: The First Use of Thyroid Extract for the Treatment of Myxoedema," in *Medicine in Northumbria*, Newcastle-upon-Tyne: Pybus Society, pp. 310–16.

Gull, William Withey (1874) *On a Cretinoid State Supervening in Adult Life in Women*. Reprinted in William Withey Gull (1896) *A Collection of the Published Writings of William Withey Gull*, London: New Sydenham Society, Vol. II, pp. 315–21.

Pearce, J.M.S. (2006) "Myxoedema and Sir William Withey Gull (1816–1890)," *Journal of Neurology, Neurosurgery, and Psychiatry* 77 (6): 639–43.

# N

## Natural Man

### Back to Nature

There is a common assumption in the twenty-first century that "natural" food is a prophylactic against obesity as well as illness. The French food writer Jean-Anthelme Brillat-Savarin could write as late as 1825 that "obesity is never found either among savages or in those classes of society, which must work in order to eat or which do not eat except to exist." But he provided a caveat, "savages will eat gluttonously and drink themselves insensible when ever they have a chance to" (Brillat-Savarin 1999: 239 and 241). This is very much in line with Immanuel Kant's view of "savages" and alcohol use in his lectures on anthropology first held in 1772–3 and published by a student in 1831 (Kant 1831: 299). Obesity, therefore, could be an illness of natural man as well as of civilization when the boundaries of power were transgressed. Christoph Wilhelm Hufeland (1762–1836), one of the first modern medical commentators on dieting, recognized this when he commented "a certain degree of cultivation is physically necessary for man, and promotes duration of life. The wild savage does not live so long as man in a state of civilization" (Hufeland 1797: 1, 169).

This notion is also reflected in the memoirs of Georg Forster (1754–94) who accompanied Captain James Cook (1728–79) around the world in the 1770s. In 1773, Cook and Forster found themselves in Tahiti, an island that they saw as the perfect natural society. Food abounded, and one did not have to work for it. Therefore, gluttony was impossible, as only in a society of inadequacy did the passion for food arise. Fat men were impossible in Tahiti. Except, Forster reports walking along the shore he saw a "very fat man, who seemed to be the chief of the district" being fed by a "woman who sat near him, crammed down his throat by handfuls the remains of a large baked fish, and several breadfruits, which he swallowed with a voracious appetite." His face was the "picture of phlegmatic insensibility, and seemed to witness that all his thoughts centred in the care of his paunch." Forster is shocked because he had assumed that obesity of this nature was impossible in a world with "a certain frugal equality in their way of living, and whose hours of enjoyment were justly proportioned to those of labour and rest." However, here was the proof that obesity and society were not linked, for Forster found a "luxurious individual spending his life in the most sluggish inactivity, and without one benefit to society, like the privileged parasites of more civilized climates, fattening on the superfluous produce of the soil, of which he robbed the labouring multitude" (Forster 2000: 1, 164–5). This contradiction caused much consternation.

The belief in the inherent absence of obesity among "natural man" still echoes in Edwin James's 1819 statement that

the Missouri Indian is symmetrical and active, and in stature, equal, if not somewhat superior, to the ordinary European standard; tall men are numerous. The active occupations of war and hunting, together perhaps with the occasional privations, to which they are subjected, prevents that unsightly obesity, so often a concomitant of civilization, indolence, and serenity of mental temperament.

(James 1905: 68)

But this is true only of men. John Wyeth observed in 1832 that among the tribes of the Northwest "the persons of the men generally are rather symmetrical; their stature is low, with light sinewy limbs, and remarkably small delicate hands. The women are usually more rotund, and, in some instances, even approach obesity" (Wyeth 1905: 307). Among "natural peoples" it is shocking to imagine a fat man then as now.

The counterpart to "natural man" in the thought of the time was the scholar. Thus there are regimens of dieting for intellectuals. In 1825, the American Chandler Robbins suggested that the "evils usually incident to sedentary and studious habits" were the result of poor diet (Robbins 1825: 56–7). Yet, the author also noted that what was an appropriate diet for one, did not always work for others (Robbins 1825: 58). The key was variety, temperature (cool was better than hot, such as food eaten in nature), frequency (three meals a day, one "liberal" and two "slight"), the avoidance of exercise (after a meal one should rest) and "chewing long and leisurely": "masticate, denticate, chump, grind, and swallow." This later becomes gospel by the end of the nineteenth century, but it is, in the end, one thing that "maintains vigour of the mind and the body, temperance becomes the parent of all other virtues," unlike what reportedly happens in the idyllic world of "natural man" (Robbins 1825: 57). In 1836, William Newnham observed in London that "over-stimulation of the brain" caused "the general health to suffer" (Newnham 1836: 3). What results is torpor, and the cure is dieting. Mastication is vital, but the diet must be "simple: animal food under dressed, roast in preference to boil'd; let vegetables be very much dressed, and bread very much baked; sauces, made dishes, and pastry to be avoided, or taken very sparingly" (Robbins 1825: 31–2). Water should be taken, rather than wine. Indeed, the cure for the scholar is the diet of "natural man."

In 1939, a Cleveland dentist named Weston Price (1870–1948) self-published *Nutrition and Physical Degeneration*, which argued that isolated cultures showed no tooth decay and less arthritis, diabetes, cancer, and heart disease than people living in urbanized, industrialized nations (Price 1939: 5). This seemed to make some sense at the time given the politics of food faddism, except that Price, as with all of the earliest advocates of "natural man," also sees such societies as better, purer, and more moral than more developed societies, which show "character changes" and are in a state of "moral deterioration" (Price 1939: 353). The communities,

including dairy farmers in Switzerland's Loetschental Valley, the Aborigines of Australia, the "Gaelics" in the Outer and Inner Hebrides, Maoris in New Zealand, and native peoples in ancient and modern Peru, as well as the Melanesians and Polynesians (remember Foster) were so varied and had such radically different food cultures that Price focused on the absence of processed foods, such as refined sugar and flour and hydrogenated oils. His goal is a "nutritional program for race regeneration" in which deficient foods for the urban dweller are the equivalent of inadequate nutrition among the "native."

The result of the poor nutrition among the "natives" is the encroachment of civilization (Price 1939: 498). For him (and his views on nutrition at least have lasted) "natural man" is healthy because *s/he* eats "natural" foods, a claim belied by the complex reality of such cultures, as observers in the eighteenth century could well have shown him. Indeed, his example comes from "the high Alps of Switzerland" where he found "an excellent state of physical development and health in adults and children living in the high valleys." This state of health persists in spite of the inroads of "refined cereals, a high intake of sweets, canned goods, sweetened fruits, chocolate; and a greatly reduced use of dairy products" among the urban Swiss (Price 1939: 43). His explanation for the innate "healthiness" of those Swiss "isolated" from the spread of modern, manufactured and, therefore, corrupting foods is the consumption of "rye . . . the only cereal that developed well for human food" (Price 1939: 509). He took a piece of the rye bread and had it analyzed, finding that "it was rich in minerals and vitamins."

A hundred years before, he would have found the valleys full of "cretins" with the stigmata of degeneration, the goiter, clearly present, as B.A. Morel (1809–73), who coined the term "degeneration" based on these cases in 1857, saw it (Morel 1857). All would be suffering from severe mental retardation—caused by the absence of iodine. Or they would have been simply gone "mad" from eating rye grain covered with ergot, a poisonous fungus. Swiss public-health officials intervened over the subsequent fifty years; they turned the verdant valleys of the Alps into Price's edenic landscape, where only healthy food is consumed. Even "natural man" needs civilization.

SLG

*See also* Brillat-Savarin; Enlightenment; Fletcher; Obesity Epidemic; Paleolithic Diet

### References and Further Reading

Brillat-Savarin, Jean-Anthelme (1999) *The Physiology of Taste or, Meditations on Transcendental Gastronomy*, trans. M.F.K. Fisher, Washington, DC: Counterpoint.

Forster, Georg (2000) *Voyage Around the World*, ed. Nicolas Thomas and Oliver Berghof, two vols, Honolulu, Hawaii: University of Hawaii Press.

Hufeland, Christopher William (1797) *The Art of Prolonging Life*, two vols, London: J. Bell.

James, Edwin (1905) *Early Western Travels, Vol. 15: Part II of James's Account of S.H. Long's Expedition, 1819–1820*, ed. Reuben Gold Thwaites, Cleveland, Ohio: A.H. Clark Co.

Kant, Immanuel (1831) *Immanuel Kant's Menschenkunde. Nach Handschriftlichen Vorlesungen*, ed. Friedrich Christian Starke, Leipzig: Die Expedition des europäischen Aufsehers.

Morel, Bénédict Auguste (1857) *Traité des dégénérescences physiques, intellectuelles, et morales de l'espèce humaine et des causes qui produisent ces variétés maladives*, Paris: Baillière.

Newnham, William (1836) *Essay on the Disorders Incident to Literary Men: And on the Best Means of Preserving Their Health, Read Before the Royal Society of Literature, Nov. 5, 1834*, London: John Hatchard and Sons.

Price, Weston (1939) *Nutrition and Physical Degeneration: A Comparison of Primitive and Modern Diets and Their Effects, etc.*, Redlands, Calif.: Published by the Author; New York and London: P.B. Hoeber.

Robbins, Chandler (1825) *Remarks on the Disorders of Literary Men, or, an Inquiry into the Means of Preventing the Evils Usually Incident to Sedentary and Studious Habits*, Boston, Mass.: Cummings, Hillard.

Wyeth, John B. (1905) *Early Western Travels, Vol. 21: Wyeth's Oregon, or a Short History of a Long Journey, 1832: Townsend's Narrative of a Journey Across the Rocky Mountains, 1834*, ed. Reuben Gold Thwaites, Cleveland, Ohio: A.H. Clark Co.

# Nidetch, Jean (1923–)

## Founder of Weight Watchers International, Inc.

Nidetch was born in Brooklyn, New York and grew up with a weight problem that continued into her late thirties. Nidetch tried various weight-loss approaches, ranging from diets to diet pills, but she seemed to always gain her weight back. Then, Nidetch joined a weight-loss program sponsored by the New York City Board of Health and followed a diet program for ten weeks. She lost about 20 pounds, but her enthusiasm to keep to the diet was slowly fading. Nidetch felt she needed support and encouragement from her friends to give her feedback on progress and keep her going. She began holding meetings with several friends, and the original group grew to about forty people within three months. Word spread rapidly about the meetings, since there were no existing self-help movements for the overweight. Within the next year, Nidetch agreed to lead similar groups throughout the area.

In May 1963, Nidetch rented a loft and held the first Weight Watchers meeting, which boasted 400 participants. As the program developed, members of Weight Watchers were required to weigh in at each meeting to keep track of weight loss progress. Nidetch's particular diet consisted of a low-fat regimen to reduce the number of calories being consumed, and she also proposed an upper limit on the total number of calories that a person could consume. Rather than have people count calories, she developed a point system to help participants keep track of how much food they were eating (Womble and Wadden 2002).

The Weight Watchers Diet is favored among nutritionists because it is not as restrictive as other commercial diet plans, making dieters more likely to maintain the lifestyle (Low et al. 2001). Today, more than 37 million worldwide have joined the Weight Watchers program, perhaps in part because the diet has been shown to reduce weight in a randomized clinic trial (Heshka et al. 2000).

However, the amount of weight that people lost on Weight Watchers was shown, in this trial, to be similar to that lost on the Zone, Ornish, and Atkins diets (Dansinger et al. 2005). Today, people interested in dieting with the help of Weight Watchers can attend meetings all over the U.S.A. and can also use the Internet rather than actually attending meetings. Due to the overwhelming success and popularity of the program, Nidetch rose from a housewife struggling with her weight to a national celebrity.

SLG/RAKHI PATEL AND SUZANNE JUDD

*See also* Atkins; Internet; Ornish; Self-help; Zone Diet

**References and Further Reading**

Anon. "Jean Nidetch: Weight Loss Therapy." Available online at <http://www.pbs.org/wgbh/theymadeamerica/whomade/nidetch_hi.html> (accessed March 15, 2007).

Dansinger M.L., Gleason, J.A., Griffith, J.L., Selker, H.P., and Schaefer, E.J. (2005) "Comparison of the Atkins, Ornish, Weight Watchers, and Zone Diets for Weight Loss and Heart Disease Risk Reduction: A Randomized Trial," *Journal of the American Medical Association* 293 (1): 43–53.

Heshka S., Greenway, F., Anderson, J.W., Atkinson, R.L., Hill, J.O., Phinney, S.D., Miller-Kovach, K., and Xavier Pi-Sunyer, F. (2000) "Self-Help Weight Loss Versus a Structured Commercial Program After 26 Weeks: A Randomized Controlled Study," *American Journal of Medicine* 109 (4): 282–7.

Horatio Alger Association (2005) "Jean Nidetch," The Horatio Alger Association of Distinguished Americans, available online at <http://www.horatioalger.com/members/member_info.cfm?memberid=Nid89> (accessed March 15, 2007).

Lowe M.R., Miller-Kovach, K. and Phelan, S. (2001) "Weight-Loss Maintenance in Overweight Individuals One to Five Years Following Successful Completion of a Commercial Weight Loss Program," *International Journal of Obesity and Related Metabolic Disorders: Journal of the International Association for the Study of Obesity* 25 (3): 325–31.

Womble, Leslie G. and Wadden, Thomas (2002) "Commercial and Self-Help Weight Loss Programs," in Christopher G. Fairburn and Kelly D. Brownell (eds) *Eating Disorders and Obesity: A Comprehensive Handbook*, New York: Guilford Press, pp. 546–50.

# Noorden, Carl Von (1858–1944)

## German Internist

Trained in Leipzig (MD, 1881), in 1894, Noorden became Director for Internal Medicine at the City Hospital in Frankfurt, where he created a private clinic for diabetes and dietetic cures. In 1906, he became the Head of the Clinic for Internal Medicine in Imperial Vienna and was as much a celebrity doctor there as his contemporary Sigmund Freud. In 1913, he returned to Frankfurt and then, in 1929, returned again to Vienna (now the capital of a republic), recalled by the new Socialist Minister of Health, Julius Tandler, as Head of the Clinic for Metabolic Diseases. His clinical reputation rested on the development of dietetic treatments for diabetes and obesity. It was, in fact, his understanding of the impact of diet on diabetes that shaped his understanding of obesity. He conceptually linked these two expressions of human metabolism, which is reflected in his view of the nature of obesity and the importance of a medically supervised diet. After Noorden, the celebrity "diet doc" becomes a fixture of the dieting culture in the twentieth century.

One of Noorden's central contributions was his categorization of different types of obesity into (a) exogenous obesity, caused by manifest overeating with less expenditure of energy and (b) endogenous obesity, caused by abnormalities within the body that may deal with endocrine function or faulty metabolism (Noorden 1907: 693). Examples of an endocrine factor causing obesity are castration and hypo-thyroidism (Noorden 1907: 703). Yet, at the core of Noorden's movement to medicalize obesity by creating classifications for its origins was the desire to reclaim this ever-expanding category of patient from the "quacks," "reduction cures have become so popular that many patients undergo a course of treatment . . . on their own accord and without consulting a physician" (Noorden 1907: 703). The legacy of Banting was clear: self-cure meant not only fewer patients but also more importantly abdicating an entire arena of medicine to the quacks.

The demographics of this self-treating patient population at the turn of the century were also clear to him. Self-treatment is found more frequently in women than in men and "more commonly in young girls and in middle-aged women than in older women" (Noorden 1903: 15). Among men, Noorden found that patients came to him for the treatment of symptoms, which he understood as the result of their obesity but "they do not understand how a reduction cure can be of any benefit nor how their trouble can be relieved by causing a loss of fat" (Noorden 1903: 15). In their own estimation, his patients were not fat and, even if they were, it had nothing to do with their complaints!

Noorden's view about the efficacy of specific diets is vague; in fact, it was clear to him that any number of diets suggested by physicians might well work. But if "the character and morals of the patient seem to indicate that they will not exercise in moderation in work and are apt to over-indulge in the good things of life" the patients should be forced onto a supervised diet and sent to a sanitarium, even if there are no overt symptoms (Noorden 1903: 22). Simply sending these people for the "water cure" to reduce their weight is useless (Noorden 1903: 28). Only medically supervised weight reduction, Noorden believed, can have the desired impact on long-term health.

Noorden was also very much attuned to the gender politics of his age. Thus, he advocates being very careful with "the whims and fancies of our lady patients" that, having given birth, are appalled at their abdominal fat. Radical reduction of such fat may lead, Noorden warns, to further medical complications even if changes of appearance are achieved (Noorden 1903: 31). In pathological cases, the general tendency towards a weakness of

will in the obese is manifest. Hysterics (who are primarily women) "are usually persons who 'cannot' or 'will not,' whose will power is small. Subjects of this kind usually eat a great deal and are at the same time lazy so that they do not get enough muscular exercise and do not develop any energy and readily grow moderately fat" (Noorden 1903: 54). Noorden placed his reduction cures in the service of a new medical science that seemed also to be answering S. Weir Mitchell's "rest cure" with its weight gain and enforced bed rest. Noorden's views impacted the later focus of obesity studies, which went on to examine factors that may regulate appetite and food consumption, such as caloric intake.

Much of Noorden's work also focused on diabetes, a disease that seemed to be increasing in late-nineteenth century Europe. The model for Noorden's insistence on medicalized diet rests on his experience with diabetics. Defined as a disease of diet in the age before Frederick Grant Banting and Charles Herbert Best discover insulin in 1921, diabetes seemed only to be controlled (if at all) through diet. As early as the work of John Rollo in 1796, it was clear that the reduction of carbohydrates would reduce the amount of sugar. As a result, Rollo urged that diabetics consume only meat and fat. In 1865, Apollinaire Bouchardat in Paris suggested that all foodstuffs should be reduced, including fats. As a result of the latter view, Edgar Allen created a radical hunger cure for the control of diabetes, which also functioned as a radical cure for overweight. Noorden supported the "Allen Cure," but in 1902 he made his own breakthrough in the dieting culture when he discovered that oatmeal (paired with a bit of butter and some plant protein) would reduce sugar levels. Ironically, it duplicated a fad diet of the time.

Noorden's understanding of diabetes rested both on his grasp of the metabolic underpinnings of the disease, which became evident during his academic life. But one must not forget that diabetes also came to be considered the disease of modern life. Only through diet could the disease be controlled, and weight came to be a symbol of that which had to be conquered. From the nineteenth century, diabetes had been seen as a disease of the obese and, in an odd set of associations, the Jew was seen as obese due to an apparent increased presence of diabetes among Jews in Central Europe. According to Noorden, mainly rich Jewish men are fat (Noorden 1910: 63). But rather than arguing for any inborn metabolic inheritance, he stated that it is the fault of poor diet among the rich—

too much rich food and alcohol, this being yet another stereotype of the Jew. For all of Noorden's reliance on the cutting edge of medical science, racial stereotypes also played a role in his view of the obese and their diseases.

SLG/RAKHI PATEL

*See also* Aboulia; Banting; Jews; Kneipp; Medical Use of Dieting; Mitchell; Murray; Pregnancy; Risks Associated with Dieting; Tarnower

## References and Further Reading

Hauk, Joachim (1980) "Carl Harko Hermann Johannes Von Noorden (1858–1944): Sein Leben und Werk unter besonderer Berücksichtigung seiner Theorien über die Ursachen des Diabetes Mellitus," PhD diss., Mainz.

Noorden, Carl von (1903) *Clinical Treatises of the Pathology and Therapy of Disorders of Metabolism and Nutrition: Obesity the Indications for Reduction Cures*, trans. Boardman Reed, New York: E.B. Treat.

—— (1907) "Obesity," in *Metabolism and Practical Medicine*, trans. I. Walker Hall, London: Heinemann Press, Vol. III, pp. 693–715.

—— (1910) *Die Fettsucht*, Vienna: Alfred Hölder.

Pawan, G.L.S. (1958) "Obesity: Some Aspects of Metabolism of the Obese," *Proceedings of the Nutrition Society* 18 (2): 155–62.

# O

## Obesity Epidemic

Obesity as a category has been the subject of much public debate over the past decades. It has become the target of public health concern and part of a rethinking of where the sources of danger for the public may lie. Such a rethinking mixes and stirs many qualities together to provide a compelling story that defines "obesity" as the "new public health epidemic." Defining where danger lies is central to a rethinking of obesity as *the* central problem of public health. Given that dieting culture today claims to "cure" obesity, the warning of George A. Bray should be taken seriously:

> The studies of diet have shown that no diet is ideal. Cannon showed that gastric contraction is a hunger signal modified by food in the stomach. Diets modifying every nutrient have been published by a gullible and optimistic public. If any of them had "cured" obesity, it is hard to see what the market would be for the next diet.
>
> (Bray 2002: 386)

Today the media is rife with warnings about the "obesity epidemic." "Epidemic" was first evoked in public health terms of the "epidemic of heart disease" for which obesity (and smoking) were seen as major causes (Moonman 1976). By 1987, the media began to evoke the specter of epidemic obesity as a problem in itself. " 'Childhood obesity is epidemic in the United States,' said Dr. William H. Dietz Jr. of New England Medical Center" (Haney 1987). Headlines such as "Obesity Epidemic Raises Risk of Children Developing Diabetes" grabbed the attention of the reader (Lawrence 2004). Even those reporters who are a bit more attuned to what the term "epidemic" may

imply tend to agree. "To describe what has happened as an epidemic may seem far-fetched. That word is normally applied to a contagious disease that is rapidly spreading. But the population that is obese has grown 400 percent in the last 25 years" (Derbyshire 2004). Even the food industry feels that they are well positioned, for who is "better suited to solve the obesity epidemic" than they are (Fusaro 2004). The "wellness" industry too is aware of the potential of the obesity epidemic: "According to a new study, Americans consider childhood obesity as serious a problem as smoking or school violence, exceeded only by substance abuse as a health threat to school-age children" (Anon. "Public Sees Childhood Obesity" 2004: 28). In both of these cases, the industries concerned will make money; obesity is a growth industry.

From the U.S.A. to Australia, the "obesity epidemic" has become a "political issue" (Anon. "Size Up Options" 2004). The British Labour Government in 2004 admitted that it had removed the tackling of this epidemic from its public health goals and belatedly published a major account of the epidemic including horror stories about the death of a three-year-old girl from obesity (National Health Service 2004). According to the press, there was no question that "her death was due to over-feeding and bad parenting" (Finnegan and Madeley 2004). The story turned out to be a poor indicator of the epidemic as the child died of a genetically transmitted disease of which obesity was only one factor.

Obesity is not itself a "disease" but rather a phenomenological category that reflects the visible manifestation of body size, which potentially can have multiple (multifactorial) causes. No one dies from "obesity." One dies from those pathologies that may result from extreme excess weight. Indeed, obesity may be a tertiary cause of morbidity or mortality; it may lead to diabetes, which may lead to vascular disease. Thus, the image of an "epidemic" of obesity demands a single, clearly defined cause for this "disease," much as has been done with other recent epidemics of infectious diseases. Indeed, it is striking that the assumptions about the causality of "obesity" as having a single cause are part of the urban myth of disease (Johnson et al. 1994).

Politicians' use of the term "epidemic" is very much in line with that of the medical profession. "Obesity and sedentary lifestyle are escalating national and global epidemics that warrant increased attention by physicians . . . and the pivotal role will be played by physicians and other health care professionals in curbing these dangerous epidemics . . ." (Manson et al. 2004). As early as 2002, *The Lancet* warned about the global "obesity epidemic" and provided a detailed account of the public health discussions of this new killer (Larkin 2002). In 2004, E.B.R. Desapriya of the British Columbia Injury Research and Prevention Centre for Community Child Health Research in Vancouver, BC (Canada) warned that

The obesity epidemic poses a public-health challenge. Obesity has a more pronounced effect on morbidity than on mortality, and an increase in its prevalence will have an important effect on the global incidence of cardiovascular disease, type 2 diabetes mellitus, cancer, osteoarthritis, work disability, and sleep apnoea. A 1% increase in the prevalence of obesity in such countries as India and China leads to 20 million additional cases. The state of childhood obesity in the U.S.A., Canada, and many other countries worldwide has reached epidemic proportions; the Canadian prevalence tripled between 1981 and 1996.

(Desapriya 2004)

We are, everyone agrees, in the middle of an obesity "epidemic."

"Epidemic" is a technical term from epidemiology meaning any "large-scale temporary increase in the occurrence of a disease in a community or region, which is clearly in excess of normal expectancy." Yet, it is "widely used to describe clusters of diseases in general [although it has] traditionally been used when infections strike a population" (Blakemore and Jannett 2001: 249). "Epidemic" maintains a powerful metaphoric connection

to contagion. It can, of course, be applied to any disease, no matter what its cause, all injury (including gunshot wounds, as the Centers for Disease Control found to its political embarrassment a number of years ago) or other health-related event. It may be global (pandemic), but it is always defined by its rate of increase, not its universality.

"Epidemic" seems to be a creation of the seventeenth century, borrowed from the French at precisely the same time as the term "obesity." In 1620, Tobias Venner's handbook of humoral good diet and health, where one of the first uses of the term obesity appears, notes that

a fat and grosse habit of body is worse than a leane, for besides that it is more subject to sicknes, it is for all corporall actions farre more unapt. They are more sickly that have grosse and full bodies, not onely because they abound with many crude and superfluous humors, but also because they lesse (by reason of the imbicillity of their heat) resist extrinsicall and intrinsicall causes that demolish their health.

(Venner 1628: 196)

"Obesity" is, according to Venner, a disease process. Thomas Lodge in 1603 needed to define this new notion of "Epidemick" for his readership: "An Epidemick plague, is a common and popular sicknesse, hapning in some region, or country, at a certaine time, caused by a certaine indisposition of the aire, or waters of the same region, producing in all sorts of people, one and the same sicknesse" (Lodge 1603: Bijb). Two decades later, Francis Bacon, in his *The Historie of the Raigne of King Henry the Seventh* (1622) can speak of the "sweating-sickness" as "was conceived not to be an epidemick disease, but to proceed from a malignity in the constitution of the air, gathered by the predispositions of the seasons; and the speedy cessation declared as much" (Bacon 1963: 6 and 33–4). "Epidemic" quickly takes on metaphoric meaning, as in John Milton's condemnation of an "epidemick whordom" in his 1643 treatise on divorce (Milton 1851: 2, 97). This movement between illness and metaphor continues in our contemporary anxiety about the epidemic of obesity.

What is seen to cause human "obesity" is varied over time. Today there seems to be a stress on a number of often conflicting causes (Chang and Christakis 2002). Central among them are social and genetic-physiological explanations:

1. A shift in "quality of life" and life expectancy. We live longer now, have less physically stressful occupations, and have easier access to more food.

2. A psychological dependency on food as a means of manipulating the immediate environment. This is an assumption that obesity is simply on a continuum with anorexia nervosa, which has been so defined by psychologists. Obesity is thus a mental illness.

3. Access to poor but abundant food and the absence of structures to engage in physical activity: the obesity of poverty argument.

4. The loss of control over our consumption of food because of our addictive behavior. Addiction is usually understood following the medical model of some type of pathological genetic predisposition in an individual or a group rather than a "weakness of will" (Miller 1980).

5. A "normal" genetic predisposition understood in terms of evolutionary biological drive to accumulate body fat in order to preclude starvation in times of famine (Kolata 2007). This is the "ob-gen" argument first put forth in the classic 1994 paper on the genetics of obesity in mice that concludes with an extrapolation about human beings (Zhang 1994, 6).

6. A disruption of normal growth because of the changes in the endocrine system though pathological changes including aging (also understood as pathological).

7. The result of infection. This had been argued by Jules Hirsch in 1982 (Lyons et al. 1982) and more recently has been advocated by Nikhil Dhurandhar (Dhurandhar 2001).

What is clear is that any single explanation maybe possible for any given individual but it is the social implications of "obesity" that have now turned it into an "epidemic."

The epidemic of obesity is actually presenting itself as a worldwide "moral panic," that is an "episode, condition, person or group of persons" that have in recent times, been "defined as a threat to societal values and interests" (Cohen 1972: 9). Thus, Stanley Cohen created the concept of a "moral panic" in the early 1970s in his work on witchcraft trials and other such "constructed" phenomena seen as "epidemic." Obesity is characterized by "stylized and stereotypical" representation by the mass media, and a tendency for those "in power" (politicians, bishops, editors, and so on) to man the "moral barricades" and pronounce moral judgments. Moral panics need not be focused on "invented" categories such as witches; they can also be associated with real health problems as a way

in which to magnify and shape their meanings. They can use "real" categories of illness to explain such health problems within the ideological focus of the time (Cohen 1972: 9).

The anxiety about "epidemics" points up the danger that seems to lie in the concept of "moral panic." Obesity is now the central "danger" to confront all aspects or all societies (as it is seen as an epidemic of poverty as well as affluence). The spread seems *like* a contagious disease. Yet each discussion of obesity seems to choose some model for the cause and nature of obesity that can be the point of intervention to end this plague: Whether it is the danger of fast food, too much sugar or fat, too little exercise, damaged psyche or weak will, too-large portions, genetic predisposition, or hormonal imbalance. It is not unpredictable that there has been a strong argument for at least some cases of obesity being the result of an infectious agency—this fulfills all of the metaphoric power of the "moral panic" about fat and limits its locus to a specific and treatable cause. In the U.S.A., this is embodied by "the Center for Science in the Public Interest. That's the advocacy group that periodically issues breathless bulletins (Food porn!) warning that one food or another (eggs, soda, shellfish, Mexican food, Chinese food, French fries, donuts, beef, salt, etc.) is bad for you" (Anon. 2005). A magic bullet can be found which is simply more difficult for most of the other imagined biological or social causes postulated for obesity.

SLG

*See also* Aboulia; Anorexia; Binge-eating; Cannon; Children; Genetics; Infectobesity; Smoking

## References and Further Reading

Anon. (2004) "Size Up Options," *MX* (Melbourne, Australia), June 30: 23.

Anon. (2004) "Public Sees Childhood Obesity As Serious Health Threat," *Fitness and Wellness Business Week*, June 30: 28.

Anon. (2005) "The Food Jihad," *St. Louis Post-Dispatch*, July 11: B6.

Bacon, Francis (1963) *The Works of Francis Bacon*, eds Robert Spedding, Leslie Ellis James, and Douglas Denon Heath, ten vols., Stuttgart: Friedrich Frommann.

Blakemore, Colin and Jannett, Sheila (eds) (2001) *The Oxford Companion to the Body*, Oxford: Oxford University Press.

Bray, George A. (2002) "A Brief History of Obesity," in Christopher G. Fairburn and Kelly D. Brownell (eds), *Eating Disorders and Obesity: A Comprehensive Handbook*, 2nd edn, New York: Guilford Press, pp. 382–7.

Chang, Virginia W. and Christakis, Nicholas A. (2002) "Medical Modeling of Obesity: A Transition from Action to Experience in a 20th Century American Medical Textbook," *Sociology of Health and Illness* 24 (2): 151–77.

Cohen, Stanley (1972) *Folk Devils and Moral Panics*, London: Macgibbon and Kee.

Derbyshire, David (2004) "Warning of 'Epidemic'," *Telegraph* (London), June 10.

Desapriya, E.B.R. (2004) "Letter: Obesity Epidemic," *The Lancet* 364 (9444): 1488.

Dhurandhar, Nikhil V. (2001) "Infectobesity: Obesity of Infectious Origin," *Journal of Nutrition 131*: 2794S–2797S.

Finnegan, Judy and Madeley, Richard (2004) "I Was So Right to Doubt the Fat Children Report," *Express Newspapers*, June 12.

Fusaro, Dave (2004) "Fear and Opportunity in Vending Machines: Who Is Better Suited to Solve the Obesity Epidemic Than the Food Industry?" *Food Processing* 65: 6.

Haney, Daniel Q. (1987) "Study Says Childhood Obesity Increasing Among Out-of-Shape Kids," *The Associated Press*, May 1.

Johnson, S.R., Schonfeld, D.J., Siegel, D., Krasnovsky, F.M., Boyce, J.C., Saliba, P.A., Boyce, W.T., and Perrin, E.C. (1994) "What Do Minority Elementary Students Understand About the Causes of Acquired Immunodeficiency Syndrome, Colds, and Obesity?" *Journal of Developmental and Behavior Pediatrics* 15 (6): 239–47.

Kolata, Gina (2007) *Rethinking Thin: The New Science of Weight Loss—and the Myths and Realities of Dieting*, New York: Farrar, Straus and Giroux.

Larkin, Marilynn (2002) "Combating the Global Obesity Epidemic," *The Lancet* 360 (9340): 1181.

Lawrence, Jeremy (2004) "Obesity Epidemic Raises Risk of Children Developing Diabetes," *Independent* (London), June 21.

Lodge, Thomas (1603) *A Treatise of the Plague: Containing the Nature, Signes, and Accidents of the Same, with the Certaine and Absolute Cure of the Fevers, Botches, and Carbuncles That Raigne in These Times: And Above All Things Most Singular Experiments and Preservatives in the Same, Gathered by the Observation of Divers Worthy Travailers, and Selected Out of the Writings of the Best Learned Phisitians in This Age*, London: Edward White and N.L.

Lyons, M., Faust, J.I.M., Hemmes, R.B., Buskirk, D.R., Hirsch, J., and Zabriskie, J.B. (1982) "A Virally Induced Obesity Syndrome in Mice," *Science* 216 (4541): 82–5.

Manson, JoAnn E., Skerrett, Patrick J., Greenland, Philip, and VanItallie, Theodore B. (2004) "The Escalating Pandemics of Obesity and Sedentary Lifestyle: A Call to Action for Clinicians," *Archives of Internal Medicine* 164 (3): 249–58.

Miller, William R. (ed.) (1980) *The Addictive Behaviours: Treatment of Alcoholism, Drug Abuse, Smoking and Obesity*, Oxford: Pergamon Press.

Milton, John (1851) *The Works of John Milton*, ed. John Mitford, eight vols, London: W. Pickering.

Moonman, Eric (1976) "Fighting the West's Man-Made Epidemic," *The Times* (London), June 14: 12.

National Health Service (U.K.) (2004) *The Government Response to the Health Select Committee's Report on Obesity*, London: Stationery Office.

Venner, Tobias (1628) *Via Recta Ad Vitam Longam: or, a Plaine Philosophicall Demonstration of the Nature, Faculties, and Effects of All Such Things As by Way of Nourishments Make for the Preseruation of Health with Diuers Necessary Dieticall Obseruations; As Also of the True Vse and Effects of Sleepe, Exercise, Excretions and Perturbations, with Iust Applications to Euery Age, Constitution of Body, and Time of Yeere: by to. Venner, Doctor of Physicke in Bathe. Whereunto Is Annexed a Necessary and Compendious Treatise of the Famous Baths of Bathe, Lately Published by the Same Author*, London: Imprinted by Felix Kyngston, for Richard Moore, and are to be sold at his shop in Saint Dunstans Church-yard in Fleetstreet.

Zhang, Y., Proenca, R., Maffei, M., Barone, M., Leopold, L. and Friedman, J.M. (1994) "Positional Cloning of the Mouse Obese Gene and Its Human Homologue," *Nature* 372 (6505): 425–31.

# Obsessive Compulsive Disorders

Is "avoidance of fat people and things they ha[ve] touched" a form of obsessive compulsive disorder (OCD) (Greist and Jefferson 1995: 106)? It sounds like it may be an eating disorder, such as anorexia nervosa. It is difficult to tell which diagnosis would be appropriate in this situation, as there seems to be relatively little information concerning the dietary and nutritional dangers associated with obsessive compulsive disorder, especially when compared to anorexia. Might there be a link between modern society's "obsession" with the "perfect" body and the clinical diagnosis of OCD?

> Anthony became very rigorous in his pursuit of weight loss ... He has been following a highly structured routine ... each morning ... he eats a breakfast consisting of 1 ounce of cereal, 1 half cup of skim milk, 1 hard boiled egg, and strawberries or blueberries. He then waits a short period of time before proceeding to the weight room, where from Monday through Friday, he spends almost exactly 2 hours performing an identical routine of weight lifting ... He skips lunch ... and has a supper consisting of a sandwich, 6 ounces of yogurt, and iced tea. He does eat salads at times but is concerned about possible ill effects from pesticides that may have been applied to the vegetables. As a result of this ritualized regimen over the past several months, Anthony has lost 75 pounds, reportedly weighing 135 pounds ... Anthony says he would prefer to weigh 145 pounds ... but is unable to eat the foods that would allow him to gain the weight.
>
> (Greist and Jefferson 1995: 25)

This case seems difficult to classify. The DSM-IV-TR definition of OCD states:

> an anxiety disorder, where it is defined as obsessions and/or compulsions that cause marked distress, are time-consuming, or interfere with functioning. Obsessions are defined as recurrent and persistent thoughts, impulses or images experienced as invasive and ego-dystonic and that cause anxiety or distress. Compulsions are defined as ritualistic behaviors or mental acts that the person feels driven to perform in response to an obsession or according to rules that must be rigidly applied. The behavior or mental act is aimed at preventing or reducing distress or preventing some dreaded event or situation and is recognized as excessive or unreasonable.
>
> (American Psychiatric Association 2000: 417)

While Anthony's obsession with weight and subsequent compulsive diet and exercise regimen clearly match parts of the DSM-IV criteria for OCD, his behavioral symptoms seem also to mimic those of an eating disorder, namely anorexia.

The DSM-IV definition of anorexia nervosa has four conditions:

> 1) Refusal to maintain body weight for age and height; 2) intense fear of gaining weight or becoming fat, even though underweight; 3) disturbance in the way in which one's body weight, size, or shape is experienced, undue influence of body weight or shape on self-evaluation, or denial of the seriousness of the current low body weight; and 4) in females, amenorrhea.
>
> (American Psychiatric Association 2000: 417–23)

This definition becomes important in understanding the relationship between anorexia and OCD, because in Anthony's case, for instance, his behaviors do superficially fit some of the DSM-IV criteria for anorexia. The DSM-IV condition that most applies to Anthony's situation is the first one mentioned above: Refusal to maintain body weight for age and height. However, when examined closely, Anthony does not truly meet these criteria, because he is not refusing to maintain healthy weight, in fact, "Anthony says he would prefer to weigh 145 pounds ... but is unable to eat the foods that would allow him to gain the weight." This is due to an obsessive fear of the foods that would allow him to gain weight, rather than the intense fear of gaining weight associated with anorexia.

The key difference between OCD and anorexia is that people suffering from anorexia actually believe that they are too fat even when they are dangerously thin and, further, believe that their dangerously restrictive diet is "healthy." A person engaging in a dangerously restrictive diet associated with OCD, on the other hand, is well aware that their actions are "crazy" and can be debilitating; however, they are unable to refrain from performing such ritualistic dieting.

After close examination of Anthony's situation and the DSM-IV criteria for OCD and anorexia, it is clear that he is suffering from OCD and not anorexia. Thus, it is clear that OCD can have just as profound an effect on one's diet, exercise, and overall nutrition as any eating disorder. So why is there a lack of literature concerning the dietary and nutritional dangers that can be associated with OCD? Perhaps the answer has a great deal to do with the superficially gray areas linked to such cases (dangerously restrictive dieting associated with OCD).

Furthermore, the stigma of anorexia as untreatable may have something to do with misdiagnoses. Many patients labeled anorexic may, in fact, be suffering from OCD and are, as a result, often treated incorrectly, likely to no avail. Cases such as Anthony's further overlap with body dysmorphic disorder, which is related to a question asked above: Is there a link between modern society's "obsession" with fat and the perfect body and such obsessive compulsive (or body dysmorphic) tendencies.

Today, body dysmorphic disorder has reappeared as a conventional means of labeling men's obesity as a problem of obsession in the clinical sense—an OCD—rather than a failure of will (Gilman 2004: 228). In conclusion, OCD and its relationship with dieting and the pursuit of the perfect body has many unanswered questions, largely due to the gray areas and overlaps (with other mental illnesses) associated with it and, therefore, a great deal of additional research is necessary.

SLG/Jason Weinstein

See also Anorexia

## References and Further Reading

American Psychiatric Association (2000) *Diagnostic and Statistical Manual of Mental Disorders DSM-IV-TR*, 4th edn, Washington, DC: American Psychiatric Publishing, Inc.

Gilman, Sander L. (2004) *Fat Boys: A Slim Book*, Lincoln, Nebr. and London: University of Nebraska Press.

Greist, John H. and Jefferson, James W. (1995) *OCD Casebook*, rev. edn, Washington, DC: American Psychiatric Publishing, Inc.

# Old Age and Obesity

In Classical Greek medicine, the elderly have, by definition, a cold and dry temperament; they were seen as melancholic and are thus in need of therapy. Youth has a sanguine complexion, as Shakespeare's Falstaff fantasizes himself as a healthy, middle-aged man: "A goodly portly man, i' faith, and a corpulent, of a cheerful look, a pleasing eye, and a most noble carriage" (*Henry IV, Part I*, Act II, Scene 4, lines 422–4). What is "happy corpulence" in youth is inherently different from "melancholic obesity" in old age (Steadman 1957). Old fat is a sign of disease. La Fontaine observes that what one wishes to achieve in life is "*embonpoint raisonnable*," not obese girth (La Fontaine 1883–92: V, 587, and I, 86).

In a 1636 translation of the Jesuit theologian Leonard Lessius's (1554–1623) autobiography is a classic account of how health flows through life, "for one kinde of proportion belongs to Youth, when it is in its flower; another to Consistencie; a third to Old Age" (Lessius 1636: 16). Lessius noted that as a young man one can eat more extensively, but old age marks the decline of such excess. One should not eat more that one can in order that one is not "made unfit for the duties and offices belonging to the Minde" (Lessius 1636: 30). A "Sober diet doth by little and little diminish this abundance of humours, and abates this ill moisture, and reduceth them to their due proportions" (Lessius 1636: 34). Central to Lessius and his Jacobean translator is the avoidance of those foods that cause illness in the elderly, which "breed cataracts, clouds, dizzinesses, distillations and coughs; and in the stomack breed crudities, inflations, gripings, gnawings, frettings, and the like ..." (Lessius 1636: 60). One must avoid these or one has no "plainer proof of his thraledom to gluttonie, than when he thus thrusts and poures in that which he knows is hurtfull unto him, onely to content his licorish appetite" (Lessius 1636: 60–61).

Such a sober diet is necessary, for it "drives away Wrath and Melancholie, and breaks the furie of Lust; in a word, replenisheth both soul and bodie with exceeding good things; so that it may well be termed the mother of Health" (Lessius 1636: 202). Everard Maynwaringe noted later in the century that such indulgence does not solely impair the individual but also the entire future of the state. He writes,

we and our posterity shall degenerate yet still into a worse and sooner fading state of life. For, as the principles of our Nature are more infirm, tainted, and debauched from our parents and Progenitors, than those of former Ages, of more vigour, soundness and integrity; are likewise more propense, and liable worse to be depraved and degenerate, and consequently of shorter duration and continuance.

(Maynwaringe 1670: 4)

"[I]ndulging Venus too much, by immoderate and too frequent acts, thereby enervating all the faculties, dispiriting and wasting the body: by wearing and fretting the mind with various passions" (Maynwaringe 1670: 6). This statement suggests that lust was just as dangerous as gluttony. The result is "the Body which was fat, or plump and fleshy; afterwards grows lean and thin; or if lean and spare bodies grow big and corpulent; here is just cause of suspicion, that all is not right" (Maynwaringe 1670: 41). Fat bodies have their own problems and they reflect the image of acedia or sloth: "Avoid day sleeps as a bad custom; [undertaken by] chiefly fat and corpulent bodies" (Maynwaringe 1670: 92). Later in the text, the soul itself is perceived as fat when the body is in distress: "The Soul is languishing, heavy and inactive, altogether indisposed to the government and tuition of the body; and perhaps desirous to be discharged and shake it off, being weary of the burthen; taking no delighted in their partnership and society, as in melancholy despair and grief" (Maynwaringe 1670: 133).

In the nineteenth century, the noted physiologist Angelo Mosso argued that older people were at risk from various pathologies if they overindulged in any area (Toye 1983: 234). Brain fatigue was the great villain of creativity, especially in the aged. Mosso, who had studied in Leipzig and later with Claude Bernard, was at the time the Professor of Physiology at Turin and a noted exponent of a materialist reading of creativity. He strongly believed that "psychic functions are . . . intim-ately united with the phenomena of nutrition and reproduction . . ." (Mosso 1906: 60). Since "mental phenomena are a function of the brain," exhaustion of the brain could be the result of inappropriate intellectual over-exertion (Mosso 1906: 62). Mosso cites Charles Darwin who claimed that he found in himself "excessive intellectual work was apt to produce vertigo . . ." (Mosso 1906: 225). Mosso, therefore, stressed that all creativity should be limited to specific periods during the day. Goethe, he notes, worked in the morning, Rousseau at night. However, in general the best work is done during limited periods of time in the morning.

Central to Mosso's presentation of the creative process is that it too is a form of work and, as such, can be debilitating, especially to those with pre-existing nervous weakness as well as the aged. He quotes the noted Dutch physiologist Jacob Moleschott (1822–93) that "in artists and scientists the material change promoted by their intellectual exertions is again moderated by their sedentary life. And it is a well-known fact that artists and scientists, in spite of their sedentary life, rarely suffer of fat" (Mosso 1906: 225). Moleschott, in his 1852 book *The Circuit of Life*, likewise noted his belief in the material basis of emotion and thought. For him, healthy artists are thin artists, as their body reflects the very work of creativity. Artists may have increased rates of urination, Moleschott claims, but this is simply a sign of the work that can in some result in intellectual fatigue. The relationship between stress and blood pressure is a relationship central to his understanding of the perils of aging. Thus, all old, creative men would be advised that they would live longer and more productively if they worked only two hours a day. Diet too is central to the preservation of life and the essence of creativity. All excess is to be avoided.

With the 1998 World Health Organization's report on the new classifications for defining obesity, much more concern has been given to old age. The statistical basis for this concern rests on the Metropolitan Life mortality tables, which ceased in 1983. Recently (1997–2000) there has been a wide range of studies that argue that obesity is the cause of a range of diseases and disabilities of aging. The Italian Longitudinal Study of Aging (1997) showed that the greater the weight in a population aged sixty-five to eighty-four, the greater the mortality. Indeed, there was a 6 percent decrease in mortality for men and a 3 percent decrease for women for every BMI unit less that people weighed. Interestingly enough, a number of these studies have been sponsored by the Seventh-Day

Adventist medical organizations, which have consistently argued for diet reform since the creation of the Church (Andres 2002).

SLG

*See also* Dublin; Greek Medicine and Dieting; White

## References and Further Reading
Andres, Reuben (2002) "Age and Obesity," in Christopher G. Fairburn and Kelly D. Brownell (eds), *Eating Disorders and Obesity: A Comprehensive Handbook*, 2nd edn, New York: Guilford Press, pp. 449–52.

Italian Longitudinal Study on Aging Working Group (1997) "Prevalence of Chronic Diseases in Older Italians: Comparing Self-Reported and Clinical Diagnoses," *International Journal of Epidemiology* 26: 995-1002.

La Fontaine (1883–92) "Le Tableau," in *Oeuvres*, twelve vols., ed. Henri de Régnier, Paris: Enoch frères & Costallat, 5, 587.

Lessius, Leonard (1636) *Hygiasticon: or, the Right Course of Preserving Life and Health unto Extream Old Age*, Cambridge: Printers of the Universitie of Cambridge.

Maynwaringe, Everard (1670) *Vita Suva & Longa, the Preservation of Health and the Prolongation of Life Proposed and Proved*, London: J.D.

Mosso, Ângelo (1891) *La fática*, Milan: Treves.

—— (1906) *Fatigue*, trans. Margaret Drummond and W.B. Drummond, London: Swan Sonnenschein.

Steadman, John M. (1957) "Falstaff's 'Facies Hippocrita': A Note on Shakespeare and Renaissance Medical Theory," *Studia Neophilologica* 29: 130–5.

Toye, Francis (1983) *Giuseppe Verdi: His Life and Works*, New York: Horizon.

# Ornish, Dean, MD

Ornish was part of the revolution in chronic disease prevention in the 1990s when he wrote *Reversing Heart Disease with Knife and Fork*. In his book, he prescribed a diet very low in saturated fat and cholesterol. In order to achieve the recommended maximum of 10 percent of calories coming from fat, people following the diet must eliminate fatty meat products, high fat dairy, and egg yolks. He claimed this dietary approach would help prevent heart disease.

He later published *Eat More, Weigh Less* (1994) in which he suggested the same diet would help a person lose weight without being hungry. He has conducted numerous clinical trials demonstrating the effectiveness of his diet and has published his findings in medical journals as well as books. Although the diet has been proven to lower weight and slow heart disease, people following the diet have a difficult time maintaining weight loss due to the restrictive nature of the diet (Womble and Wadden 2002).

Ornish is currently a professor in the medical school at the University of California, San Francisco. At the time of publication, there was continued debate in the scientific community about the effectiveness of low-fat diets like the Ornish diet (Johnston et al. 2004).

SLG/SUZANNE JUDD

## References and Further Reading
Johnston, C.S., Tjonn, S.L., and Swan, P.D. (2004) "High-Protein, Low-Fat Diets Are Effective for Weight Loss and Favorably Alter Biomarkers in Healthy Adults," *Journal of Nutrition* 134 (3): 586–9.

Ornish, Dean (1990) *Dr. Dean Ornish's Program for Reversing Heart Disease: The Only System Scientifically Proven to Reverse Heart Disease Without Drugs or Surgery*, New York: Random House.

—— (1993) *Eat More, Weigh Less: Dr. Dean Ornish's Life Choice Program For Losing Weight Safely While Eating Abundantly*, New York: HarperCollins.

Womble, Leslie G. and Wadden, Thomas (2002) "Commercial and Self-Help Weight Loss Programs," in Christopher G. Fairburn and Kelly D. Brownell (eds) *Eating Disorders and Obesity: A Comprehensive Handbook*, New York: Guilford Press, pp. 546–50.

# P

## Paleolithic Diet

According to the modern reconstructions by anthropologists, the Neolithic revolution began in the Middle East at about 10,000 BCE. It is defined as marking the change from hunter-gatherer groups to agricultural societies and brought about a drastic change in the nature of human diets, but, it is claimed, not in our genes. The shift to agriculture was a gradual one; however, by 7,500 BCE, most people in the Middle East had switched to an agrarian way of life, and the first state was born by 5,500 BCE. The Industrial Revolution in eighteenth-century Europe brought about another major shift in human diets without any alteration in our underlying genetic makeup.

The Paleolithic Diet is based on the premise that these shifts in diet without shifts in genetics or anatomy that have caused the "diseases of civilization" such as high blood pressure, Type 2 diabetes, obesity, and even cancer (Eaton et al. 1988a). The promoters of the Paleolithic Diet base these claims on evidence gathered on the few remaining hunter-gatherer groups who have almost no occurrence of these diseases (Eaton et al. 1988a). This is in direct contrast to developed and developing nations where these diseases are becoming more and more rampant (Dehghan et al. 2005; King et al. 1998). Thus, the "Paleolithic Prescription" claims that if we shift back to our ancestral diet, we can once again be healthy.

The claims of the Paleolithic Diet are simple; with a return to a preagricultural diet and an increase in exercise, the "diseases of civilization" would decrease, people would live longer and healthier lives, and there would be no more obesity in the world. This, however, is the claim of almost all diets. Nevertheless, this diet is special for two reasons: It is scientifically supported, and many popular diets today, such as Atkins, have used this science as a justification for their diets. While, thus far, the diet appears sound, there are important factors to consider.

The diet's claims rest on correcting two misconceptions concerning life expectancy and stature. The average life expectancy for Paleolithic humans was much lower than that of Americans today, though this was mostly due to the very high infant-mortality rate. If a child actually lived through childhood, its life expectancy was actually much higher than the average. There has even been evidence from some Neanderthal fossils of a social network that helped the elderly survive. Stature is an important indicator of dietary quality because without proper nutrition in one's childhood and adolescence, growth will be stunted. Interestingly, most of our Paleolithic ancestors were not radically shorter than the average for modern Americans about 177.8 cm (70 inches) for males and 147.8 cm (58.1 inches) for females. Fossil evidence has even shown that some individuals were as tall as 188 cm (74 inches) (Eaton et al. 1988a). This means that the nutritional quality of the diet in Paleolithic times was very close to what it is now and that people had enough to eat. It is also important to ask how we know what foods our Paleolithic ancestors were eating.

The ideal diet of Paleolithic humans was extrapolated from data collected from living hunter-gatherer groups. This data shows that most (73 percent) of these groups ate far more meat than the average American does with more than 50 percent of their energy coming from meat. This, combined with the lower carbohydrate content of wild plants, means that these groups derive about 19–35 percent of their energy from protein and about 22–40 percent from carbohydrates (Cordain et al. 2000). Also, most of these groups consume little to no dairy products

(Eaton 2006). Although modern hunter-gatherer groups rely heavily on meat, like the Paleolithic hunters and gatherers most likely did, they strike a balance between protein, fats, and carbohydrates. As Cordain explains this balance must occur because human beings cannot process food which is excessively high in protein (Cordain et al. 2000: 682). This is especially important to note because of the popularity of low-carbohydrate diets, such as Atkins and South Beach. It is also important to look at the food pyramid put out by the United States Department of Agriculture, which is very different from our ancestral diet.

*The Paleolithic Prescription* also blames the heavy increase of sodium, refined sugars, and drugs, most especially alcohol and tobacco, for the rise in obesity in the modern world. Humans today are the only mammals that actually consume more sodium than potassium. The increased availability of sodium today is one of the reasons for this, but the decrease in potassium-rich foods in the modern diet is also partly responsible. In Paleolithic times, the only source of refined sugar was honey, and this accounted for only about 2 percent of the caloric intake of Paleolithic humans. This is in stark contrast to the 15 percent that refined sugars now add to our caloric intake. Alcohol, though not necessarily completely lacking from Paleolithic times as "some fruits and grains do naturally ferment" (Eaton et al. 1988b: 23), would have been scarce; it now makes up a significant part of the diet of the average American at 7–10 percent of the daily caloric intake. This is even more amazing when it is factored in that many Americans do not drink. Tobacco, although not usually consumed to provide caloric intake, does affect a person's metabolic rate and thus can contribute to obesity.

The authors of *The Paleolithic Prescription* do not advise a return to the Paleolithic way of life but instead recommend picking and choosing the healthier aspects of the Paleolithic way of life. To give up the advances of modern medicine and the battles that humans have won against microbes would be foolish, but the authors claim that these victories have come with a price: our overall fitness. The human body, which has not substantially changed in about 35,000 years, was designed to be energy efficient when walking long distances in order to acquire food, but humans in developed nations today rarely do more than walk around the supermarket to acquire their food. Evidence shows that Paleolithic humans would routinely travel about 5 miles in their search for food. Walking

5 miles is double the USDA's current recommendation for daily physical activity (the USDA Food Pyramid). However, it is also true that Paleolithic people most likely only did this about three to four times per week. Exercise is a key foundation of this diet and one that many other diets today tend to overlook.

This diet is based on science; however, the science is highly speculative. The world that modern hunter-gatherers live in is much different from the world our Paleolithic ancestors lived in. Thus, it is hard to determine exactly what resources would have been available to our ancestors; so much of this evidence must be questioned. No clear first-hand evidence exists for what Paleolithic people actually looked like; what we do have is based on cave paintings and forensic reconstructions. Moreover, forensic reconstructions are one of the most controversial parts of anthropology because of their subjective nature. Though life expectancy was much longer if one matured to adulthood, the quality of adult life in the Paleolithic is questionable. The same Neanderthal fossil used to show social care for the elderly also has clear evidence of arthritis.

Much of what is said about the Paleolithic diet is based solidly in good science, but there are parts of it that are nothing more than speculation. There is the underlying assumption that our problems with obesity stem from our diets not our genes. Humans are hyper-omnivorous, meaning we can eat just about anything, but the authors of *The Paleolithic Prescription* seem to ignore this evolutionary fact and concentrate on the information gathered from a few ethnographic studies of a very small number of modern people. This data does nothing to answer the question of why did humans develop as hyper-omnivores and maintain this trait into modern times.

SLG/JOE BAUER

*See also* Atkins; Food Pyramid; Natural Man; Smoking

## References and Further Reading
Cordain, L., Miller, J.B., Eaton, S.B., Mann, N., Holt, S.H.A., and Speth, J.D. (2000) "Plant-Animal Subsistence Ratios and Macronutrient Energy Estimations in Worldwide Hunter-Gatherer Diets," *American Journal of Clinical Nutrition* 71 (3): 682–92.
Dehghan, Mahshid, Akhtar-Danesh, Noori, and Merchant, Anwar T. (2005) "Childhood Obesity,

Prevalence and Prevention," *Nutrition Journal* September 2 (4): 24.

Eaton, S.B. (2006) "The Ancestral Human Diet: What Was It and Should It Be a Paradigm for Contemporary Nutrition?" *Proceedings of the Nutrition Society* 65 (1): 1–6.

Eaton, S.B., Konner, M., and Shostak, M. (1988a) "Stone Agers in the Fast Lane: Chronic Degenerative Diseases in Evolutionary Perspective," *American Journal of Medicine* 84 (4): 739–49.

—— (1988b) *The Paleolithic Prescription*, New York: Harper & Row.

King, H., Aubert, R.E., and Herman, W.H. (1998) "Global Burden of Diabetes, 1995–2025: Prevalence, Numerical Estimates, and Projections," *Diabetes Care* 21 (9): 1414–31.

Kottak, C.P. (2006) *Anthropology: The Exploration of Human Diversity*, 12th edn, New York: McGraw-Hill.

United States Department of Agriculture (2006) "The USDA Food Pyramid." Available online at <http://www.mypyramid.gov> (accessed March 15, 2007).

# Peters, LuLu Hunt MD (1873–1930)

## American physician credited with first suggesting calorie counting as a means of gaining and losing weight

Peters served as chairman of the Public Health Committee of the California Federation of Women's Clubs in Los Angeles. She is the author of the first bestselling American diet book, *Dieting and Health: With Key to the Calories*, published in 1918. Framed as a response to World War I (and dedicated to Herbert Hoover, whose claim to fame at that point was that he "fed starving Belgium") it set out obesity as a "crime to hoard food" for which one would be fined or imprisoned. "How dare you hoard food when our nation needs it?" (Peters 1918: 12). The book is said to have sold 2 million copies and was published in more than fifty-five editions by 1939. As the model for recent modern diet books, it was directed and marketed primarily to women, written in a popular style, and included testimonials of successful weight loss. Unlike modern diet books, however, Peters included suggestions for weight gain as well as beauty tips, such as how to eliminate wrinkles.

Dr. Peters was "overweight" herself, apparently 220 pounds at her heaviest, and claimed to have lost 70 pounds following her own plan. She writes,

All my life [I fought] the too, too solid. Why, I can remember when I was a child I was always being consoled by being told that I would outgrow it, and that when I matured I would have some shape. . . . I was a delicate slip of one hundred sixty-five when I was taken [in marriage].

(Peters 1918: 13)

Her "key to the calories" was an extensive list of food portions adding up to 100 calories. On a 1,200 calorie per day diet, a dieter could have twelve 100-calorie units of food. Much of her book consisted of lists of foods and their caloric content. Her system was premised on the idea of an ideal weight, for which she provided tools of measurement. The formula consisted of taking the number of inches over 5 feet of one's height, multiplying that number by 5.5 and adding 110. The equation was meant to yield the ideal weight, in pounds, of a "normal" woman. The number of calories a dieter was meant to consume depended upon how far their actual weight exceeded the ideal for their height. Peters dismissed the notion that fat people (women) were overindulgent or lazy; rather, she divided the world into those whose metabolism quickly or slowly burned fat. She argued that even eating a bird seed if your metabolism was slow would add fat to your body. She admitted that there were those with pathologies, such as those of the thyroid, who became fat and could be cured by curing their illness, but most fat people became fat from "overeating and under-exercising" (Peters 1918: 16). This destigmatizing position stressed the difference of obese bodies from those of individuals who were "naturally thin."

SLG/Angela Willey

*See also* Calorie

## References and Further Reading

Bryn, Austin S. (1999) "Fat, Loathing, and Public Health: The Complicity of Science in a Culture of Disordered Eating," *Culture, Medicine and Psychiatry* 23 (2): 245–68

Fangman, Tamara D., Ogle, Jennifer Paff, Bickle, Marianne C., and Rouner, Donna (2004) "Promoting Female Weight Management in 1920's Print Media: An Analysis of Ladies' Home Journal and Vogue Magazines," *Family and Consumer Sciences Research Journal* 32 (3): 213–53.

Korda, Michael (2001) *Making the List: A Cultural History of the American Bestseller, 1900–1999*, New York: Barnes and Noble.

Peters, Lulu Hunt (1918) *Diet and Health, with Key to the Calories*, Chicago, Ill.: Reilly and Lee.

# Pets

Obesity occurs in about one out of every four pets. Just as Americans are gaining more weight, pets are as well. Weight gain in pets occurs for the same reasons that it does in humans: Not enough exercise and too much food. Obesity can pose health risks to pets, and, therefore, it is important for pet owners to watch what their pets eat. A pet is considered to be obese when it weighs more than 15 percent over the healthiest weight for its sex and breed. Some problems associated with obesity are: heart disease, orthopedic issues, skin problems, increased risk during surgery, lung and liver problems, hip problems, digestive issues, arthritis, and diabetes. Obesity can reduce a pet's life by two to three years.

Dieting suggestions for pets mirror those of humans. For example, veterinarians suggest the best way to change a pet's diet is to do it gradually. A sudden diet does not work for pets, especially for cats, as they can develop liver problems. In addition, pets can have hormonal imbalances, which may lead to weight gain. Occasionally, veterinarians will test animals for thyroid function and can even recommend placing the animal on hormone replacement therapy in order to help them lose weight. While the causes and treatments of pet obesity may be similar to those in humans, animals do have dietary requirements very different to those of humans. Dogs do not have to eat a meal every day. In fact, a dog can go without food for five days before any negative health effects occur.

Cats are also at risk for weight problems. Many veterinarians report that over 70 percent of cats are obese, and obese cats are especially at risk for diabetes. A healthy weight for cats is 8 to 10 pounds for females and 9 to 11 pounds for males. Because cats are carnivores, they need protein, fat, water, and minerals in their diet, so they have some specific dietary requirements. One important study examined the relationship between diabetic cats and their diet. It showed that cats can benefit from a high-protein diet called the "Catkins" diet, a play on the human Atkins diet. Many cats on the "Catkins" diet no longer needed insulin shots for their diabetes. Cat treats should be treated like desserts, and most have many calories; therefore, it is best to refrain from these. Pet owners should feed their cats small amounts two to six times a day. Cats should not eat as many carbohydrates because they do not have any of the carbohydrate-digesting enzymes in their saliva that most mammals do. This makes it harder to break down carbohydrates. It is also recommended that pet owners not feed their cats too much dry cat food because it has too many carbohydrates. Canned diets are healthier because they provide more water, and it is easier for pet owners to control how much their pets are eating.

While dietary changes at home are usually the first recourse for owners of obese pets, some companies even market dieting food for animals. According to the National Research Council of the National Academy of Sciences, obesity is the top health problem for the nation's dogs. Pet Ecology Brands, Inc. has created the first 100-percent fat-free dog treat. The dog treats are made from rice, garlic, and meat flavors. The treats are also sodium and cholesterol free. Pet Ecology Brands, Inc. also introduced a fat-free cat treat due to an influx of obese felines.

SLG/MARY STANDEN

*See also* Atkins; Metabolism

**References and Further Reading**

Acosta, Tracy (2006) "Preventing Obesity for the Life of Your Pet," *Sun Herald* (Biloxi, Miss.), February 15.

Anon. (2005) "The Overweight Pet," the PetCenter.com, available online at <http://www.thepetcenter.com/imtop/overweight.html> (accessed March 15, 2007).

Jeter, Heidi (2004) "Study Shows 'Catkins' Diet Helps Cats Beat Diabetes." Available online at <http://www.medicalnewstoday.com/medicalnews.php?newsid=16452> (accessed March 15, 2007).

Pet Ecology Brands, Inc. (2006) "First to Bring 'Fat Free' to Pet Industry," market wire, available online at <http://www.marketwire.com/mw/release_html_b1?release_id=114594> (accessed March 23, 2007).

Soule, Jan (2006) "Cats (and Other Animals Too): Obesity Is Growing Problem, and Not Just with People. About One-Quarter of Family Pets Are Also Drastically Overweight," *Barrie Examiner* (Ontario), March 18: C1.

# Phytochemicals

In addition to nutrients, plant foods consist of phytochemicals, which may affect human health. Phytochemicals are the nonnutritive plant components with biological activity (Bennick 2001: 11). Fruits, vegetables, beverages, and several herbs and plant extracts contain these phytochemicals. There are numerous phytochemicals including carotenoids, flavonoids, indoles, and protease inhibitors, among others (Watson 2001: 3). Many research studies have determined that such chemicals have health benefits, naturally aiding the body in disease prevention and neutralizing chemical and hormonal imbalances. One study conducted estimated that plant based diets prevent 20–50 percent of all cancers (Nestle 1997: 11149). This medical research prompted doctors to begin prescribing diets rich in foods containing these phytochemicals. It did not take long until these ideas caught on in the fad-dieting and dietary-supplement worlds. Due to the new popularity of diets rich in phytochemicals, individuals are consuming these chemicals not only for health benefits but also for the prospect of losing weight and stubborn fat. Interestingly, the popularity of phytochemicals began among medical professionals due to results of medical research. However, more recently they have gained popularity with the public as a result of only partially or wholly unsubstantiated claims made by the creators of fad diets and supplements.

As a result of medical research, about thirty classes of phytochemicals have been described as having cancer-preventative effects (Watson 2001: 4). Several epidemiological studies suggest, "that micro chemicals present in our diet could be the most desirable agents for the prevention and/or intervention of human cancer incidence and mortality due to stomach, colon, breast, esophagus, lung, bladder, and prostate cancer" (Watson 2001: 3). The specific mechanisms of these phytochemicals that aid in cancer prevention are not yet fully known. However, there are many plausible reasons being investigated. For example, it is recognized that "phytochemicals can inhibit carcinogenesis by induction of phase II enzymes and inhibiting phase I enzymes, scavenge DNA reactive agents, suppress the abnormal proliferation of early preneoplastic lesions, and inhibit certain properties of the cancer cell" (Watson 2001: 3).

Much recent research has focused on the anticancer activity of phytochemicals found in soy products (Bennick

2001: 11). Early observations of the role of soybeans in prevention of human cancer developed from correlative investigations that were seeking explanations for the global differences in cancer between the Western and Asian countries (Birt 2001: 4). Research has shown that the Asian diet, which is richer in soy products and contains fewer fatty products than the typical Western diet, decreases incidence of cancer (Riulin 2001: 256). In addition, a large number of animal investigations have provided strong evidence for the role of soy in cancer prevention (Birt 2001: 5).

A subgroup of phytochemicals, phytoestrogens or plant estrogens, have been implicated as having additional disease-preventative and healthful effects. A high intake of these phytoestrogens may help alleviate the symptoms associated with the low estrogen levels that plague menopausal women. Phytoestrogens also may reduce the risk for diseases, such as cancer, associated with estrogen (Scholten 2006). For example, resveratrol, a phytochemical in the skins of grapes and peanuts, was found to limit the growth and proliferation of human breast cancer cell lines, by inhibiting the binding sites of estrogen receptors in human breast cancer cells (Diamondis and Goldberg 2001: 173).

Since the discovery of these disease-preventative characteristics, many people have altered their diets for a healthier lifestyle. Doctors have strongly recommended that their patients incorporate more fruits and vegetables, which contain such nutrients and phytochemicals, into their diets. Foods that include these phytochemicals, other than soy, are dark green, leafy vegetables like spinach, kale and collards; citrus fruits, such as oranges, grapefruit and tangerines; and other red, yellow, and orange fruits and vegetables as well as their juices (Anon. (2005) "Phytochemicals"). Diets rich in phytoestrogens consist of soybeans, black cohosh, whole grains, legumes, tempeh, and flax seed (Scholten 2006).

These doctor-recommended healthful diets that incorporate phytochemicals have become the basis for fad diets that proclaim they promote health and weight-loss. For example, the Mediterranean Diet has become increasingly popular as people have become aware that good health is linked to a good diet (Watson 2001: 217). This diet is based on the "historic" food intake in the Mediterranean region, which includes larger amounts of vegetables, fruits, beans, and grains, as well as olive oil as the main source of fat and moderate amounts of protein, primarily from fish and poultry. Such views of "traditional"

cuisine as being innately healthy have their historical rationale in the claims that "natural" foods are consumed by "natural" society and therefore show the innate superiority of such groups over "modern," globalized society and its production and consumption of foods. The Mediterranean Diet prescribes that people eat certain proportions and combinations of these foods, each with their own phytochemicals, throughout the day. The fad diet also uses cooking methods similar to those used several decades ago around the Mediterranean Sea. It is considered the model of a healthful diet and has attracted attention because of the low rates of chronic diseases and the high life expectancy noted in countries of the Mediterranean region. This diet is found to produce beneficial effects on blood lipid profiles and protect against oxidative stress and carcinogenesis (Watson 2001: 217).

Additionally, some cuisine of the Mediterranean diet is believed to contain minor metabolites, like limonene, that are thought to speed weight loss. This diet is easily accepted by most people due to this possibility of weight loss combined with the hundreds of recipes that conform to the rules of the diet (Watson 2001: 224). It has gained vast popularity, for it provides the best chance for influencing people to abandon unhealthy foods in favor of fresh and less saturated-fatty foods (Watson 2001: 217).

Although the diet in the Mediterranean region has been linked with reduced frequency of disease among inhabitants of the lands around the Mediterranean Sea, the Mediterranean Diet sold as a fad diet. The diet has not been sufficiently studied or proven to reduce disease or induce weight loss. It is based on the author's perception of the diets of inhabitants of the Mediterranean and, thus, is not an exact replica of their eating practices. For instance, Watson argues that "there is no single typical Mediterranean diet. Defining and understanding the Mediterranean diet is not easy because there are several countries that border the Mediterranean Sea" (Watson 2001: 218). Also, prescribing the diet of a certain region alone is not necessarily enough to mimic the lifestyles of the people of that region. The diet fails to take into account other factors in Mediterraneans' living, such as their physical activity level. Because this fad diet does not account for the differences between it and the precise diet and activities of the Mediterraneans, it may be mistaken in claiming that its prescription of certain foods and their associated phytochemicals actually reduce the incidence of diseases and overweight as they actually do in the Mediterranean region.

Phytochemicals have also justified the "science" behind some dietary supplements that claim their products help individuals achieve leaner bodies and/or increase disease prevention. For example, the makers of a supplement called EstroX, containing naturally occurring estrogen inhibitors, claim that their product along with a diet rich in natural estrogen-inhibiting foods, such as certain vegetables, whole grains, and fatty fish, will help individuals lose weight. The product advertisement claims that individuals who have been subject to hormone therapy or who have been exposed to the "unhealthy estrogenic environment" of everyday life have too much estrogen in their bodies. The makers claim that too much estrogen, rather than playing its usual role as an antioxidant and anticancerous compound at normal levels, instead converts into toxic compounds that are stored as fat and are thought to contribute to the formation of breast, ovarian, and prostate cancers. Therefore, by taking their supplement, which contains the "superior" proportion of three estrogen inhibitors derived from bee propolis, broccoli, tobacco, passiflora, and chamomile, the makers of EstroX claim that individuals suffering from excess estrogen will decrease their estrogen levels and thus achieve leaner bodies and healthier lives (Hofmekler 2006).

It at first seems as though the makers of EstroX have done their medical research. However, the creators use vague language about the extent to which their claims are scientifically supported. As with all supplements, ExtroX is not required to pass FDA or any other government regulations in order to make certain claims or break into the supplement market.

Phytochemicals can be found in a wide variety of foods and beverages people consume. Considering their abundance, it is no wonder that these phytochemicals have become famous as a result of the medical discoveries tying their consumption to a healthier lifestyle. However, much of their popularity has grown due to the unsubstantiated claims of the more public fad dieting and dietary supplement worlds that have embraced phytochemicals as a new phenomenon in health and weight loss. There is no question that it will take more years of research into phytochemicals and the effects of the phytochemical products claiming miraculous results, before these non-established declarations are proven.

SLG/Caroline A. Bugg

*See also* Natural Man; Risks Associated with Dieting

## References and Further Reading

Anon. (2005) "Phytochemicals," Medline Plus: Medical Encyclopedia (September 2), available online at <http://www.nlm.nih.gov/medlineplus/ency/imagepages/19303.htm> (accessed March 15, 2007).

Bennick, Maurice R. (2001) "Dietary Soy Reduces Colon Carcinogenesis in Humans and Rats," *Advances in Experimental Medicine and Biology: Nutrition and Cancer Prevention: New Insights into the Role of Phytochemicals* 492: 11–17.

Birt, Diane F. (2001) "Soybeans and Cancer Prevention: A Complex Food and a Complex Disease," *Advances in Experimental Medicine and Biology: Nutrition and Cancer Prevention: New Insights into the Role of Phytochemicals* 492: 1–10.

Diamondis, Eleftherios P. and Goldberg, David M. (2001) "The World of Resveratrol," in *Nutrition and Cancer Prevention: New Insights into the Role of Phytochemicals*, 492, 173, New York: Plenum Publishing Corporation.

Hofmekler, Ori (2006) "Excess Estrogen and Weight Gain (Belly Fat): The Problem and the Solution," Defense Nutrition, available online at <http://www.defensenutrition.com/article/excess-estrogen-and-weight-gain> (accessed March 15, 2007).

Nestle, Marion (1997) "Broccoli Sprouts as Inducers of Carcinogen-Detoxifying Enzyme Systems: Clinical, Dietary, and Policy Implications," *Proceedings of the National Academy of Sciences of the United States of America* 94 (21): 11149–51.

Riulin, Richard S. (2001) "Nutrition and Cancer Prevention: New Insights into the Role of Phytochemicals," in *Nutrition and Cancer Prevention: New Insights into the Role of Phytochemicals*, 492, 256, New York: Plenum Publishing Corporation.

Scholten, Amy (2006) "Menopause," New York Medical Center, available online at <http://www.med.nyu.edu/patientcare/library/article.html?ChunkIID=11676> (accessed March 15, 2007).

Watson, Ronald R. (2001) *Vegetables, Fruits, and Herbs in Health Promotion*, New York: CRC Press.

# Post, Charles William (1854–1914)

## Health food provider and cereal tycoon

Post was the commercial genius who built the Postum Cereal Company as one of the major players in the American food reform movement of the late nineteenth century and, incidentally, made a 17-million-dollar fortune. In 1890, Post, a self-taught inventor and salesman, arrived at the Battle Creek sanitarium in Michigan because of his own failing health. The sanitarium was run for the Seventh-day Adventist Church by Dr. John Harvey Kellogg. The town had been a major center for religion-based health reform since the arrival of the founders of the Church, James and Ellen Gould White, in the 1850s. During his visit, Post became exposed to the food reform movement and its claims about human health. Here he experienced the use of breakfast cereals as the basis for health therapies, using the double idea of a "modern" health regime with a "religious" foundation.

Here, Post, like all of the cereal manufacturers of the time, followed the lead of Henry Perky (1843–1906) who had developed the "wheat shredding process" and created shredded wheat. Post called on "science" with his advocacy of a "true domestic science" that "should be taught in all our schools" (Perky 1902: 86), but he also condemned American Protestantism with its lack of a strict dietary regime as one of the causes of American ill health. In contrast, he praised the strict regimes of Judaism and Islam for their attention to diet.

Post left the sanitarium after nine months and purchased a farm in Battle Creek, where he began experimenting with grain-based health foods and beverages, which he was introduced to at Kellogg's sanitarium but found almost uneatable due to the bland taste. Post then founded La Vita Inn at Battle Creek. He also advocated a mind cure for bodily illness in his tract *I Am Well! The Modern Practice of Natural Suggestion as Distinct from Hypnotic Unnatural Influence* (1895), positioning himself in the "New Thought" movement dominated by figures like William James and Mary Baker Eddy, who argued, "Disease is entirely a mental picture" (Post 1895: 4). His views echoed the Social Darwinism of his day, seeing such health advocacy as improving the "race." But underlying all was the need to sell a notion of health. In 1908, he explained,

I studied psychology, dietetics, hygiene and medi-

cine in this country and Europe. I have been through psychology from the book by Mrs. Eddy to the clinics of Charcot in mental therapeutics at Paris. What we say in our advertising is a popular expression of things I believe to be vitally important to many others.

(Paxson 1993: 36)

By 1895, Post abandoned his foray into mental healing and planned to create an alternative to coffee and tea, as well as to develop a ready-made breakfast cereal that would be enjoyable and affordable. His model here was clearly Kellogg and the Seventh-Day Adventist vegetarian diet, but, unlike them, he rejected a "theological" rationale for the power of his food to heal. This was the triumph of science in the warfare between "theology" and "science" (the title of a major book of 1896 by the historian and President of Cornell, Andrew Dickson White). His food was seen as "modern," as it incorporated arguments about science and evolution in its claims for cure. Post developed and produced his first product, Postum Cereal Beverage, and a caffeine-free coffee substitute. "If Coffee Don't Agree, try Postum," stated the ads. They also pictured "the coffee fiend saved at the last gasp by changing to Postum" (Paxson 1993: 193).

In 1897, Post developed Grape-Nuts, the first cold cereal, and, in 1899, he created a brand of cornflakes, to compete with Kellogg's Corn Flakes®. When he brought his to the market he called it "Elijah's Manna," only changing the name in 1908 to Post Toasties. The outrage by ministers across the country at the appropriation of the biblical name by someone who had little interest beyond marketing caused the change. The Kellogg cereal had been developed by Will Keith Kellogg (1869–1951), who was employed by his older brother at the sanitarium, as an attempt to bring health food to the masses. He received a patent for a corn-flaking process in 1895. In 1906, W.K. Kellogg was excommunicated by the Seventh-Day Adventist Church for adding sugar to his cornflakes in violation of the Church's dietary principles. Post had no such principles.

Post's advertising and marketing was his genius, and yet he too made distinct gestures to the religious culture of Battle Creek. By 1900, Battle Creek was the center of cereal production, but Post and Kellogg dominated the field. Post promoted his products by creating appealing phrases in language he believed appealed to the working class. He demanded that his salesmen "must use plain words, homely illustrations and more or less of the vocabulary of the customer ... In other words talk to your customer in a way that he will instantly grasp what you have to say, and believe it" (Paxson 1993: 191). As a leader of the National Association of Manufacturers, however, Post took a hard, antilabor line in his conflicts with Samuel Gompers, the labor leader. Labor advocates were, according to him, "mongrels, prostitutes, and the most poisonous enemies of the common people" (Paxson 1993: 203).

Post committed suicide in 1914, and within days the alternative physician E.H. Pratt at a convention of the Illinois Eclectic Medical Society interpreted his death as the result of "intestinal problems" (Paxson 1993: 325). Post might well have agreed with an explanation of mental illness resting on poor food and digestive disorders. Perhaps his life would have been saved had he only stuck to Postum and Grape-Nuts. His only daughter, Marjorie Post, inherited the Post Cereal Company and turned it into one of the most successful and recognizable food brands in the world, General Foods Company. She donated the land for the C.W. Post Campus of Long Island University, which was founded in 1954, the 100th anniversary of Post's birth.

SLG

*See also* Fat Camp; Ibn Sina; Jews; Kellogg; White

## References and Further Reading

Anon. "Charles William Post." Available online at <http://www.kraft.com/100/founders/CWPost.html?> (accessed March 15, 2007).

Anon. "C.W. Post Campus. Long Island University." Available online at <http://www.cwpost.liu.edu/cwis/cwp/pr/events/post/index.html> (accessed March 15, 2007).

Breen, Bill (2005) "The Three Ways of Great Leaders," *Fast Company* 98: 50.

Paxson, Peyton John (1993) "Charles William Post: The Mass Marketing of Health and Welfare," Ph.D. diss., Boston University.

Perky, Henry (1902) *Wisdom Vs. Foolishness*, Worcester, Mass.: The Perky Publishing Co.

Post, C.W. (1895) *I Am Well! the Modern Practice of Natural Suggestion As Distinct from Hypnotic Unnatural Influence*, Boston, Mass.: Lee and Shepard.

# Pregnancy

A healthy diet is essential for both the mother and the fetus during pregnancy (Brown 1998). Proper maternal nutrition is important for the development of fetal cells, organs, and central nervous system, as well as allowing the fetus to store essential nutrients for optimum growth. This is especially important in the last seven months of pregnancy when the fetus's weight increases from about 1 ounce to 8 pounds. Since the time of Hippocrates, there have been many diets proposed for pregnant women. When a woman is pregnant, her needs for calories, minerals, water, vitamins, and protein all increase, so Judith Brown recommends the following: sufficient fluid (eight to ten cups per day), no restriction of salt, no alcohol, and enough fiber to prevent constipation. A pregnant woman should follow the suggested food group distributions of the Food Guide Pyramid and consume about 300 more calories per day than she did before pregnancy. It is also important for pregnant women to have specific additional nutrients. The table, referred to as the recommended dietary allowances (RDAs) for pregnancy, provided by the National Academy of Sciences, recommends certain amounts of nutrients important for pregnant women. The key nutrients include folate, vitamin D, iron, zinc, calcium, and vitamin C. There have not been any studies of the effects of low-carbohydrate diets on the fetus. Therefore, it is safest to eat foods from all groups of the Food Guide Pyramid.

The debate about weight gain in pregnancy has been

heated. In 1990, the U.S. Institute of Medicine liberalized its suggested maximum weight. General recommendations are that pregnant women should gain between 25 and 35 pounds during the nine months that they are carrying a baby. Average weight gain is distributed across each of the three trimesters as follows: 3–5 pounds in the first three months, 12–14 pounds in the second trimester, and 1–2 pounds per week in the final three months of pregnancy (Murkoff et al. 2002: 169–71). Recent studies have shown that there seems to be little ill effect to fetus or mother until the weight gains exceed 33 pounds. Low maternal weight has always been seen as an indicator of potential risk for infant mortality, disability, and mental retardation (Rössner 2002).

While it is not recommended for pregnant women to radically lose weight during pregnancy because it can deprive both the fetus and mother of essential nutrients, there has not been much research on the effects of eating disorders and pregnancy. The research that has been done, however, indicates that there can be negative effects on the fetus as a result of an eating disorder in the mother. It has shown that pregnant women with eating disorders often experience hyperemesis gravidarum (a disorder that includes severe nausea and vomiting during pregnancy), miscarriage, vaginal bleeding, hypertension, and radical weight gain or weight loss. The following are the most common fetus complications: low birth weight, cesarean section, and preterm delivery. Complications also include stillbirth, cleft palate, breech delivery, fetal abnormality, and prenatal mortality.

Poor nutrition, specifically folic-acid deficiency, has also been shown to cause brain and spinal cord defects in fetuses known as neural tube defects (NTDs). A study conducted found that women who reported dieting, defined as restricting food intake, throughout the first trimester of pregnancy were more likely to have babies with NTDs (Carmichael et al 2003). This study also showed that women who reported dieting three months before they were pregnant did not generally have infants with NTDs. However, another study found that women who used laxatives, barbiturates, and diuretics before or around the time of conception were more likely to have babies who had NTDs. It is believed that the increased risk of NTDs is due to the impact of dieting on consumption, absorption, and metabolism of nutrients, such as folic acid (Carmichael et al. 2003). Therefore, proper nutritional practices by the mother are essential for the brain and spinal cord in fetal development. Research indicates that women should be very careful if they diet during pregnancy. It is essential that these women consume enough nutrients to provide for themselves as well as the child that they are carrying. Neglecting to do so can lead to many health problems for both the mother and the baby.

Once the baby has been born, many women are concerned with losing the weight they gained while pregnant. There is much literature focused on techniques of how to lose the "baby fat." Weight Watchers, in particular, has many tips for new mothers. Some of these include:

Eat healthy foods.

Set realistic goals.

Reduce portions.

Eat small meals frequently rather than fewer large meals.

Drink plenty of water.

Exercise frequently.

Set a positive example of eating habits for your children.

Pregnancy can be a major mitigating factor in clinically obese women deciding to lose weight. The fear of "heavier infants, increased likelihood of cesarean sections, [and] prolonged labor" seems to encourage weight reduction (Rössner 2002: 445). The counterargument has now officially been made by the British National Health Service, which, in August 2006, has banned funding any invitro-fertilization procedures for morbidly obese women as a risk to the health of mother and child. Smokers can, however, have the procedures (Waheed 2007).

## Recommended Allowances (RDAs) for Pregnancy

| Nutrient | RDA |
| --- | --- |
| Protein | 60 g |
| Vitamin A | 800 RE (4,000 IU) |
| Vitamin D | 10 mcg (400 IU) |
| Vitamin E | 8 mg (24 IU) |
| Vitamin K | 65 mcg |
| Vitamin C | 70 mg |
| Thiamin | 1.5 mg |
| Riboflavin | 1.6 mg |
| Niacin | 17 mg NE |
| Vitamin B6 | 2.2 mg |

| | |
|---|---|
| Folate | 400 mcg |
| Vitamin B12 | 2.2 mcg |
| Calcium | 1,200 mg |
| Phosphorus | 1,200 mg |
| Magnesium | 320 mg |
| Iron | 30 mg |
| Zinc | 15 mg |
| Iodine | 175 mcg |
| Selenium | 65 mcg |

National Academy of Sciences, 1989

SLG/MARY STANDEN

*See also* Food Pyramid; Greek Medicine and Dieting; Nidetch; Smoking

### References and Further Reading

Anon. (2005) "Pregnancy: Eating Right While Pregnant," The National Women's Health Information Center, available online <http://www.webmd.com/content/article/51/40816.htm> (accessed March 15, 2007).

Anon. (2006) "About Pregnancy Weight Gain," The American Pregnancy Association, available online at <http://www.americanpregnancy.org/pregnancy-health/aboutpregweightgain.html> (accessed March 24, 2007).

Anon. (2006) "Bye-Bye Baby Fat: Weight Watchers Offers Tips on Losing Weight Successfully After Baby," PR Newswire Association, available online at <http://www.lexisnexis.com>, April 28 (accessed April 19, 2006).

Anon. (2006) "Hyperemesis Gravidarum," National Organization for Rare Disorders, available online at <http://www.rarediseases.org/search/rdbdetail_abstract.html?disname=Hyperemesis%20Gravidarum%20> (accessed March 15, 2007).

Brown, Judith (1998) "The Right Diet for Pregnancy." Available online at <http://www.webmd.com/content/Article/4/1680_51792.htm?pagenumber=1> (accessed March 20, 2006).

Carmichael, Suzan L., Shaw, Gary M., Schaffer, Donna M., Laurant, Cecile, and Selvin, Steve (2003) "Dieting Behaviors and Risk of Neural Tube Defects," *American Journal of Epidemiology* 158 (12): 277–319.

Crandall, Carolyn J. (2002) "Weight Control After Pregnancy." Available online at <http://www.medicinenet.com/script/main/art.asp?articlekey=20244> (accessed March 15, 2007).

Franko, Debra L. and Spurrell, Emily B. (2000) "Detection and Management of Eating Disorders During Pregnancy," *Obstetrics and Gynecology* 95 (6): 942–6.

Murkoff, Heidi, Eisenberg, Arlene, and Hathaway, Sandee (2002) *What to Expect When You're Expecting*, New York: Workman Publishing.

Rössner, Stephan (2002) "Pregnancy and Weight Gain," in Christopher G. Fairburn and Kelly D. Brownell (eds), *Eating Disorders and Obesity: A Comprehensive Handbook*, 2nd edn, New York: Guilford Press, pp. 445–8.

Waheed, Zulehkha (2007) "Ban on fertility treatment for obese women proposed", Progress Educational Trust (10 April 2007). Available online at http://www.ivf.net/ivf/index.php?id=2632&page=out (accessed September 20, 2007).

# Pritikin, Nathan (1915–85)

## Creator of the Pritikin Diet

Pritikin initially developed the Pritikin Diet as a way to combat his own heart disease. A self-taught inventor, Pritikin held over two dozen patents in fields from engineering to photography and aeronautics. He had observed that the results of the famines of war reduced the onset of heart disease and diabetes in Europe during World War II. Lester Morrison, a Los Angeles cardiologist, had given half of a group of cardiac patients a diet mimicking the low-fat wartime food rations. By 1955, the cholesterol levels of the experimental low-fat, low-cholesterol group had dropped from an average of 312 to 220. Morrison's control remained at their higher level (Morrison 1960). In 1956, Morrison discovered that Pritikin, then forty-one, had a cholesterol count of over 300. As such, Pritikin adopted a form of the Morrison Diet, became a vegetarian, and added intensive exercise in the form of jogging. In four years, his cholesterol was lowered to 120, and his heart function had become normal. As with many cases of dieting self-cure, beginning with William Banting, Pritikin's cure became his cause.

Pritikin's self-treatment became known as the "Pritikin Diet," which was developed in the 1970s. In his book, Pritikin makes the case that the diet is "natural": "For centuries the hardiest, most long lived peoples in the world have thrived on these foods" (Pritikin and McGrady 1979: xvi). The goal of the diet plan was to provide a means for people to battle health conditions similar to those from which Pritikin suffered. It also claimed to enable diabetics to regulate their blood sugar without the help of insulin. As such, the diet includes eating foods "low in fats, cholesterol, protein, and highly refined carbohydrates, such as sugars; . . . high in starches, as part of a complex, most unrefined carbohydrates, and are basically 'food as grown,' eaten raw or cooked" (Pritikin and McGrady 1979: 3). These claims are a fascinating mix of the rhetoric of vegetarianism and "science." In general, though, this diet falls on the side of the "fat makes fat" school of the nineteenth century, which was pioneered by Banting.

Not surprisingly, foods that are highly processed such as pasta, animal protein, and white bread are not allowed. The diet prescribes mostly vegetables, fruits, grains, seafood containing Omega 3s, lean meat, and nonfat dairy foods. It also contains less than 10 percent of daily calories from fat, and it is low in saturated fat, total fat, and cholesterol. The suggested intake of nutrients includes 5–10 percent from fat, 10–15 percent from protein, and 80 percent from carbohydrates (mostly complex carbohydrates). Exercise is also an important component of the diet: "Jogging does more for you because it stresses the heart more and makes more demands upon your heart" (Pritikin and McGrady 1979: 66). Here Pritikin follows the fad for jogging advocated by Jim Fixx (1932–84) in his 1977 best-selling book *The Complete Book of Running.*

In 1976, Pritikin created the Pritikin Longevity Center in Santa Barbara, California, which later moved to Santa Monica. Since this center opened, over 70,000 people have visited to learn how to eat healthily and exercise regularly. In 1979, Pritikin also wrote a bestselling diet book with Patrick M. McGrady called *The Pritikin Program for Diet and Exercise.*

In 1985, his son Robert Pritikin took on the task of managing the Pritikin Longevity Center after his father died that year. Robert has kept many of the same aspects of his father's "Pritikin Diet." However, over time, he also altered it as market expectations shifted. As with the older program, the new program, articulated in his 1990 book *The Pritikin Principle,* is based on a "science plus fitness" model. In it, Robert Pritikin stresses how close the recommendations of the American Heart Association and other health groups have become to the original Pritikin Diet (Pritikin 1990: 26). Yet, he also notes that his approach is "natural weight loss" (Pritikin 1990: 31). Like his father, Robert Pritikin stresses the importance of foods from plants and the reduced intake of fat: "the Pritikin diet won't assault your body the way that crash diets do. A low-fat diet high in unrefined carbohydrates and fiber enables you to reach your ideal weight by shedding pounds gradually but steadily" (Pritikin 1990: 43). This approach answered the extreme popularity of the Atkins' high-protein/fat diet. To stress the difference, he added a new concept called the Calorie Density Solution. Robert Pritikin argues that the density of calories in different types of food is very important in losing weight. He claims that eating more foods with fewer calories per pound will help people lose weight.

The Pritikin diet remains one of the gold standards for American dieting success. While numerous medical studies have documented the success of the Pritikin diet, its impact has been equally felt in the athletic and fitness communities. The *London Business Times* recently called the diet program "arguably the most effective diet, exercise, and lifestyle-change program in the world" and, one can add, one of the most visible.

SLG/Mary Standen

*See also* Atkins; Banting; Vegetarianism; Wigmore

## References and Further Reading

Anderson, James W., Konz, Elizabeth C., and Jenkins David J.A. (2000) "Health Advantages and Disadvantages of Weight-Reducing Diets: A Computer Analysis and Critical Review," *Journal of the American College of Nutrition* 19 (5): 578–90.

Anon. (2004) "Diets: A Primer," CBC News Online, available online at <http://www.cbc.ca/news/background/food/diets.html> (accessed March 15, 2007).

Anon. (2006) "What is Pritikin?" The Pritikin Longevity Center and Spa, available online at <http://www.pritikin.com/pritikin/pritikin_Overview.shtml> (accessed March 15, 2007).

Anon. "The Pritikin Principle: 1996–2004," WebMD Inc. Available online at <http://www.webmd.com/content/pages/7/3220_282.htm> (accessed March 15, 2007).

Fixx, Jim (1977) The Complete Book of Running, New York: Random House.

Hubbard J.D., Inkeles, S., and Barnard, R.J. (1985) "Nathan Pritikin's Heart," New England Journal of Medicine 313 (1): 52.

Mandell, Terri (2000) "The Living Laboratory," American Fitness (March), available online at <http://findarticles.com/p/articles/mi_m0675/is_2_18/ai_60589338> (accessed March 24, 2007).

Morrison L.M. (1952) "Results of Betaine Treatment of Atherosclerosis," American Journal of Digestive Diseases 19 (12): 381–4.

—— (1960) "Diet in Coronary Atherosclerosis," Journal of the American Medical Association 25 (173): 884–8.

Morrison, Lester M. and Morrison, Nugent (1983) Dr. Morrison's Heart-Saver Program: A Natural, Scientifically Tested Plan for the Prevention of Arteriosclerosis, Heart Attack, and Stroke, New York: St. Martins Press.

Pritikin, Nathan and McGrady, Patrick M. (1979) The Pritikin Program for Diet and Exercise, New York: Grosset & Dunlap.

Pritikin, Robert (1990) The New Pritikin Program: The Easy and Delicious Way to Shed Fat, Lower Your Cholesterol, and Stay Fit, New York: Simon & Schuster.

Walls, Ken R. (2001) "Pritikin Diet." Available online at <http://www.findarticles.com/p/articles/mi_g2603/is_0006/ai_2603000605> (accessed March 15, 2007).

# Processed Foods

Human beings have been confronted with the need to preserve food ever since the first hunter killed the first mammoth and wondered what to do with all that meat! From drying and salting to smoking, fermenting, and covering the off-flavor of spoiling foods with exotic spices and peppers, the search for means of preserving food became a search both for the ability to store food in times of scarcity and to conserve its nutritional value. Such attempts led (if the legend is correct) to the exploration of Asia and the discovery of the Americas—and certainly to the centrality of salt mining in all cultures (Kurlansky 2003). Processing was the first step in controlling diet (Shephard 2000). By the eighteenth century, the traditional forms of processing foods gave way to the notion of "manufactured" food that was both accessible and healthy. Indeed some of these methods, such as the use of vinegar to pickle foods, which became wildly popular in England in the sixteenth century, quickly were appropriated for dieting purposes. Vinegar as food preservative quickly became vinegar as dieting aid.

Canning, the first modern method of food processing, was invented in France by the cook Nicolaus Appert (1750–1841) in 1795 to solve the problem of feeding Napoleon Bonaparte's troops. Napoleon's army had one seemingly insurmountable problem, bringing sufficient food with them to match the speed of their march. Malnutrition was so rampant among his troops that he was losing men much faster to scurvy and starvation than to enemy bullets. In desperate need of a way to preserve food for their army, the French Government offered a sizable reward of 12,000 francs to anyone who could invent a method of keeping food fresh. At this point, Appert, an obscure Parisian chef and winemaker proposed that the processes commonly used to preserve wine should also work for food, so he began experimenting. After years of work, Appert perfected his preservation process of sealing food in glass bottles with pitch (a tar-like substance), then heating it to high temperatures. Appert's canned food was quickly put through field-testing, and it passed with flying colors. In 1810, the Parisian chef received his cash prize from Napoleon himself. This was an extremely powerful military development, and the French attempted to keep it a secret, but it inevitably leaked across the English Channel. By the time of the Battle at Waterloo in 1815, nearly all of the troops on both sides were eating canned rations.

The first vacuum-packing plant in France opened in 1804, and in 1810 an Englishman named Peter Durand patented the use of metal cans which were far more durable than their French glass predecessors (Shephard 2000: 226ff). Although canning started off as a military development, refrigeration in this time period was primitive at best, and canned food was just as appealing to civilians as it was to military forces. As people realized that the risk of becoming sick from foods preserved by canning was dramatically lower than from fresh foods that were constantly threatening to spoil, the civilian demand for canned foods skyrocketed.

Parallel to this development, food concentrates as a health aid and health food presented highly processed food as a means of improving the diet of the working class. While concentrates were known as early as the sixteenth century, it was only with the rise of food chemistry and "modern notions" of processed food and health that they became a staple. In 1848, the German food chemist Justus von Liebig (1803–73), then working at Liverpool University, developed his "Beef Extract" when the daughter of a friend developed typhus. This "new Soup for Invalids" became a standard medication for illness but also a new foodstuff to feed the "craving multitudes" of workers who could not afford meat. Thereafter, Liebig's *Fleischextract* competed with Oxo and Bovril for the world health food market (Shephard 2000: 175ff).

A century later, Clarence Birdseye (1886–1956) duplicated a food-preservation technique he had seen in Arctic cultures, creating the first processed quick-frozen foods. Birdseye built on a new technology of generating cold air by the use of compressed gas. This led to a whole new industry of safe and fresh-tasting processed foods. Birdseye developed this process based on his own experiences living in Labrador as a fur trapper. In 1917, he returned to the U.S.A., where he began to advocate "quick frozen" foods as a healthier alternative to fresh foods. In the 1920s, Majorie Merriweather Post arranged to purchase

Birdseye's process for 22 million dollars, and the Postum Company became General Foods. It was seen as the salvation of the modern family's health: "The potential of . . . the family-sized food freezer, is its power, when ably used to make us really free; free from want, free from the usual fears of security—and I dare say free from envy" (Smith 2001: 186). Thus, one generation of processed foods as health foods gave way to the next.

Yet as early as 1942, Philip Wylie in his *Generation of Vipers* condemned the collapse of social relations in America, which he blamed on the unholy alliance of women seeking leisure time and big business, which markets to them. By the 1950s, his target was the frozen TV dinner, which he included in his 1954 attack article "Science has Spoiled My Supper" (Wylie 1954). He saw the collapse of the family, its cohesion, and its health, as promoted by the quick fix of frozen foods. Today, the World Health Organization shares his pessimistic attitude toward processed foods. In fact, it recommends that people reduce their intake of processed foods as much as possible. What caused this change in the perception of processed foods?

For most of human history, the majority of sickness and death in the human population was caused by infectious disease. Most diseases were the result of bacteria, viruses, and parasites, and people commonly became infected by eating contaminated food. However, with improved sanitation, better healthcare, and safer food-preservation techniques developed in the past fifty years, the risk of catching a serious infectious disease has dropped dramatically. The reduction in the incidence and severity of infectious diseases, when combined with improved access to food and increasingly sedentary lifestyles, has paved the way for a new kind of health problem: chronic diseases. These diseases, often referred to as "diseases of affluence," include heart disease, cancer, diabetes, and obesity. The main difference between infectious and chronic diseases is that most chronic diseases result from a lifestyle of poor health choices rather than chance infections. The Centers for Disease Control and Prevention rank poor diet, namely with an excess of calories, high levels of sodium, and unhealthy fats (a major characteristic of many processed foods), as a major risk factor for many chronic diseases. Dieting means, in part, eliminating such foods from one's daily consumption.

Processed foods traditionally were considered healthier than fresh foods because they are sterile and do not spoil or become contaminated easily. When eating contaminated food was a significant cause of disease, this was a very legitimate argument for increased consumption of processed foods. However, with the recent improvements in food transportation and sanitation, the risk of becoming sick from eating fresh food in the Western world is very low. Therefore, processed foods are no longer advantageous for their sterility, and the high levels of sodium and transfats used in processing are far more threatening to health than the negligible risk of becoming sick from fresh foods. From the praise of canning and concentrates in the eighteenth century as the source of health and longevity, processed foods in the current "Fast Food Nation," have come to represent illness and early death.

SLG/SARAH GARDINER

*See also* Behavior; Brillat-Savarin; Fast Food; Hopkins; Medieval Diets; Post; Spurlock

## References and Further Reading

Anon. (2005) "Preventing Chronic Diseases and Obesity through Good Nutrition and Physical Activity," Centers for Disease Control and Prevention, available online at <http://www.cdc.gov/nccdphp/publications/factsheets/Prevention/obesity.htm> (accessed March 15, 2007).

Anon. (2005) "A Short History of Processed Foods," Food Products Association, available online at <http://www.fpa-food.org/content/consumers/history.asp> (accessed March 15, 2007).

Anon. (2006) "Obesity and Overweight," World Health Organization, available online at <http://www.who.int/dietphysicalactivity/publications/facts/obesity/en/index.html> (accessed March 15, 2007).

Derven, Daphne L. (2003) "Preserving," in Solomon H. Katz (ed.), *Encyclopedia of Food and Culture*, Vol. III, New York: Charles Scribner's Sons.

Kurlansky, Mark (2003) *Salt: A World History*, New York: Penguin.

Shephard, Sue (2000) *Pickled, Potted, and Canned: How the Art and Science of Food Preserving Changed the World*, New York: Simon & Schuster.

Smith, Christopher Holmes (2001) "Freeze Frames: Frozen Foods and Memories of the Postwar American Family," in Sherrie A. Inness (ed.), *Kitchen Culture in America*, Philadelphia, Pa.: University of Pennsylvania Press, pp. 175–209.

Wylie, Philip (1954) "Science Has Spoiled My Supper," *Atlantic* (April): 45–7.

# Professionalization of Dieting

In the history of dieting, various groups and individuals have been responsible for handing out dieting advice. From the 1860s to the 1950s, the church and religious groups, as well as celebrity and socialites from Lord Byron to Upton Sinclair, emphasized the importance of keeping the body pure (Griffith 2004: 50). In the 1960s, people shifted from following traditional diet advice of keeping the body clean to conforming to a thinness campaign (Bordo 2003: 102–3). Restrictive diets became popular and, thus, the average American looked to supermodels like Twiggy for "advice." Again, in the 1980s, celebrity figures and fad doctors published the bulk of dieting books and gave out dieting tips on how they were able to achieve a slim figure. Celebrities like Jane Fonda and Oprah, among others, provided their personal dieting stories for Americans to follow. Currently, the research-driven food and dieting industry has caused a shift in dietary advice, which emphasizes the expertise of medical doctors with university degrees in diet and nutrition.

In order to understand to whom people are turning for advice at the beginning of the twenty-first century, it is important to understand the difference between a nutritionist and a dietitian. A dietitian is a healthcare professional who has received specialized accredited tertiary education and training. Dietitians are also required to adhere to regulatory rules and guidelines. A nutritionist, on the other hand, advises people on dietary issues related to health, well-being, and proper eating. Even though no formal organization regulates the work and advice of a nutritionist, these specialists often write dieting books and appear on television programs publicizing their advice (Anon. "Dietitian/Nutritionist" 2007).

The shift from individuals following the advice from diet gurus to diet professionals is evident in the increasing number of members of the American Dietetic Association (ADA). As of 2006, the ADA had 65,000 members and was the U.S.A.'s largest food and nutrition organization. The ADA was founded in 1917 in Cleveland, Ohio by a group of women who wanted to enhance America's health and nutrition during World War I. Since the early 1900s, the ADA has evolved into an organization of people with diverse practice areas (ADA). Whether dieters actually check to see if their dietitian or doctor is a member of the ADA is unknown; however, as in other professions, belonging to the national organization is important. According to the ADA's vision statement, its "members *are the most valued source of food and nutrition services,*" because of their extensive training.

However, becoming a professional dietitian is not easy. In order to join the ADA, one must hold one of numerous degrees. Most common among members of the ADA are registered dietitians (RD), who are food and nutrition experts. RDs are required to meet extensive academic and professional requirements, including holding a bachelor's degree with coursework approved by ADA's Commission on Accreditation for Dietetics Education (CADE). Courses typically focus on food and nutrition sciences, food-service systems management, business, economics, computer science, sociology, biochemistry, physiology, microbiology, and chemistry. Seventy-five percent of the ADA is comprised of registered dietitians, and the remaining members are made up of dietetic technicians, food-service managers, educators, researchers, and other dietetic professionals. As of November 2006, there were approximately 228 bachelors and masters programs all over the U.S.A. approved by CADE in which one could begin one's career in dietetics. In addition, potential candidates for licensing must complete a CADE-accredited supervised program at a healthcare facility, community agency, or food-service corporation. Such a practice program typically lasts six to twelve months. In addition, one must take and pass the national exam given by CADE. Lastly, registered dietitians must complete continuing educational requirements to maintain registration. The ADA believes that such a rigorous

program guarantees expertise and quality advice which consumers now demand.

After completing their degree, about half of all registered dietitians work in clinical settings, private practice, or healthcare facilities. Others work in community and public health settings, academia and research, business, journalism, sports nutrition, and wellness programs. According to the U.S. Department of Labor Bureau of Labor Statistics, heightened public interest in nutrition and health has increased the job market in areas such as food manufacturing and advertising where dietitians analyze aspects of foods and report on their nutrition value. The employment of dietitians is expected to grow through the next ten years as disease prevention and nutrition are growing public concerns and as people are continuing to live longer. Specifically, the Department of Labor predicts that employment will increase in nursing homes, residential care facilities, and physician clinics. The growth for dietitians and nutritionists, however, may be sustained by limitation on insurance and reimbursement for dietetic services. Nevertheless, the diversity of jobs available for graduates with degrees in dietetics reflects the growing demand for professionals to give diet advice.

Clearly, there are many trained dietitians in the U.S.A.; however, can average Americans actually afford a dietitian? Several years ago, the cost of seeing a dietitian was considered an unnecessary visit and thus not insured by healthcare companies. However, a recent survey of twenty-three healthcare plans in the U.S.A. conducted by the *Journal of the American Dietetic Association* found that more healthcare companies are covering a visit to a dietitian (Tufts Health and Nutrition Letter 2004). In other words, when a primary-care physician refers a patient to a dietitian, a growing number of health-insurance companies are beginning to pay for the 100-dollar session. While the restrictions are tight, such as one must seek "medical nutrition therapy" or the dietary treatment should be medically necessary to treat a chronic illness, the ball is rolling for more coverage. Health-insurance companies have recognized that correcting one's dietary problems can help general illness, prove more cost effective, and even prevent future conditions (Tufts Health and Nutrition Letter 2004).

Now that more and more people are looking to professionals for dieting advice, and people can actually afford the care, those who hand out diet advice are being held to higher standards. People who claim to be "diet experts" may have to seek the advice of legal counsel because of faulty claims of their dieting regimens. In the case of television's Dr. Phil McGraw, three irate dieters from Los Angeles sued Dr. Phil for claims made in his "Shape Up!" diet plan (Casewatch 2007). In both his television program and book, Dr. Phil promotes his Shape Up! plan by recommending dieters to take twenty-two herbal supplements and vitamin pills daily at a cost of 120 dollars a month in addition to exercising regularly. According to the product label, the pills "contain scientifically researched levels of ingredients that can help you change your behavior to control your weight." Disgruntled dieters were sure that the plan was useless as they found themselves losing money, not weight (Roope 2005). Their dissatisfaction led the Federal Trade Commission to investigate McGraw's advertising.

In late 2004, the *Los Angeles Times* reported that CSA Nutraceuticals discontinued Shape Up! products amid the FTC's investigation. A settlement of 10.5 million dollars came in September of 2006, and customers will be able to choose either replacement products or small cash reward as part of the settlement. Luckily for McGraw, CSA Nutraceuticals' insurance will cover the cost of the settlement, and he will have no personal responsibility for his unsubstantiated claims. Dr. Phil has since denied all allegations (American Broadcasting Corporation). A class action lawsuit such as this may illustrate how some consumers are changing whom they trust for such advice.

However, it is hard to hold those who give out dieting advice accountable because it is inherently difficult to prove or disprove the effectiveness of their plans. First, it is tough to prove which diets work because there are no double blinds; only dieters know what they are eating, and thus studies cannot accurately report whether weight changes occur because of the plan and not other factors. In addition, when it comes to dieting, people feel embarrassed about their eating habits and thus misreport unhealthy meals and choices. Also, each dieter's body functions in a unique way, and genetics and exercise play important roles that are difficult to measure. Therefore, there is no real mechanism to resolve the problems that lie in the way of studying diet.

While there is a growing movement that prefers professional advice, there are limits on this trend. The limits are that consumers want cheap and convenient advice that will provide "quick fixes" to their dieting dilemmas. Some Americans may see no need in paying high prices to a professional when they can buy a dieting book or surf the Internet for advice. Professionals usually require more long-term commitments and cost much more. The overwhelming amount of dieting advice available in accessible and inexpensive ways is evident when the word "diet" is entered into amazon.com's book search and more than 183,000 results pop up. In addition, at any one time, a diet book is on the charts on the *Publisher's Weekly* National Bestseller list (Dahlin and Hix 2006). Moreover, the dieting community continuously changes who is admitted into the professional crowd or quack doctor circle. With the rise of dieting books, internet advice, and more and more diet gurus making faulty claims, it is hard to predict where the next wave of dietary advice will rise.

SLG/JESSICA SAWHNEY

*See also* Byron; Fonda; Hornby; Internet; McGraw; Self-help; Sinclair; Winfrey

## References and Further Reading

American Broadcasting Corporation (2006) "Settlement Reached on Dr. Phil Diet Plan," September 26, available online at <http://abcnews.go.com/Entertainment/wireStory?id=2493931&CMP=OTC-RSSFeeds0312> (accessed January 25, 2007).

American Dietetic Association "Commission on Accreditation for Dietetics Education." Available online at <http://www.eatright.org/cps/rde/xchg/ada/hs.xsl/CADE.html> (accessed January 30, 2007).

—— "For Registered Dietitian." Available online at <http://www.eatright.org/cps/rde/xchg/ada/hs.xsl/CADE_748_ENU_HTML.htm> (accessed January 29, 2007).

Anon. (2007) "Dietitian/Nutritionist," The Thompson Corporation, available online at <http://www.delmarhealthcare.com/pdf/careers/Dietitian%20Nutritionist.pdf> (accessed January 25, 2007).

Bordo, Susan (2003) *Unbearable Weight: Feminism, Western Culture, and the Body*, 10th edn, Berkeley, Calif.: University of California Press.

Casewatch, "Your Guide to Health Fraud-and Quackery-Related Legal Matters, 'Dr. Phil' Mcgraw Facing Class-Action Suit." Available online at <http://www.casewatch.org/civil/drphil/classactioncomplaint.shtml> (accessed January 25, 2007).

Dahlin, Robert and Charles Hix (2006) "Diet and Fitness

Books," *Publishers Weekly* (November 13). Available online at <http://www.publishersweekly.com/article/CA6390047.html?industryid=23590&industry=Diet+%26+Health+Books> (accessed January 25, 2007).

Griffith, R. Marie (2004) *Born Again Bodies: Flesh and Spirit in American Christianity*, Berkeley, Calif.: University of California Press.

Roope, Jim (2005) "Class Action Sought for 'Dr. Phil' Diet Suit," Cable News Network, October 7, available online at <http://www.cnn.com/2005/LAW/10/04/dr.phil> (accessed January 25, 2007).

*Tufts Health and Nutrition Letter* (2004) "More Health Insurance Plans Covering Visits to Dietitians." Available online at http://healthletter.tufts.edu/issues/2004-03/dietitian.html (accessed September 20, 2007).

U.S. Department of Labor, Bureau of Labor Statistics (2007) "Dietitians and Nutritionists." Available online at <http://stats.bls.gov/oco/ocos077.htm> (accessed January 10, 2007).

# Psychotherapy and Weight Change

**P**sychotherapy has regularly been used in conjunction with exercise and dieting to help with weight loss. Certain forms of psychotherapy, such as behavioral therapy have been more recently employed in order to facilitate weight loss. Indeed "body image treatment" through "cognitive behavioral therapy" has become commonplace in the self-treatment of both over- and underweight individuals since the development of Jonathan Butters and Thomas Cash's approach in the mid-1980s (Butters and Cash 1987). Cash's audiotape program *Body-Image Therapy: A Program for Self-Directed Change*, while aimed at mental-health practitioners, set the stage for self-treatment for women who desired to change their own negative body image. Other nonclinical settings like weight-loss support groups also use a psychotherapeutic model to enable the loss of weight (Jeffery et al. 1998). Experts suggest that behavioral therapy is a good non-surgical alternative when it comes to weight loss; the results, however, are not always long-lived. While there is an average weight loss of 7–10 percent of initial body weight during the first twenty-four weeks of treatment, further treatment seems to offer no more weight loss. Indeed, there seems to be a pattern of relapse attributed by behavioral therapists to their patient's inability to sustain the practices they learn in therapy. Given that such strategies are designed to change behavioral patterns, long-term efficacy is disproved (Wilson and Brownell 2002).

Behavioral techniques rest on the claim that obese people gain weight either as a response to conditioned learning or environmental stimuli or as a coping mechanism in response to stress and arousal. Thus, therapy can include stimulus control (controlling the presence of certain "trigger" foods in the home and increasing the presence of exercise cues), problem-solving strategies, social assertion (figuring out ways to assert one's dietary philosophy in an uncongenial environment), setting short-term goals to enhance positive thinking, cognitive reconditioning to help alter negative thought patterns, relapse prevention (learning to gauge which situations are detrimental to weight loss commitments), and building a support network.

Therapy for eating disorders has now reached into the online world of the Internet. There is the claim that internet-driven intervention combined with individual therapy is more effective than therapy alone. Such online activities tend, it is claimed, to reduce clients' anxiety about how they appear and being judged when they are unseen by the therapist. The use of online behavioral therapy together with online virtual reality has been claimed to modify the body awareness and thus impact on problematic social and eating behaviors (Derrig-Palumbo and Zeine 2005: 117–18).

A comparative study that assigned some participants to Weight Watchers and others to a self-help group for weight loss found that clients who attended Weight Watchers had a greater tendency to lose weight (Lowe et al. 1999: 51–9). The researchers concluded that this was due to the behavioral component of the program, which was actively reinforced through group meetings and weekly weigh-ins. Dieting, they found, could only have long-term results if it was part of a larger lifestyle philosophy instead of a compartmentalized activity one undertook merely to lose weight. Another study conducted by scientists at Baylor analyzed the difference between two types of treatment for women engaged in binge-eating: One involved dieting and behavioral therapy, while the other consisted only of behavioral therapy measures (Goodrick et al. 1998: 363–8). What the research team found six months after the treatment program was that the women who dieted and had therapy had lost about 1.32 pounds, while those who only had therapy had gained about 1.86 pounds. What these women had experienced was a marked reduction in their binge-eating patterns. An eighteen-month follow-up examination revealed that both groups had once again gained weight, but that there had been an overall reduction in binge-eating. The researchers once again concluded the ineffectuality of dieting as a weight-loss measure but saw that other behavioral patterns, such as binge-eating had undergone a significant change.

When weight gain or loss is considered to be a psychological illness rather than a behavioral aberration, very different approaches are used. Certainly, the use of "talk-therapy," whether in the form of classic psychoanalysis or short-term psychotherapy, has a long history. Indeed, family therapy remains a mainstay for the treatment of eating disorders such as bulimia and anorexia nervosa, but it is used relatively rarely as a treatment for obesity. Alternative psychoanalytic explanations, such as libido theory, have been offered to explain the presence of obesity (Friedman 1972: 364–83). The effectiveness of interpersonal psychotherapy has been claimed by Christopher Fairburn as an answer to the lack of long-term effectiveness of behavioral therapy (Fairburn 1997). One large-scale study in 1977 tracked the treatment of eighty-four obese patients (paired with sixty-three normal-weight patients) treated with a wide range of psychoanalytic approaches. The resultant (short-term) weight loss was seen to be approximately the same as those patients treated specifically for weight loss (Rand and Stunkard 1977: 459–97).

With the reappearance of "Body Dysmorphic Disorder" as a major diagnosis for certain forms of mental illness in the standard American handbook of mental illnesses (DSM-IVR) and the championing of this by American psychiatry, the relationship between eating disorders (also a psychiatric category) and body dysmorphic disorder has been raised. "Dysmorphophobia" is a diagnostic category coined by the Italian psychiatrist Enrico Morselli (1852–1929) in 1891. Given that the treatment of choice of the latter is the prescription of serotonin reuptake inhibitors, a class of psychotropic drugs, one can imagine the use of such interventions in the treatment of eating disorders (Phillips 2002: 113–17). Thus, weight loss (and gain) comes to be understood as a somatic rather than a psychological disorder.

Even in the application of alternative approaches to weight loss, such as mental imagery, there is a neurological claim for efficacy. Imaging is " 'seeing' in the absence of actual visual sensory imputs" and is claimed to activate the dopamine reward pathway and thus enhance weight loss (Heinkel et al. 2003: 226). The creation of "aversive imagery," such as "disgusting images" of "rat droppings in chocolate chip cookies," seems to be effective in weight reduction (Johnson and Karkut 1996: 664). Such approaches have a wide range of therapeutic modalities. As early as 1843, hypnotism was used to "control a female patient's appetite for certain foods which exacerbated dyspepsia in her" (Gravitz 1988: 68–9). By the 1960s, hypnotism (now restored to clinical acceptability) reappeared for the treatment of overweight.

SLG/SHRUTHI VISSA

*See also* Anorexia; Binge-eating; Bruch; Internet; Nidetch; Self-help

## References and Further Reading

Butters, J.W. and Cash, T.F. (1987) "Cognitive-Behavioral Treatment of Women's Body Image Dissatisfaction," *Journal of Consulting and Clinical Psychology* 55 (2): 889–97.

Derrig-Palumbo, Kathleene and Zeine, Foojan (2005) *Online Therapy*, New York: Norton.

Fairburn, C.G. (1997) "Interpersonal Psychotherapy for Bulimia Nervosa," in D.M. Garner and P.E. Garfinkel (eds), *Handbook of Treatment for Eating Disorders*, New York: Guilford Press, pp. 278–94.

Friedman, Stanley (1972) "On the Presence of a Variant Form of Instinctual Regression: Oral Drive," *Psychoanalytic Quarterly* 41 (3): 364–83.

Goodrick, G. Ken, Kimball, Kay T., Reeves, Rebecca S., and Foreyt, John P. (1998) "Non-Dieting Versus Dieting Treatment for Overweight Binge-Eating Women," *Journal of Consulting and Clinical Psychology* 66 (2): 363–8.

Gravitz, M.A. (1988) "Early Uses of Hypnosis in Smoking Cessation and Dietary Management: A Historical Note," *American Journal of Clinical Hypnosis* 31 (1): 68–9.

Heinkel, Colleen, Rosenfeld, Michelle and Sheikh, Anees A. (2003) "Imagery in Smoking Cessation and Weight Management," in Anees A. Sheikh (ed.) *Healing Images: The Role of Imagination in Health*, Amityville, NY: Baywood Publishing, pp. 223–54.

Jeffery, R.W., Wing, Rena R., Thorson, Carolyn, and Burton, Lisa R. (1998) "Use of Personal Trainers and Financial Incentives to Increase Exercise in a Behavioral Weight-Loss Program," *Journal of Consulting and Clinical Psychology* 66 (5): 777–83.

Johnson, D.L. and Karkut, R.T. (1996) "Participation in Multicomponent Hypnosis Treatment Programs for Women's Weight Loss with and Without Overt Aversion," *Psychological Reports* 79 (2): 659–68.

Lowe, Michael R., Miller-Kovach, Karen, Frye, Nema, and Phelan, Susan (1999) "An Initial Evaluation of a Commercial Weight Loss Program: Short-Term Effects on Weight, Eating Behavior and Moods," *Obesity Research* 7 (1): 51–9.

Phillips, Katharine A. (2002) "Body Image and Body Dysmorphic Disorder," in Christopher G. Fairburn and Kelly D. Brownell (eds), *Eating Disorders and Obesity: A Comprehensive Handbook*, 2nd edn, New York: Guilford Press, pp. 113–17.

Rand, Collen S. and Stunkard, Albert J. (1977) "Psychoanalysis and Obesity," *Journal of the American Academy of Psychoanalysis* 5 (4): 459–97.

Wilson, G. Terence and Brownell, Kelly D. (2002) "Behavioral Treatment for Obesity," in Christopher G. Fairburn and Kelly D. Brownell (eds), *Eating Disorders and Obesity: A Comprehensive Handbook*, 2nd edn, New York: Guilford Press, pp. 524–8.

# R

## Religion and Dieting

The history of fasting extends far into the past and is powerfully connected to religious ideas about contamination and rituals of devotion and purification (Douglas 2002). Many groups of people today still fast for religious reasons, but fasting is now also used by people to lose weight. There is, even today, a large body of religious literature on the evils of overeating, which suggests that fasting and weight loss will bring an overweight person back into God's graces. However, secular materials on fasting and diet also express many of the same ideas about contamination, cleansing, and salvation (or at least health). Ritual fasting remains a feature of Judaism (on Yom Kippur and other fast days), Christianity (during Lent), and Islam (during the days of Ramadan). The Enlightenment transformed fasting into dieting as a means of affecting the material body rather than providing some metaphysical relationship between the godhead and human beings. Fasting itself comes to be seen as a form of dieting.

The origins of the association between dieting and religious practice in America may be traced back to William Metcalfe (1788–1862), the first public advocate of vegetarianism in the U.S.A. and its mass popularization by Sylvester Graham (1794–1851), a Presbyterian minister and an advocate of dietary reform. Although Graham had no medical background or training, he was convinced that a vegetarian diet was a cure for alcoholism and, more importantly, would alleviate the impure thoughts associated with lust and sexual urges.

In modern-day America, dieting culture is still articulated through a Protestant Christian idiom and lexicon so that fitness culture now bears the characteristics of a religious movement (Griffith 2004: 8). Contemporary diet and fitness jargon is glutted with religious metaphors, conversion narratives and testimonials (Griffith 2004: 11). A corollary to this is seen in the medical field where eating disorders are often diagnosed as a "spiritual crisis." In today's culture, marketers have profited greatly by combining two things that sell, *diet* and *religion*. The emergence of many religious-based diets has become quite popular, some of these including: the Maker's Diet, the Body by God Plan, the What would Jesus Eat Program, and the Hallelujah Diet. The dieting regimen with prayer is exemplified in books such as Deborah Pierce's *I Prayed Myself Slim* and Charlie Shedd's *Pray Your Weight Away*. Shedd believes that our bodies do not belong to us, but instead belong to the Creator. He claims, "Your body is the temple of the Holy Spirit . . . Inside, outside, God made you for His Glory" (Shedd 1957: 41). The concept of sin in these books is associated with gluttony and unattractiveness. Prayer is a means by which the desired result of attractiveness can be achieved; in doing so, one can be taken away from gluttony and ill health and be brought closer to God. This is an indication that sin and guilt have become a gauge of fat.

Evidence of the relationship between religion and dieting is also present in support groups like Overeaters Anonymous (OA), which is a nonprofit organization, originally founded to help those who suffer from compulsive eating but now also includes anorexics, bulimics, and compulsive eaters. The structure and philosophy of OA is based on the model of Alcoholics Anonymous (AA). AA, founded in 1935, involves a "twelve-step" program for "recovery from alcoholism." This social movement has had a considerable impact on therapy across all levels of society. Central to its message, rooted in the Judeo-Christian tradition, is the need for a particular relationship between God and oneself. The "Secular Organization for Sobriety" (also known as "Save our Selves") was created as an answer to AA. OA feels that compulsive eating is an "emotional and spiritual disease" and is "progressive and incurable," unless one turns their individual control over to God, the higher power, and asks for his help to aid in his or her reevaluation of life (Sobal and Maurer 1999).

It is not just religious diets, however, that emphasize the need for spiritual purpose in dieting. Indeed, many contemporary dieting books suggest that either dieters need to find peace in order to achieve dieting success or that the diet proposed will actually bring the reader peace. From wherever the peace originates, modern science has shown that religion can be a powerful factor in dietary success. One of the reasons suggested by researchers is that the church group can be a good support system for someone looking to improve his/her health. In addition, the Sunday morning service can be a good platform to distribute information on dietary changes for healthy weight maintenance. Therefore, some investigators have used people who attend church as research subjects to test dietary interventions.

In contrast to the use of diet as a representation of austerity and reverence to God in the time of Sylvester Graham, dieting in contemporary society has a very different relationship to religion. From the use of church groups as support groups for those coping with diabetes to the OA model based on curing the spirit, dieting is intrinsically linked to a higher power in many diets.

SLG/RAKHI PATEL

*See also* Binge-eating; Christianity; Enlightenment Dietetics; Graham; Ibn Sina; Jews; Metcalfe; Self-help; Sinclair

### References and Further Reading

Douglas, Mary (2002) *Purity and Danger*, London and New York: Routledge.

Griffith, R. Marie (1997) "The Promised Land of Weight Loss." Available online at <http://www.religion-online.org/showarticle.asp?title=249> (accessed March 12, 2007).

—— (2004) *Born Again Bodies: Flesh and Spirit in American Christianity*, Berkeley, Calif.: University of California Press.

Pierce, Deborah (1960) *I Prayed Myself Slim: The Prayer-Diet Book*, New York: Citadel Press.

Resnicow, Ken, Jackson, Alice, Braithwaite, Ronald, DiIorio, Colleen, Blisset, Dhana, Rahotep, Simone, and Periasamy, Santhi (2002) "Healthy Body/Healthy Spirit: A Church-Based Nutrition and Physical Activity Intervention," *Health Education Research* 17 (5): 562–73.

Sabate J. (2004) "Religion, Diet and Research," *British Journal of Nutrition* 92 (2): 199–201.

Shedd, Charles (1957) *Pray Your Weight Away*, Philadelphia, Pa.: J.B. Lippincott.

Sobal, J. and Donna Maurer (eds) (1999) *Interpreting Weight: The Social Management of Fatness and Thinness*, New York: Aldine de Gruyter.

# Risks Associated with Dieting

Every year, many people are encouraged to diet by their physicians. These physicians prescribe diets for many reasons, including weight loss (the main reason), Type 2 diabetes, hypertension, and various other ailments. Another large group of people diet without doctor recommendations. These people use dieting to maintain a certain lifestyle, whether it is physical, mental, religious, or otherwise. The hope is that a proper diet will facilitate a longer healthier life. There are many different dieting options available to the consumer. Many of these dieting practices can take a toll on the human body, with consequences ranging from mild rashes or headaches to severe cardiac problems and even death.

One of the problems with most dieting techniques is

that although they may provide a period of weight loss, this loss is rarely permanent, and, in some cases, their weight will even increase. Fluctuations in weight have been shown to be unhealthy. Diet is regularly prescribed to patients with hypertension. Occasionally, however, a hypertensive obese person may attempt dieting to lower blood pressure, fail, and, consequently, be more likely to die from cardiovascular disease than before (Campos 2004). One study also found a positive correlation between weight fluctuation and the development of renal cell cancer (Lindblad et al. 1994). It is important to be conscious of all aspects of health during dieting because something as simple as weight fluctuation can be dangerous.

In addition, there is a whole category of diets considered "fad" diets. A fad is a practice or interest that is very popular for a short time and is followed with exaggerated zeal. This obviously describes a fad diet. An even more complete definition of fad diet includes its promise to help people lose large amounts of weight in short periods of time. Fad dieting consists of eating very little or cutting certain food groups out altogether. Fad diets are currently popular in the U.S.A., and the most popular of all in recent years is the Atkins Diet, which suggests a low-to-no-carbohydrate, high-fat, high-protein diet.

This type of diet may indeed show an initial period of weight loss, but most of the weight loss "is not due to the miracle of 'switching the body's metabolism over to burning fat stores.' It is due to a diet-induced diuresis" (Denke 2001: 59). A diet low in carbohydrates changes some of the metabolic processes in the body, leading to an increase in the production of urine by the kidneys. Furthermore, these diets calling for elevated quantities of protein may not be healthy because "[h]igh levels of animal protein intakes have been linked to higher risks for [coronary heart disease] and cancer … and also have been linked to higher risks for osteoporosis, and renal disease, but both of these areas are controversial" (Anderson et al. 2000: 586). High-protein, low-carbohydrate diets also recommend no intake of fruits, vegetables, or grains, which contain many of the important nutrients needed by the body for daily processes. The loss of these foods can cause unwanted health problems, such as headaches, constipation, muscle cramps, halitosis, diarrhea, weakness, and rashes among other things. More importantly, long-term nutrient deficiencies "might pose a second-line increased risk of cardiovascular disease and cancer" (Astrup et al. 2004: 898). Nevertheless,

fad diets are increasing in popularity and seem to be neverending; when one fades, another will replace it, claiming the same quick weight-loss benefits.

Other weight-loss methods, such as weight-loss/diet pills, anorexic and bulimic behavior, and various surgical options pose an even greater risk to health than general diet. Prescription diet pills with the combination of fenfluramine and phentermine were proven to have dangerous side effects; the most worrisome problem was the development of leaky heart valves. A study reported by the FDA in 1997 found that one-third of all patients on the fenfluramine, phentermine combination developed a leaky heart and another 25–30 percent displayed an abnormal echocardiogram (Berg 1999: 279). More commonly used diet pills are sold over the counter (OTC). These can be dangerous because they are not regulated in the same fashion as prescription drugs by the FDA. OTC diet pills are usually classified as dietary supplements and not drugs, though "drug manufacturers may claim that their product will diagnose, cure, mitigate, treat, or prevent a disease. Such claims may not legally be made for dietary supplements" (National Women's Health Resource Center).

Most OTC diet pills contain the ingredient phenyl-propanolamine (PPA), which is now being pulled from the market by the FDA because it is linked with an increased risk of hemorrhagic stroke. Another weight-loss ingredient is ephedrine, which is found in many pills and has also proven to be dangerous. One study found "evidence to conclude that ephedrine and ephedra are associated with two to three times the risk of psychiatric symptoms, autonomic symptoms, upper gastrointestinal symptoms, and heart palpitations" (Shekelle et al. 2003: 1544). Another study done on the effects of ephedrine found a link between its use and adverse cardiovascular events, including acute myocardial infarction, severe hypertension, myocarditis, and lethal cardiac arrhythmias, leading them to conclude that the use of "supplements that contain ephedra alkaloids pose a serious health risk to some users" (Haller and Benowitz 2000: 1836).

Bariatric (branch of medicine that deals with the treatment of obesity) surgeries are aimed at helping people lose weight. These surgeries, as all surgeries, can be dangerous and should be utilized only as a last resort. A report published in 2005 found that 17 percent of 219 gastric-bypass patients had major complications, including gastric leaks, hemorrhages, and obstructions. One patient even died from complications of a gastric leak. The same report found that 6 percent of 154 gastric-band patients had major complications, including stomach perforations, blood clots, and one death from complications during surgery (Anon. "Surgically Slim" 2006: 26). Another study found a drastic increase in the amount of hospitalizations following the surgery. These visits were for various complications after surgery. The study "found significant and sustained increases in the rates of hospital admission for morbidly obese patients after RYGB [Roux-en-Y bypass]. Annual rates of hospital admission after RYGB are double that prior to operation and are sustained beyond a year . . . " (Zingmond et al. 2005: 1921). These surgeries have consistently shown great benefits to obese patients, but safety remains an issue to be resolved.

Eating disorders can also be considered a form of dieting as the basis of the practice is to either maintain or lose weight. Eating disorders are generally the most dangerous of all dieting techniques and are usually accompanied by a psychological problem, which only makes them worse. Anorexia nervosa is characterized by very unusual eating habits, where people may eat very little or obsessively control their food portions. The eating pattern may be combined with other practices, such as compulsive exercise and the use of laxatives or diuretics. Anorexia is a very dangerous condition that can lead to extremely poor health and even death.

Anorexia shares its infamy with another eating disorder, bulimia nervosa, which is characterized by a period of extreme binge-eating followed by a period of equally extreme practices to prevent weight gain. These compensatory practices include self-induced vomiting, use of diuretics, laxatives, fasting, and extreme exercise. These behaviors are truly unhealthy as they affect all aspects of the human body. Eating disorders are disproportionately practiced by younger people, usually "develop[ing] in girls between age 12 and 25. Age 17 is the average age that an eating disorder develops, and between five percent and 10 percent of young people have eating disorders" (National Women's Health 2004). This is extremely dangerous, as there is a real risk of life altering trauma to the body due to early eating disorders.

Research has routinely shown that diets do hold many beneficial qualities when used in the correct manner and when overall health is monitored by a professional. What is important to remember is that there are many unproven, unhealthy diet programs promising

weight loss. The human body is an amazing machine capable of dealing with many circumstances, but if it is not maintained in the right manner, it can and will falter. It is imperative to pay attention to the needs of the human body when choosing a weight loss method.

SLG/DARREN JOHNSON

*See also* Anorexia; Atkins; Bariatric Surgery; Binge-eating

## References and Further Reading

Anon. (2006) "Surgically Slim: A Cure for Obesity, and Why It's Risky," *Consumer Reports* February 71 (2): 24–8.

Astrup, A., Larsen, T. and Harper, A. (2004) "Atkins and Other Low-Carbohydrate Diets: Hoax or an Effective Tool for Weight Loss?" *Lancet* 364 (9437): 897–9.

Anderson J.W., Konz, E.C., and Jenkins, D.J. (2000) "Health Advantages and Disadvantages of Weight-Reducing Diets: A Computer Analysis and Critical Review," *Journal of the American College of Nutrition* 19 (5): 578–90.

Berg, Frances M. (1999) "Health Risks Associated with Weight Loss and Obesity Treatment Programs," *Journal of Social Issues* 55 (2): 277–97.

Campos, Paul (2004) *The Obesity Myth*, New York: Gotham Books.

Denke, M. (2001) "Metabolic Effects of High-Protein, Low-Carbohydrate Diets," *American Journal of Cardiology* 88 (1): 59–61.

Fisher, M.C. and Lachance, P.A. (1985) "Nutrition Evaluation of Published Weight-Reducing Diets," *Journal of the American Dietetic Association* 85 (4): 450–4.

Haller, Christine A. and Benowitz, Neal L. (2000) "Adverse Cardiovascular and Central Nervous System Events Associated with Dietary Supplements Containing Ephedra Alkaloids," *New England Journal of Medicine* 343 (25): 1833–8.

Lindblad, P., Wolk, A., Bergström, R., Persson, I. and Adami, H.O. (1994) "The Role of Obesity and Weight Fluctuations in the Etiology of Renal Cell Cancer: A Population-Based Case-Control Study," *Cancer Epidemiology, Biomarkers & Prevention* 3 (8): 631–9.

National Women's Health Resource Center (2004) "Eating Disorders: Overview." Available online at <http://www.accessmylibrary.com/coms2/sum-

mary_0286–4655431_ITM> (accessed March 12, 2007).

Shekelle, P., Hardy, M.L., Morton, S.C., Maglione, M., Mojica, W.A., Suttorp, M.J., Rhodes, S.L., Jungvig, L. and Gagné, J. (2003) "Efficacy and Safety of Ephedra and Ephedrine for Weight Loss and Athletic Performance," *Journal of the American Medical Association* 289 (12):1537–45.

Zingmond, David S., McGory, Marcia L., and Ko, Clifford Y. (2005) "Hospitalization Before and After Gastric Bypass Surgery," *Journal of the American Medical Association* 294 (15): 1918–24.

# Roman Medicine and Dieting

Early Roman medicine, following the lead of classical Greek medicine, saw obesity as a sign of illness. This was best articulated in the works of the Alexandrian physician Celsus (fl. 30 CE). He argued, however, that the body tended toward fat naturally. Nevertheless, too much weight was a sign of disease. "The obese, many of them, are throttled by acute diseases and difficult breathing; they die often suddenly, which rarely happens in the thinner person" (Celsus 1935: I: 97). In treating extra weight, he suggests tepid saltwater baths, hard exercise, food of an austere kind, and restricted sleep (Paulus Aegineta 1844: I, 81).

More important is the shift in Roman medicine, which takes place in the first century when Galen (129–c. 216 CE) began to rethink the basic categories of Hippocratic medicine. He dismissed mere "empiricism" as per the Hippocratic method and demanded that there be a theoretical underpinning to medical knowledge. While the Hippocratic physicians used foodstuffs to treat the imbalance of the humors, Galen saw the natural world as the very source of the illness from which human beings suffer. The core concept remains the humors; Galen's dictum is that "it is always the case that everything superfluous in the body runs to the weakest site and produces effect in them according to its own nature" (Galen 2003: 45). For Galen what is common in all the diseases is "plethos," an excess of bad blood, blood mixed with "residues," which, if not excreted, would wander about the body, settle in weak parts, and there cause "putrefaction" (Galen 2003: 45).

Yet, it is the external world that provides the source of such residues. It is not the weak will of the phlegmatic individual that leads to *polysarkia* (too much skin), but the very nature of the food itself. For Galen in his *On the Fat and Lean Mode of Life*, the causes of illness lie in those things that are "non-natural," (i.e., not the humors) *res contra naturum*: *aer* (light and air), *cibus et portus* (food and drink), *motus et qies* (movement and rest), *somnux et vigilia* (sleeping and waking), *exkreta et sekreta* (metabolism), and *affectus animi* (affect). This was an argument that made "nurture" equivalent to "nature." In his *De alimentorum facultatibus* (*On the Nature of Foods*) Galen suggests "quick exercise" as a cure for obesity. He provides food, "but not of a very nourishing description," to be consumed only after exercise. He argued that a "sufficiently stout patient [could become] moderately thin in a short time by running and massages" (Paulus Aegineta 1844: I, 81). The cause of obesity lies in the natural products of the world consumed in excess. His work was as much for the educated lay reader as for the medical professional. Galen provides clear guidance about what is good to eat and what is not. His first book deals with "starchy" products of nature and what foods result from them, the second with fruits and vegetables, and the third with animal products. Galen's approach is culinary as well as medical; he suggests how food should be best and most tastefully prepared. His focus is both on treating the ill and preserving the healthy. All foods, according to Galen, are necessary and natural, but, used improperly, they can create illness.

Following Galen, the Alexandrian physician Paul of Aegina in the seventh century saw obesity as a problem only when it is "immoderate." Since "warm temperament renders the body lean," it is this state that should be created in fat people. "Active exercise, an attenuated regimen, medicines of the same class, and mental anxiety bring on the dry temperament, and thereby render the body lean." He also recommends that diuretics and small amounts of food (in proportion to exercise taken and preferably only once a day) should be undertaken (Paulus Aegineta 1844: I, 81).

The Romans incorporated diet as a classical therapy along with exercise to treat obesity. The key to all of the diets suggested was the Greek concept of a moderate reduction of foodstuffs complemented by exercise and some herbal treatments. In general Galenic medicine saw "food as therapy," but it also was concerned with questions of food as preserving health and life.

SLG

*See also* Greek Medicine and Dieting

### References

Celsus (1935) *De medicina*, trans. W.G. Spencer, Cambridge, Mass.: Harvard University Press, Vol. I.

Galen (2000) *Galen on Food and Diet*, trans. Mark Grant, London: Routledge.

—— (2003) *Galen on the Properties of Foodstuffs*, trans. Owen Powell, Cambridge: Cambridge University Press.

Oribasius (1997). *Dieting for an Emperor: A Translation of Books 1 and 4 of Oribasius' Medical Compilations.* Trans. Mark Grant, Leiden; New York: Brill.

Paulus Aegineta (1844) *The Seven Books of Paulus Aegineta*, trans. Francis Adams, London: Sydenham Society.

Wilner, Ortha L. (1931) "Roman Beauty Culture," *The Classical Journal* 27 (1): 26–38.

# Russell, Lillian (1861–1922)

## American singer and actress

Born Helen Louise Leonard, she changed her name upon entering show business in 1879. She was considered by many "a transcendent national beauty" (Fields 1999: 216) and was one of the first modern "celebrities" whose image so captivated the public that they wished to emulate her. In fact, her photograph was so prized that early manufacturers of mass-produced tobacco products included them as an attraction in the 1890s. Russell, however, was so appalled by this use of her likeness that she went to court to prevent her image being given away "to induce customers to purchase boxes of cigars and packages of chewing and smoking tobacco" (Fields 1999: 67). What made Russell unique as a beauty may, however, surprise contemporary readers.

Russell was corpulent: her weight topped at 160 pounds over her lifetime, but she was referred to in the public press as the "American Beauty," the title of one of her hit musicals. In fact, young women coveted her looks so much that they padded their clothes in order to look more "well rounded" like the actress. In contrast to today's desire to be ever thinner, girls of Lillian Russell's era frantically wrote to the *Ladies' Home Journal* for weight-gain advice in order to more closely resemble her. In the 1890s, plumper bodies were not only considered fashionable, they were considered a symbol of success.

Russell was also an advocate of the health benefits of bicycle riding. When she was given one of the first "modern" bicycles, gold-plated nonetheless, by "Diamond Jim" Brady in 1895, she rode it all over New York and was regularly interviewed about its health benefits. Riding a bicycle was a sign of liberation, health, and temperance, as the anti-alcohol spokesperson Frances E. Willard noted in her *A Wheel within a Wheel, or How I learned to Ride a Bicycle*. To ride it she wore a "split-skirt," one of the reform clothing innovations, which made it possible for women to ride a bicycle without being indecent. It quickly became a national fad because she wore it (Fields 1999: 104). Despite riding, her friend Brady was infamous as a gourmand, eating huge meals, and Russell joined him regularly in these fourteen-course extravaganzas, "pounds and pounds . . . accumulating on her already stuffed figure" (Morell 1940: 172). Her hourglass figure, she believed, would never go out of style (Morell 1940: 172). Yet, the *New York Journal* commented "she has no beauty below the chin . . . and moves with the soft heaviness of a nice white elephant" (Morell 1940: 185). After the introduction at the same time of Charles Dana Gibson's (1867–1944) tall, slim-hipped "Gibson Girls," Russell realized that riding her bicycle was a means of weight control.

After 1912, she wrote a column in the *Chicago Tribune* and the *Chicago Herald*, as well as other newspapers, providing beauty tips for women. She lectured widely on health and exercise with a talk entitled "How to Live 100 Years." In Chicago she was hailed as "the priestess of the art of living sanely, correctly, and preserving health and beauty" (Fields 1999: 180). But still "the living, breathing Lillian was at all times a cure for sore eyes," according to the *New York Sun* (Fields 1999: 181). Russell remained an icon of beauty even as she aged.

She was considered an expert in this field because she was, for her generation, deemed the feminine ideal incarnate. In addition to acting as an ambassador of celebrity debutantes in her column, Russell discussed women's health, love, and, most provocatively, women's suffrage, a cause to which her mother had been devoted. After World War I broke out, she was a recruiter for the Marine Corps and raised money for the American Legion. In 1922, she acted as a special investigator on immigration for President Warren G. Harding in Europe. After her death, she was buried with full military honors because of her contributions to the war effort.

SLG/Jessica Rissman

*See also* Smoking

## References and Further Reading

Anon. (2006) "Russell, Lillian," Encyclopaedia Britannica premium service, available online at <http://www.britannica.com/eb/article-9064472>M/ (accessed February 20, 2006).

Fields, Armond (1999) *Lillian Russell: A Biography of "America's Beauty,"* Jefferson, NC: McFarland.

Morell, Parker (1940) *Lillian Russell: The Era of Plush*, New York: Random House.

# S

## Scales and Public Weighing

Weighing the body is definitely a marker of the twentieth century; however, there is some evidence that people started to weigh themselves using various instruments in previous centuries. The first public weighing machines were developed in France in the seventeenth century and first appeared in 1760 in London. The medical theory regarding physical weight had been developed by the Venetian Sanctorius Sanctorius in late sixteenth-century Padua. Sanctorius monitored his body weight for thirty years. He announced in his *De statica medicine* (1614) that what he consumed weighed more than what he excreted and assumed that the missing weight had been perspired, a sign of health. He, therefore, recommended the regular weighing of the body to promote health. In his aphorisms, he also argued against too rapid weight gain or loss, for "when the body is one day of one weight, and another day of another, it argues an introduction of evil qualities" (Sanctorius 1806: 129). But he implied that too great a weight gain is itself pathological: "That weight, which is to any one such as that when he goes up some steepy place, he feels himself lighter that he is wont, is the exact standard of good health" (Sanctorius 1806: 129). Consistent weight and mobility define health, and the act of weighing oneself in public became a measure of public accountability for one's health. Sanctorius discovered that some amount of weight was not accounted for and figured out that this weight was lost by "insensible perspiration." Today, this loss is explained by human metabolism. The energy from the food is turned into heat to maintain body temperature around 98 degrees Fahrenheit.

Throughout history, the two most common weighing instruments (scales) were the balance and the steelyard. Both of these types of instruments were structurally similar, consisting of weights of a known value, a load of unknown value, and a lever in between to reach equilibrium. The difference between a balance and a steelyard is that a balance consists of two equal arms and a suspension from the middle. At each end of the arm is a pan. The idea is to weigh an object of known weight against an object of unknown weight to compare the difference. A steelyard is comprised of a beam with unequal arms, a pan on one side, a weight on the other, and a fulcrum or pivot located somewhere on the beam. The weight can be moved around until the longer part of the beam reaches equilibrium with the shorter beam. The position of the weight on the beam represents the weight of the object in the pan.

Weighing instruments (scales) have evolved to better meet the needs of measuring body weight. The scale has been modified to include a platform, which makes it easier to weigh awkward, large objects such as a human body. Today many people have digital scales in their bathrooms that can record their weight in a matter of seconds. More advanced scales are always being created that can measure more than overall body weight. Recently, Tanita Corporation of America came out with the first consumer scale passed by the Food and Drug Administration that measures body water as well as body fat.

Measuring body weight has become more popular as the obsession with obesity has increased. Consequently, weighing devices have been altered to make it easier to weigh human bodies. They will continue to evolve as the population demands to know more about their body composition and its relation to obesity.

SLG/MARY STANDEN

*See also* Metabolism

237

## References and Further Reading

Anon. (2004) "Weighing Instruments," Institute and Museum of the History of Science, available online at <http://brunelleschi.imss.fi.it/catalogo/genappr.asp?appl=SIM&xsl=approfondimento&lingua=ENG&chiave=204101> (accessed May 8, 2006).

Anon. (2005) "National Grid for Learning," Timelinescience.org, available online at <http://www.timelinescience.org/index.php> (accessed May 8, 2006).

Anon. (2006) "The World's Heaviest People," *Dimensions Magazine*, available online at <http://www.dimensionsmagazine.com/dimtext/kjn/people/heaviest.htm> (accessed March 3, 2007).

Anon. (2006) "Weighing Scale," *Wikipedia*, available online at <http://en.wikipedia.org/wiki/Weighing_scale> (accessed May 8, 2006).

Rabinowtich, I.M. (1930) "Pitfalls in the Clinical Application and Interpretation of the Basal Metabolic Rate." Available online at <http://www.pubmedcentral.gov/picrender.fcgi?artid=381992&blobtype=pdf> (accessed May 8, 2006).

Sanctorius, Sanctorius (1806) "*De statica medicine*," in John Sinclair (ed.) *The Code of Health and Longevity*, four vols, Edinburgh: Arch. Constable & Co, Vol. III, pp. 122–230.

Wolinsky, Howard (2004) "New Water-Weight Scale Shows What You Are Made of," *Chicago Sun Times*, November 9.

# Schwarzenegger, Arnold (1947–)

## Noted body builder, actor, and politician

Schwarzenegger's scope of influence extends outside the obsessive muscle-building sport in which he made his initial mark. He is also a successful entrepreneur, actor, and politician. His lifestyle and discipline has made him the model of fitness enthusiasts for over thirty years (1979). Unlike the strongmen of earlier years who epitomized health through exercise, Schwarzenegger has become an ideal of the modern perception of masculinity, one of those individuals that have, "advance billing as leaders, dominators, controllers—in short, masters of the universe" (Klein 1993: 9).

In the past, masculinity, as defined by exercise, was not as much a symbol of success as it was a symbol of health. For most of the nineteenth and early twentieth centuries, the ideal masculine male was defined in terms of his strength and fitness, rather than his size. For example, for most of the early twentieth century, Charles Atlas was the ideal male form. Unlike the past characterizations of masculinity associated with exercise and health as embodied by men such as Atlas, modern males exercise to achieve the stature and dominance that they believe is associated with masculinity today. Historian

Alan Klein claims that bodybuilding "exploits grandiosity" of the male body for the purpose of "compensation; the bodily fortress protected the vulnerability inside." He asserts that this internal vulnerability stems from insecurity and that "the powerful arms and chests are a bodybuilder's way of working out a range of personal issues" and believes that a man measures his success in life through the development of his body (Klein 1993: 3). He argues, in addition, that

bragging about the size of grants won or the numbers of publications one has is the same thing, in this respect [measuring success/masculinity], as showcasing a massive chest or arms with a skin-tight T-shirt. It matters not how a man resolves this issue, but resolve it he must by coming to terms with societal notions of masculinity that best suit him.

(Klein 1993: 4)

Therefore, men will attempt to adhere to a symbolically representative form of a masculine body in order to form a dialogue as they seek a sense of masculinity. This form to which men attempt to conform is often the traditional view of masculinity that associates heavily muscled men with, among other "manly" traits: virility, attractiveness, and prowess. Critics argue that men, and bodybuilders in particular, find it necessary to become "stacked" with muscles in order to assert their masculinity and ultimately be successful in all areas of life, particularly in roles of leadership that traditionally were only considered positions for men (Klein 1993: 9).

Arnold Schwarzenegger represents this modern "overcompensating" masculinity, and, indeed, began his successful career through earning notoriety as a weight-training fanatic. It may be difficult to imagine it now, but Schwarzenegger began as a "sickly child" who improved his health by playing soccer. When he reached the age of fifteen, however, Schwarzenegger began studying physiology and developing training routines designed to maximize his workout results. In his autobiography, he explains,

> It was the summer I turned fifteen, a magical season for me because that year I'd discovered exactly what I wanted to do with my life. . . . I knew I was going to be a bodybuilder. It wasn't simply that either. I would be the best bodybuilder in the world, the greatest, the best-built man.
>
> (Schwarzenegger and Hall 1977: 13)

His goals were initially met with skepticism and concern in his family. Schwarzenegger was raised in a Roman Catholic household and was "reared under strict paternal discipline" (Anon. 2000). His father favored nutrition and athletics and instilled these values in his family. Yet, despite the fact that he lived in a "physical family," as Schwarzenegger's workouts became more intense, his parents became concerned that he was overexerting himself. In his autobiography, he recollects "my father was baffled by my eagerness." In particular, he notes a conversation between his parents when his father said, "I think we better go to the doctor with this one, he's sick in the head." Schwarzenegger explains that his family was "genuinely worried about me" because they "felt I wasn't normal." Admitting that they were right, he points out that his desire and drive to achieve bodybuilding fame were not normal but that they, nonetheless, propelled him to the success that he enjoys today (Schwarzenegger and Hall 1977: 19).

In 1965, Schwarzenegger enlisted in the Austrian Army and "continued his strenuous training regimen" (Anon. 2005). That same year, he won Mr. Europe Junior, his first bodybuilding competition (Schwarzenegger and Hall 1977: 37). Years later Schwarzenegger would admit that "a career in the Army was my last choice"; instead, he wanted to leave Austria and "get to America" (Schwarzenegger and Hall 1977: 33–4). Nevertheless, he admits that joining the army helped him on his way to bodybuilding success. "Many people regret having to serve in the Army," he writes, "But it was not a waste of time for me. When I came out I weighed 225 pounds. I'd gone from 200 to 225 pounds. Up to that time, this was the biggest change I'd ever made in a single year" (Schwarzenegger and Hall 1977: 39).

Continuing his hard work, in 1966 Schwarzenegger won the Mr. Europe title and began preparing for the Mr. Universe competition (Schwarzenegger and Hall 1977: 45–7 and 51). In 1967, Schwarzenegger reached his ultimate goal when he won the Mr. Universe title as the youngest champion in the history of the event; he was just nineteen years old. In his autobiography, Schwarzenegger recalled his feelings at hearing his name called as the victor and the appeal of fame that would drive him throughout his career: "I looked out at the audience. They were screaming, flashbulbs were going off, I was caught up in the strange, unreal splendor of it. I thought, This is what you have been training for, this moment" (Schwarzenegger and Hall 1977: 77–8).

Over the next decade, Schwarzenegger went on to win thirteen more professional bodybuilding titles and appeared in the documentary *Pumping Iron* (1977), directed by George Butler and Robert Fiore and based on the book of the same name. The film "follows world-class body-builders preparing for competition, depicts bodybuilding as an artistic endeavor, bringing audiences into the gym where 'sculpting' takes place and Schwarzenegger is the main figure" (Anon. 2005).

After leaving the army, Schwarzenegger worked at a health and bodybuilding club for some time, where he truly established his legacy in the bodybuilding community. He spent most of his time at the gym developing "many of the innovative training techniques that were to win him wide respect and emulation among bodybuilders." This included his trademark split-routine "in which the upper and lower parts of the body are trained in two separate sessions" (Anon. 1979).

In addition to his success and influence in the gym and

bodybuilding culture, Schwarzenegger was successful at many other endeavors as well. While training for competitions in California, he earned a bachelors degree in business administration. Schwarzenegger "used his initial popularity as a sportsman to start businesses including real estate, gyms, and diet products" (Anon. 2000). He also engaged in many different business initiatives including mail-order training courses in bodybuilding and physical fitness and food supplements and other products endorsements (Anon. 1979). His influence on the pop-culture aspect of fitness has increased the popularity of protein bars and GNC shops among amateur fitness enthusiasts of our day.

The next phase of Schwarzenegger's rising business career included film stardom, which he reached in the 1980s. At the dawn of his career, Schwarzenegger was most suited playing himself on the big screen (Anon. 2000). Like the book, the film *Pumping Iron* appealed to audiences and helped to introduce Schwarzenegger to the film business (Anon. 1979). The film itself would have been only moderately intriguing had it not been for the charismatic and Greek-god-like image of Schwarzenegger. His charm and humor was a great balance to his imposing physique, which served to humanize him. Capitalizing on his unbelievably muscular body, Schwarzenegger became a movie star after appearing in *Conan the Barbarian* (1982) and in his most recognizable role as the murderous cyborg in the *Terminator* (1984).

Later in his career, Schwarzenegger's notoriety in physical fitness earned him political success as well. In 1990, he was named by George H.W. Bush to chair the President's Council on Physical Fitness and Sports. Schwarzenegger traveled throughout the U.S.A., in an effort to instill new values in America's youth. He has been quoted as saying that the lack of physical fitness among young people is "America's secret tragedy," and that schools and parents should take a greater initiative in getting children to exercise regularly (Anon. 2005).

Recently, Schwarzenegger took his life and career to yet another level, after being elected Governor of the State of California in a historic recall election. He has used his position of power as a bodybuilder, businessman, actor, and politician to launch numerous health initiatives and programs in this new position. As Governor, he partnered with the California Endowment, a foundation that seeks to increase healthy choices at the community level, to launch the Get Healthy California: Governors Summit on Health, Nutrition, and Obesity. This meeting brought together business leaders, educators, public-health experts, and government officials to work toward essential reforms for combatting obesity in the state (Belshe 2006).

Throughout his entire life, Schwarzenegger has used his powerful influence to promote physical fitness and health. He has coauthored many books on bodybuilding, fitness, and health, even writing on more specialized topics like children's fitness and women's body-shaping. Schwarzenegger appears to be the ideal example of modern-day masculinity. Through his incredibly muscular physique, he not only gained fame, fortune, and power in the bodybuilding world but in many other areas of life as well. However, there are a number of critics, Klein included, who do not believe that "stacking" will bring ALL men success. Rather than trust that all bodybuilders will be as successful in all their endeavors as Schwarzenegger, Klein argues that society would likely be better to "recognize those hypercompetitive, mondo-macho, self-centered tendencies that often inform our masculinity, recognize them for their imprisoning properties," that is their push for conformity to restrictive notions of masculinity, and "recast them or reject them" (Klein 1993: 8). With such an overemphasis on exercising for success and dominance, many men, unlike Schwarzenegger, lose sight of proper reasons for exercise, such as increased strength and health. As a result, unfortunately more and more men, particularly bodybuilders, are turning to unhealthy methods, such as injecting themselves with steroids, to achieve bigger bodies that they believe will bring them success. Hopefully, a time will come when masculinity through exercise is again associated primarily with health, rather than success, so that such unhealthy practices to gain body mass at any cost cease, and exercise is again used to improve well-being.

SLG/CAROLINE A. BUGG

*See also* Atlas; Hormones Used in Dieting; Men; Trall

## References and Further Reading

Anon. (1979) "Schwarzenegger, Arnold," *Current Biography Yearbook*, H.W. Wilson Company. Available online at <http:// vnweb.hwwilsonweb.com.proxy.library.emory.edu// hww/shared/shared_mainjhtml?_requestid=11526> (accessed June 25, 2007).

Anon. (2000) "Schwarzenegger, Arnold," in Tom Pendergast and Sara Pendergast (eds), *St. James Encyclopedia of Popular Culture*, five vols, Detroit, Mich.: St. James Press.

Anon. (2005) "Schwarzenegger, Arnold," *Authors and Artists for Young Adults*, Vol. LIX, Detroit, Mich.: Thompson Gale.

Belshe, Kim (2006) "Health. Office of the Governor: State of California." Available online at <http://www.gov.ca.gov/index.php?/blog/issue/blog-a-year-after-the-obesity-summit/health> (accessed February 3, 2007).

Klein, Alan M. (1993) *Little Big Men: Bodybuilding Subculture and Gender Construction*, Albany, NY: State University of New York Press.

Schwarzenegger, Arnold and Hall, Douglas Kent (1977) *Arnold: The Education of a Bodybuilder*, New York: Fireside, Simon & Schuster.

# Self-Help

In the West, we have long been concerned with how as individuals we can properly manage our lives and bodies. This concern, some argue, has developed since the Enlightenment into a "makeover culture," that is, a culture obsessed with transforming the self through managing the body. The makeover culture, like much in the modern world, emphasizes the importance of aesthetics and promises people with eating and weight problems that they can become more successful and happy if they just have the right tools and the right attitudes.

Today, our diverse tools for self-transformation include plastic surgery, designer diet drugs, and high-powered life coaches. Self-help often implies the intervention by others, whether physicians, psychologists, lifestyle coaches, or the authors of self-help guides. Such self-help books and programs remain a mainstay in the self-improvement industry. While many researchers express skepticism about the efficacy of self-help treatments for obesity and eating disorders, others argue that they provide important tools to help people transform their bodies and their lives. Despite uncertainty about the efficacy of self-help treatments for weight and eating disorders, people continue to buy diet-advice books and join for-profit and non-profit guided programs, spurred on by the promise of total self-transformation.

Popular culture has always been a powerful tool for transmitting narratives about how to act (or not to act) in order to be successful in society, and our contemporary self-help literature is a modern descendant of older didactic traditions in print and oral culture (Dolby 2005: 26–7). The central idea of self-help culture, that it is pos-sible to manage one's life through reflection, discipline, and routine is not new either. Judeo-Christian anxieties about bodily disorder extend back to Paul, and his Corinthian epistles are some of the earliest advice literature, explaining how to combat physical temptations to achieve spiritual salvation. Paul, of course, was not interested in the "seven habits of highly effective people" or in losing weight. He was, however, determined that the Corinthians would "glorify God" in the body as well as in the spirit (1 Cor. 6:19–20).

A concern with spiritual development and collectivity were understood as integral to self-help until the late twentieth century. Self-help interventions were generally "cooperative efforts for mutually improved conditions on the part of a community of peers," and much of the early work was done by religious groups (McGee 2005: 18). Grassroots efforts and community improvement typified the self-help model prior to the 1970s, and mutual aid is still an important part of self-help groups (Katz 1981: 135–6). However, in the past thirty years, self-help has come to be associated primarily with individual efforts at self-improvement. Books give advice on how to win friends and influence people, how to get noticed at work, and how to improve our appearances all in an effort to get ahead.

This increasingly competitive culture is fueling a growing self-help industry based on the myth that success and happiness can be achieved through proper life management, and consumers, it appears, are buying in with big dollars. In 2005, one historian reported that "the self-improvement industry, inclusive of books, seminars, audio and video products, and personal coaching, is said to constitute a $2.48 billion-a-year industry" (McGee 2005: 11). A large portion of these profits, no doubt, are from diet and weight-loss books. A 2005 study of commercial weight-loss programs, in particular, reported that "Each year, millions of Americans participate in commercial and self-help weight loss programs" (Tsai et al. 2005: 171).

Because of the proliferation and popularity of self-help weight-loss methods, research on the uses and effectiveness of self-help for weight and eating problems has been increasing since the late 1970s (Katz 1981; Hartley 1994). Many of these studies distinguish between "pure" and "guided" self-help interventions. Pure self-help programs use books that include all of the instructions for completing the program and are undertaken by individuals without therapeutic assistance. Buying a weight-loss manual or other book, reading it, and attempting to follow that program at home alone is pure self-help. Guided self-help, on the other hand, is carried out in contact with a therapist or other "expert." Guided programs may also use manuals, but they supplement individual work with one-on-one counseling and, in the case of self-help groups, group leaders, and peer support (Perkins et al. 2006: 4).

Pure self-help materials are probably the most familiar and accessible. Consumers who want to help themselves recover from weight or eating problems have access to literally hundreds of books on dieting, weight loss, and eating disorders (Santrock et al. 1994: 195–201). Many self-help authors derive their authority as experts from their experiences with food and dieting, and they seek to establish a connection with the reader, who they assume has a similar problem with food. In their books, they combine spiritual and secular traditions of body management and promise to provide the overweight individual with all of the tools he or she needs to transform their lives and bodies. These self-help books (or manuals) range from medical and scientific-based resources to confessional and personal narratives and, as such, vary widely in their content and suggestions for treatment.

Like many diet gurus of the past two centuries, the authors of contemporary self-help diet books frequently use their own experiences with weight loss as a platform for selling their program. For example, Susan Powter, whose confessional diet book *Stop the Insanity!* and concomitant television infomercial were widely popular in the 1990s, explained in an interview, "I'm not a nutri-

tionist, I'm not a doctor, I'm not a dietician. I'm a housewife that figured it out" (Fraser 1997: 75). Powter makes clear that her only expertise comes from her own experiences of being fat and losing weight. She uses her own experiences to speak from a place of aggressive authority (Powter is known for yelling at her audience) and motivate people to lose weight the way that she did. Similarly, Richard Simmons has marketed his brand of diet and exercise based largely on his personal experiences with weight and the connection that he feels that shared experience creates between him and his customers (Fraser 1997: 70–1).

Self-help diet books like those by Powter and Simmons almost invariably contrast the disorderly, overweight person (before) with the successful and happy person (after) who has gained self-control by learning to "flip the switch" or "stop the insanity." Jim Karas, for example, speaks to his imagined readers about their dieting history, which he suggests has been a disordered mess of yo-yo diets and disappointments. About their body image and motivation to lose weight, he assumes, "Right now, you are probably comfortable *not* believing in your ability to flip [successfully complete the program]. You are, however, unhappy with your weight." He immediately follows his comment about body image with, "Holding this book in your hands indicates that you have a desire to change" (Karas 2002: 10). Buying Karas's book, it seems, it the first step in real and lasting weight loss, and he assures his readers that following the written exercises and visualization techniques in his book will "pave the way to successful weight loss" and, it is implied, a more successful life overall (Karas 2002: 3–4).

Like many self-help diet books, Karas also uses metaphors of healing and nourishing to talk about overcoming eating and weight disorders. He advocates starting at "*your* beginning; that is, your childhood" in order to understand how one's individual weight and eating problems developed (Karas 2002: 13). Karas's method is fairly typical of self-help diet books, most likely because overeating and obesity are often attributed to untreated emotional pain in popular culture. The literature on emotional overeating includes books like *Feeding the Hungry Heart* (Roth 1982), *When Food is Love* (Roth 1992), *Healing the Hungry Self* (Price 1996), and *Conquering Compulsive Eating* (Katz 1986), which posit the neglected internal self as the root cause of overweight and eating disorders.

Much of this literature views overeating as an addictive

behavior because, as Geneen Roth explain, "compulsions, though they manifest themselves differently according to personality, spring from a common source: the hunger of the heart—attempting to satisfy, express, and, at the same time, numb itself" (1982: 5). The compulsion to overeat, according to this model, results from feelings that are "too painful to bear, so, as a way of coping with the discomfort, you resort to binging or grazing on food or starving yourself" (Price 1996: 116). Repressed emotions cause anxiety and discomfort, which the compulsive person assuages by eating. In order to treat the physical weight problem, these self-help authors believe that the dieter must heal emotional and spiritual pain first.

This philosophy of healing emotional pain in order to lose weight also appears in explicitly religious self-help literature. For example, the *Weigh to Go: Self-Help Weight Loss Manual*, which rightly disclaims in its prefatory pages that it is not "an exhaustive treatise" on the subject of weight loss, quotes Corinthians 1 and 2 and provides spiritual advice about how to lose weight. Overeating, according to the authors, is attributable to "shame issues," which will be healed by God "as you begin to deepen your spiritual life and grow in this area" (McLain et al. 1998: 65). In this view, overeating is a temptation, which may be overcome by turning to God. Following a "one day at a time" program, the overeater should pray to God for self-control because "nothing helps like prayer" (McLain et al. 1998: 37). With faith, the overeater finds the strength to take control of the disorderly behavior and reform his or her life. The best way to lose weight, according to these authors is, "surrendering your care to God first, and then to a physician with experience in weight loss" (McLain et al. 1998: 32–3).

Despite their rhetorical differences, these and other self-help books promise to give readers all of the tools that they need to understand, control, and transform their thoughts and behavior. However, it is difficult to measure the real success of self-help diet books. Despite high sales, there have not been many studies undertaken to measure the effectiveness of individual programs. The research that has been done comparing "pure" self-help efforts with structured weight loss programs suggests that dieters who go it alone in their self-help are less likely to lose weight than those who participate in a program like Weight Watchers or the Trevose Behavior Modification Program (Hellmich 2003: 80d; Heshka et al. 2003: 1793; Heshka, et al. 2000: 285; Latner et al. 2002). The

regular structure and personal contact provided by structured programs, which frequently include group meetings, has been cited as one factor in the greater success that group dieters have at losing weight.

Like self-help literature, most for-profit weight-loss groups are nonmedical, meaning that they are not carried out under the supervision of a physician (Tsai et al. 2005: 173). Unlike diet books, however, group programs use guided self-help methods in which dieters receive one-on-one help from group leaders or nutrition counselors. Jenny Craig and LA Weight Loss, for example, use instructional materials and individual meetings with dietary counselors to help clients lose weight. Weight Watchers also combines pure and guided self-help techniques, providing programs for members to follow on their own at home as well as weekly group meetings (Tsai et al. 2005: 173–4; Womble and Wadden 2002: 547–8). Group leaders and counselors in these programs have varying levels of expertise and education; some are professionally trained in nutrition or kinesiology, but most have little if any training outside of the company that they work for (Fraser 1997: 146–7). At Weight Watchers, for example, the authority and expertise of many group leaders is based, as with diet gurus, on their own experiences with weight loss.

The improved success of dieters in these programs may not, however, rest on the authority (or lack thereof) of the group leader. Research shows that simply being a member of a peer group provides support and motivation that may not be as readily available for the individual dieter. Early research into self-help weight-loss groups indicated, for example, that "identification with a group of peers contributes to the effectiveness of the group" (Bumbalo and Young 1973: 1590). In this view, groups allow people to exchange stories about their struggles and triumphs, which help them to learn from one another how to manage their compulsions. The presence of others who share similar compulsions to overeat, it seems, allows people with eating and weight problems to more objectively understand and control thought and behaviors.

In addition, the ritual weighing-in at groups like Weight Watchers and Taking Off Pounds Sensibly (TOPS) allows members to publicly measure their progress and receive praise and encouragement (Bumbalo and Young 1973: 1590; Stinson 2001: 145–6). The support and accountability provided by the group, researchers argue, may provide increased motivation for dieters to stick to their program each week. The ritual power of the weigh-in is, however, also based on competition and fear of being shamed in front of the group. For example, TOPS, a nonprofit weight-loss support group that was popular in the 1970s, was organized around the premise that "women needed to keep an eye on each other" in order to lose weight. At TOPS weigh-ins, "Good Losers" were cheered, and the "Turtles" (slow losers) and "Pigs" (gainers) were derided. At the end of the weigh-in, members who lost the most weight pinned cardboard pigs on the people who gained weight while the rest of the group booed or cheered (Fraser 1997: 150; Latner 2001: 91–2). This ritual of praise and punishment was designed to deter "bad" dietary behaviors and keep members "honest."

Honesty and progress coupled with spiritual rhetoric and healing exercises are also important in Overeaters Anonymous (OA), perhaps the most well-known self-help group for overweight people. OA is a nonprofit twelve-step program that differs considerably from both Weight Watchers and TOPS in its emphasis on spiritual and emotional "recovery." In its online promotional material, OA deliberately sets it apart from other weight-loss support groups, claiming that "Unlike other organizations, OA is not just about weight loss, obesity or diets; it addresses physical, emotional and spiritual well-being" (Anon. 2006). Like print-based self-help, OA sees overeating as an addictive behavior and focuses on healing the emotional and spiritual problems that underlie the compulsion to overeat. In order to work on these problems individually, members read instructional and inspirational materials at home. However, "food addicts" also work with a sponsor, who provides guided self-help, and attend regular group meetings where they support one another to achieve their goal of abstinence from overeating (Wasson and Jackson 2004: 340).

While OA claims that it is not a religious group because it does not adhere to any specific doctrine, it is highly spiritual and faith is a cornerstone of the program. OA literature, like that of Alcoholics Anonymous and other twelve-step groups, assumes that the reader will believe in the existence of a "higher power," who will take on their suffering and heal them (Weiner 1998: 165–6). The first three steps of the program require that food addicts:

1. admit that they are powerless over food and their lives have become unmanageable;
2. believe that a Power greater than ourselves could restore us to sanity;

3. make a decision to turn their will and their lives over to the care of God *as they understand Him.*

While the compulsory spirituality of OA may turn off some potential members, others see spirituality as central to their success in the program. Participants in a 2004 study of OA and recovering bulimics overwhelmingly cited this spirituality as a key element in their ability to overcome the disorder. Another important element cited in aiding recovery was the food plan (Wasson and Jackson 2004: 352), which is developed individually through guided interactions with sponsors. Weight loss may result from using this twelve-step program; however, spiritual healing and "surrender" are the foremost goals of OA (Anon. 1981: 563; Wasson and Jackson 2004). When a person's internal pain is healed, it is assumed that they will stop overeating, and their weight will no longer be an issue. This assumption may be idealistic, but the few studies which have been done of OA suggest that twelve-step support groups may be useful in supplementing more traditional treatments for obesity.

Self-help ideologies are deeply rooted in Western culture and history, and, while much has changed since the time of Paul, self-improvement messages continue to emphasize discipline and bodily management. Today, a person may choose "pure" self-help by following a diet book, opt for a structured program with guided self-help, or join a support group like Overeaters Anonymous. While reviewers of self-help diet materials argue that "evidence to support the use of the major commercial and self-help weight loss programs is suboptimal" (Tsai and Wadden 2005: 56; Wilson 2005; Womble and Wadden 2002), there is other evidence supporting the efficacy of self-help treatments for eating and weight disorders. In particular, several studies of the role of self-help and guided self-help in treating bulimia nervosa have indicated that both support groups and self-help manuals may aid patients in managing their binging and purging behaviors (Carter et al. 2003; Ghaderi 2006; Pritchard et al. 2004). If this preliminary research is any indication, self-help interventions may provide at least a partial solution to the eating and weight problems that plague consumer culture.

SLG/C. Melissa Anderson

*See also* Banting; Binge-eating; Brillat-Savarin; Christianity; Nidetch; Peters; Psychotherapy and Weight Change; Religion and Dieting

## References and Further Reading

Anon. (1981) "Overeaters Anonymous as Self-Help," *The American Journal of Nursing* 81 (3): 560–3.

Anon. (2006) "The Twelve Steps of Overeaters Anonymous," Overeaters Anonymous, available online at <http://www.oa.org/twelve_steps.html> (accessed January 2, 2007).

Bumbalo, Judith A. and Young, Dolores E. (1973) "The Self-Help Phenomenon," *The American Journal of Nursing* 73 (9): 1588–91.

Carter, J.C., Olmsted, M.P., Kaplan, A.S., McCabe, R.E., Mills, J.S. and Aimé, A. (2003) "Self-Help for Bulimia Nervosa: A Randomized Controlled Trial," *American Journal of Psychiatry* 160 (5): 973–8.

Dolby, Sandra K. (2005) *Self-Help Books: Why Americans Keep Reading Them*, Urbana, Ill.: University of Illinois Press.

Fraser, Laura (1997) *Losing It: America's Obsession with Weight and the Industry That Feeds It*, New York: Dutton.

Ghaderi, Ata (2006) "Attrition and Outcome in Self-Help Treatment for Bulimia Nervosa and Binge Eating Disorder: A Constructive Replication," *Eating Behaviors* 7 (4): 300–8.

Gilman, Sander L. (1999) *Making the Body Beautiful: A Cultural History of Aesthetic Surgery*, Princeton, NJ: Princeton University Press.

Hartley, Pat (1994) "Research: Can Self-Help Groups Make Meaningful Contribution?" *European Eating Disorders Review* 2 (2): 1–5.

Hellmich, Nanci (2003) "Weight Watchers Beats Self-Help Diets," *U.S.A. Today*, April 9: 80d.

Heshka, Stanley, Anderson, James W., Atkinson, Richard L., Greenway, Frank L., Hill, James O., Phinney, Stephen D., Kolotkin, Ronette L., Miller-Kovach, Karen and Pi-Sunyer, F. Xavier. (2000) "Self-Help Weight Loss Versus a Structured Commercial Program After 26 Weeks: A Randomized Controlled Study," *American Journal of Medicine* 109 (4): 282–7.

—— (2003) "Weight Loss with Self-Help Compared with a Structured Commercial Program," *Journal of the American Medical Association* 289 (14): 1792–8.

Karas, Jim (2002) *Flip the Switch: Discover the Weight-Loss Solution and the Secret to Getting Started*, New York: Harmony Books.

Katz, Alfred A. (1981) "Self-Help and Mutual Aid: An Emerging Social Movement?" *Annual Review of Sociology* 7: 129–55.

Katz, Alice (1986) *Conquering Compulsive Eating: A Complete Self-Help Guide*, Vancouver: International Self-Counsel Press.

Latner, J.D. (2001) "Self-Help in the Long-Term Treatment of Obesity," *Obesity Reviews* 2 (2): 87–97.

Latner, J.D., Wilson, G.T., Stunkard, A.J. and Jackson, M.L. (2002) "Self-Help and Long-Term Behavioral Therapy for Obesity," *Behaviour Research and Therapy* 40 (7): 805–12.

McGee, Micki (2005) *Self-Help, Inc.: Makeover Culture in American Life*, New York: Oxford University Press.

McLain, Judi G., McLain, Patrick G. and Andreacchio, Russell W. (1998) *Weigh to Go: Self-Help Weight Loss Manual*, Puckett, Miss.: Aweigh Publishing Company.

Perkins, S.J., Murphy, R., Schmidt, U. and Williams, C. (2006) "Self-Help and Guided Self-Help for Eating Disorders," *The Cochrane Database of Systematic Reviews* 3 (4): 1–67.

Price, Dierdra (1996) *Healing the Hungry Self: The Diet-Free Solution to Lifelong Weight Loss*, New York: Plume.

Pritchard, Briony J., Bergin, Jacqueline L., and Wade, Tracey D. (2004) "A Case Series Evaluation of Guided Self-Help for Bulimia Nervosa Using a Cognitive Manual," *International Journal of Eating Disorders* 36 (2): 144–56.

Roth, Geneen (1982) *Feeding the Hungry Heart: The Experience of Compulsive Eating*, New York: Signet Books.

—— (1992) *When Food Is Love: Exploring the Relationship Between Eating and Intimacy*, New York: Plume.

Santrock, John W., Minnett, Ann M., and Campbell, Barbara D. (1994) *The Authoritative Guide to Self-Help Books*, New York: The Guilford Press.

Stinson, Kandi (2001) *Women and Dieting Culture: Inside a Commercial Weight Loss Group*, New Brunswick, NJ: Rutgers University Press.

Tsai, A.G. and Wadden, T.A. (2005) "Systematic Review: An Evaluation of Major Commercial Weight Loss Programs in the United States," *Annals of Internal Medicine* 142 (1): 56–66.

Tsai, Adam Gilden, Wadden, T.A., Womble, L.G. and

Byrne, K.J. (2005) "Commercial and Self-Help Programs for Weight Control," *Pediatric Clinics of North America* 28 (1): 171–92.

Wasson, Diane H. and Jackson, Mary (2004) "An Analysis of the Role of Overeaters Anonymous in Women's Recovery from Bulimia Nervosa," *Eating Disorders* 12 (4): 337–56.

Weiner, Sydell (1998) "The Addiction of Overeating: Self-Help Groups As Treatment Models," *Journal of Clinical Psychology* 54 (2): 163–7.

Wilson, Stephen A. (2005) "Review: Little Evidence Supports the Efficacy of Major Commercial and Organized Self-Help Weight Loss Programs," *ACP Journal Club* 143 (1): 36–7.

Womble, Leslie G. and Wadden, Thomas A. (2002) "Commercial and Self-Help Weight Loss Programs," in Christopher G. Fairburn and Kelly D. Brownell (eds), *Eating Disorders and Obesity: A Comprehensive Handbook*, 2nd edn, New York: Guilford Press, pp. 546–50.

# Sex

Sex and dieting are linked everywhere. Our increasingly transnational contemporary popular culture is saturated with sexualized images of ever-thinner folks. Advertisements for everything from perfume to cars rely on sexualized images of the female body which are very much a product of (and themselves publicity for) a culture obsessed with dieting and slimness. That sexiness, more than health, strength, or long life, is the promise of the dieting industry. This is classically true for women and increasingly the case for men. So the logic of dieting culture says that weight loss makes women (and men) more appealing to "the opposite sex." Dieting on the whole holds out the promise of more sex, sex appeal, or sex with "sexy" partners, but there is also a market for diets that promise *better* sex.

Some diets are designed to improve a dieter's sex life, not through weight loss, but rather by making sex more enjoyable. These include foods thought to have either desire or performance-enhancing properties, are often faddish, and frequently turn up in articles and editorials in the weeks before Valentine's Day. Lynn Fisher's *The Better Sex Diet*, for example, suggests a diet high in soy to keep the vagina well lubricated and ginger and chili peppers for good circulation. Eating more fruits, vegetables, whole grains, and nuts is recommended along with classic aphrodisiacs such as oysters and chocolate. Oysters are high in zinc, which aids in testosterone production, and chocolate contains a chemical compound that releases dopamine (the chemical released in the brain during an orgasm). Eating these foods, it is suggested, will increase sexual desire and pleasure.

SLG/ANGELA WILLEY

*See also* Advertising; Celebrities; Globalization; Media

## References and Further Reading
Fisher, Lynn (1999) *The Better Sex Diet*, New York: St. Martin's.

Kamhi, Ellen (2004) *The Natural Guide to Great Sex: Improve Your Love Life with Nature's Alternatives to HRT and Viagra*, Alresford: Godsfield Press.

# Sexual Orientation

Body image and dieting patterns differ both interculturally as well as intraculturally. Subcultures built around sexual orientation and/or sexual practices possess varying corporeal aesthetics. The gay and lesbian community in the industrialized West, for example, is a multilayered subculture that has developed a specific set of body ideals and a definitive politics of consumption, of which dieting forms a part. Nancy Barron, lesbian founder of Ample Opportunity (AO), a size-positive organization, asks "Are lesbians more size acceptant?" (Atkins 1998: 10). The answer to this question appears to be yes. Bisexual freelance writer Greta Christian is convinced that "dykes are far more tolerant and appreciative of other women's bodies than straight men are" (Atkins 1998: 76). Whatever one's opinions, the embrace of sexual marginality has also meant to some extent an embrace of other kinds of marginality, such as having an "overweight" body.

Studies conducted to measure the relationship between sexual orientation and body expectations are slightly less conclusive, however. Christine A. Smith and Shannon Stillman of the University of Minnesota conducted a study of personal advertisements in alternative newspapers and the Internet to gauge how the level of emphasis the ads placed on physical attributes differed based on the sexual orientation of the women placing the ads. Out of the ads analyzed, 357 had been placed by lesbians, 135 by bisexual women, and 334 by heterosexual women. The study concluded that while bisexual women required the most physical descriptors, lesbians required the least, revealing the role that community and culture can play in determining beauty and desirability (Smith and Stillman 2002: 337–42). However, another research article published in 1996 stated that lesbians had similar concerns as straight women when it came to questions of appearance, weight, and dieting (Heffernan 1996: 127–38).

A comparative study of forty-one gay and forty-seven straight men conducted in Britain in 1998 disclosed that young gay men were more prone to body dissatisfaction and eating disordered behavior. The authors of the study found that "gay participants revealed strong correlations between levels of eating disturbance, self-esteem, and body dissatisfaction whilst these relationships did not achieve significance for heterosexuals" (Williamson and Hartley 1998: 160–70). Instead of viewing dieting as a neutral practice that occurs within sexual and gender-subversive subcultures, Cressida Heyes argues that anyone who engages in dieting, straight or gay, trans or non-trans, is attempting to alter their body to fit heteronormative specifications of gender. Dieting, to her, is assimilable to queer culture because it is about configuring and changing identity (Heyes 2007).

SLG/SHRUTHI VISSA

*See also* Anorexia; Fat-Positive; Men

## References and Further Reading

Atkins, Dawn (ed.) (1998) *Looking Queer: Body Image and Identity in Lesbian, Gay, Bisexual and Transgender Communities*, New York: Harrington Park Press.

Heffernan, K. (1996) "Eating Disorders and Weight Concern Among Lesbians," *International Journal of Eating Disorders* 19 (2): 127–38.

Heyes, Cressida J. (2007) *Self Transformations: Foucault, Ethics, and Normalized Bodies*, New York: Oxford University Press.

Smith, Christine A. and Stillman, Shannon (2002) "What Do Women Want? the Effects of Gender and Sexual Orientation on the Desirability of Physical Attributes in the Personal Ads of Women," *Sex Roles* 46 (9–10): 337–42.

Williamson, Iain and Hartley, Pat (1998) "British Research into the Increased Vulnerability of Young Gay Men to Eating Disturbance and Body Dissatisfaction," *European Eating Disorders Review* 6 (3): 160–70.

# Sigler, Jamie Lynn (1981–)

## American actress

Sigler is known for playing Meado, mobster Tony Soprano's daughter on the HBO show *The Sopranos*, is one of a few actresses who has publicly recounted her personal battle with anorexia. Sigler's illness started during the filming of the first season of the show and almost cost her the role. The show's producers voiced concern about Sigler's condition, letting her know that if she did not recover, her role would be terminated. Sigler got help and, through hard work, changed her life and recovered from her condition. In an interview on *The Oprah Winfrey Show*, Sigler stated,

> I fell into the trap of looking in magazines and seeing . . . how someone's make-up is done, or hair, or how they're dressed, and say "oh! I want to look that way" . . . I don't think that girls really have to worry so much about how they look, and trying to look like other people. Be yourself, and that will make you more beautiful than anything.
>
> (Sigler 2006)

Sigler has used her fame to educate millions of teenage girls who suffer from similar disorders. At age twenty, she wrote a memoir of her life, *Wise Girl: What I've Learned About Life, Love, and Loss* (2002), which included an in-depth revelation of her battle and recovery from anorexia. Currently, Sigler is a spokesperson for National Eating Disorders Association.

SLG/Laura Goldstein

*See also* Anorexia

### References and Further Reading
Sigler, Jamie-Lynn (2006) "Learning to Love Yourself," *The Oprah Winfrey Show*, available online at <http://www.oprah.com/rys/journeys/rys_journeys_20010105.jhtml> (accessed June 24, 2007).
Sigler, Jamie-Lynn and Berk, Sheryl (2002) *Wise Girl: What I've Learned About Life, Love and Loss*, New York: Pocket Books.

# Simmons, Richard (1948–)

## Self-proclaimed fitness expert and central fitness icon of the 1980s

Simmons, himself, was once obese, but after losing weight, he became a "motivator" and revolutionized the modern fitness movement to include those not already in shape. In 1974, he opened one of the first aerobic studios in the country called Slimmons in Beverly Hills. According to his own website, he consulted with doctors and nutritionists in order to ensure that the weight-loss program he created was safe for all potential clients (people of various ages, weights, and physical health). In addition to his studio, Simmons produced numerous weight-loss videos, in which he displays his notorious enthusiasm about losing weight and exercising. Following the success of these videos, Simmons had his own Emmy Award-winning talk show, which was nationally syndicated between 1980 and 1984. Additionally, Simmons has written books and has even created his own meal plan program (which includes food) to help people shed pounds. He is known for preaching in his classes and videos that people must "love themselves" before they can find themselves worthy of being healthy and losing weight.

SLG/Jessica Elyse Rissman

**References and Further Reading**
Anon. "A Biography of Richard Simmons,"
Richardsimmons.com, available online at <http://
www.richardsimmons.com/bio.php> (accessed March
3, 2007).

Carney, Kat (2003) "Simmons still 'Sweatin' to the
Oldies'," *CNN Headline News*, January 3, available
online at <http://edition.cnn.com/2002/HEALTH/
diet.fitness/10/10/hln.bio.richard.simmons> (accessed
March 3, 2007).

# Sinclair, Upton (1878–1968)

## American social reformist and author

Sinclair had been living on fried foods and sweets when he was afflicted with indigestion and headaches. These ailments tended to occur when he was focused on his writing and didn't spend much time exercising. He attempted such treatments as Horace Fletcher's diet and the diets practiced at John Harvey Kellogg's Battle Creek Sanitarium (including vegetarianism). After Sinclair met a woman who used fasting to cure her and her friends' various illnesses, he, too, began fasting and became a staunch supporter. He describes the benefits of such abstention from food in his book *The Fasting Cure* (1911), where he also repudiated the diet claims he made in his earlier co-authored book *Good Health and How We Won It* (1909). In *The Fasting Cure*, Sinclair rejects the classic American emphasis on rich and plentiful food like "fried chicken and rich gravies and pastries, fruit cake and candy and ice-cream," seeing it as socially unacceptable and as unhealthy.

Sinclair claimed that by the second day of his first fast, he no longer had headaches, by the third stopped feeling hungry and weak, and on the fifth began feeling mentally and physically strong again. He lost 14 pounds in the first four days and 2 pounds afterwards, believing this excess weight was "a sign of the extremely poor state of [his] tissues" (Sinclair 1911: 21). He broke his fast on the twelfth day with fruit juice and Bernarr Macfadden's milk diet. After the fast, he gained the desire for physical activity, which resulted in the development of a more athletic build. Feeling the need to "prove" that fasting really worked, Sinclair included before and after photographs of himself in *The Fasting Cure*, and the efficacy of his "diet" was, therefore, based on his personal experience.

Sinclair is also the author of *The Jungle* (1906), which exposed the unsanitary conditions of the meatpacking industry. His novel was influential in the establishment of the Pure Food and Drug Act, which later led to the creation of the United States Food and Drug Administration. Given the vivid and disturbing image of the slaughterhouse presented in his book, it is of little surprise that Sinclair espoused vegetarianism, as did thousands of other Americans who read him. Later in life, he switched to a diet of broiled meat and hot water.

Today, there are many diet books, which claim that fasting is the way to cleanse the body of impurities and simultaneously lose weight. Paul and Patricia Bragg claim in *The Miracle of Fasting* that fasting is a cleansing period to purge the body of the waste: "You know you are fasting to purify the body of the accumulated toxic poisons and waste" (Bragg and Bragg 1999: 51). They both believe about 75 percent of Americans are obese and these people will never know the "thrill of wellness" because fat is a psychological burden as well as a health risk and fasting is the key to improving health. Purifying the body of supposed "toxins" and reducing weight remains linked by most advocates of fasting, as if the body trapped by modernity in impurity cannot cleanse itself.

SLG/DOROTHY CHYUNG

*See also* Fletcher; Kellogg; Macfadden; Milk; Vegetarianism

**References and Further Reading**
Anon. "Sinclair, Upton: About the Famous Faster: Upton
Sinclair, History and Biography of the Author of the

Jungle," in David Wallechinsky and Irving Wallace (eds) *The People's Almanac*, available online at <http://www.trivia-library.com/b/famous-feasts-in-history-upton-sinclair.htm> (accessed March 3, 2007).

Arthur, Anthony (2006) *Radical Innocent: Upton Sinclair*, New York: Random House.

Bragg, Patricia C. and Bragg, Paul (1999) *The Miracle of Fasting: Proven Throughout History for Physical, Mental & Spiritual Rejuvenation*, Santa Barbara, Calif.: Health Science.

Gale, Robert L. (2000) "Sinclair, Upton," *American National Biography Online*, available online at <http://

/www.anb.org/articles/16/16–01510.html> (accessed February 27, 2006).

Harris, Leon A. (1975) *Upton Sinclair, American Rebel*, New York: Crowell.

Sinclair, Upton (1906) *The Jungle*, New York: Doubleday, Page and Co.

—— (1911) *The Fasting Cure*, New York and London: M. Kennerley.

Sinclair, Upton and Williams, Michael (1909) *Good Health and How We Won It*, New York: F.A. Stokes Company.

# Smoking

Both overeating and dieting have been framed in different moments and arguments as (at least potential) addictions. Beyond the metaphor of food/diet as a drug, cigarettes have historically played and continue to play a part in dieting culture. A number of both illicit and legal drugs—including speed, nicotine, opium, cocaine, caffeine, Ritalin, and MDMA ("Ecstasy") among others—are widely acknowledged to be used as appetite suppressants. Some findings suggest that, at least in the case of smoking, this effect is largely mythical and that smoking does not in fact affect food intake (Perkins 1992: 193–205; Zancy and de Witt 1992). Research indicates that there may, however, be physiological reasons for weight gain after quitting, though it is highly variable by age and socioeconomic status (Filozof et al. 1992).

Cigarettes are prominently linked in dieting practice and in the popular imagination to weight loss. Marketing of cigarettes to women beginning in the 1920s made the claim explicit and initiated an image of smoking as a smart and effective weight-loss strategy. American Tobacco advertisers Edward Bernays and George Washington Hill famously launched the slogan "Reach for a Lucky instead of a Sweet" in 1928. Other Lucky ads from the same era showed the face of a thin, young woman with the shadow of a larger face with double chins in the background. These images were accompanied by alarmist text, such as "THE MENACING SHADOW that threatens the modern figure!" and "WARN HER ere her bloom is past" (Segrave 2005).

Since then, Lucky Strikes, Capri, Misty, More, and Virginia Slims have all used similar campaigns that highlight the pro-metabolic effects of nicotine more or less overtly (Boyd et al. 1999–2000: 19–31).

Recent anti-smoking initiatives have had to contend with this association in a culture obsessed with slimness. Weight concerns have been cited in numerous studies as a factor (especially for younger women) in the decision to smoke and/or to continue smoking (Silberstein 2002; Strauss and Mir 2001: 1381–5; Tomeo et al. 1999: 918–24). Some say concern about weight gain is the number one factor in the decision not to quit (Filozof et al. 1992: 149–57). Another study found that among female smokers, dieters (smokers concerned with weight gain), had shorter periods of cessation of smoking and were less likely to finally quit (Jarry et al. 1998: 53–64). Interestingly, dieters were also more likely than non-dieters to gain weight upon quitting. Indeed, as one self-confessed sufferer from anorexia nervosa stated, she "learned 'diet tricks' from older dancers [when she was a teenager]. Coffee and cigarettes soon became my staple diet. . . . I was dieting like everyone else" (Rose 2002: 101).

Weight gain is addressed explicitly in antismoking research and advertising, which increasingly includes diet and exercise tips (like munch on carrot sticks when you have a craving) for avoiding the gain associated with quitting. While the Food and Drug Administration (FDA) cracked down on the marketing of "Trim Reducing-Aid

Cigarettes" (containing tartaric acid) as a treatment for overweight in 1959, the move away from explicit medicalization has clearly not quelled the powerful association of smoking and weight loss.

Yet there is an argument that the combination of smoking and overweight increases the risk for a wide range of diseases. While, in general, it is impossible to make an absolute correlation between weight and illness, it is clear that even individuals who have a lower weight and smoke are at greater risk for illness (Björntorp 2002: 377–81). As with other illnesses that reduce weight but increase mortality and morbidity, such as depression or alcoholism, smoking is a major co-factor in shortening the life span. Yet, even for smokers, the greater the weight, the higher the risk for fatal illnesses. A thin smoker will, at least statistically, outlive a fat smoker (Manson et al. 2002: 422–8).

SLG/ANGELA WILLEY

*See also* Anorexia; Binge-eating; Socioecomomic Status

## References and Further Reading

Björntorp, Per (2002) "Definition and Classification of Obesity," in Christopher G. Fairburn and Kelly D. Brownell (eds), *Eating Disorders and Obesity: A Comprehensive Handbook*, 2nd edn, New York: Guilford Press, pp. 377–81.

Boyd, C., Boyd, T., and Cash, J. (1999–2000) "Why Is Virginia Slim? Women and Cigarette Advertising," *International Quarterly of Community Health Education* 19: 19–31.

Brandt, Allan M. (2007) *The Cigarette Century: The Rise, Fall, and Deadly Persistence of the Product That Defined America*, New York: Basic Books.

Filozof, C., Fernández Pinilla, M.C., and Fernández-Cruz, A. (1992) "Smoking Cessation and Weight Gain," *Addictive Behaviors* 17 (2): 149–57.

Jarry, Josée L., Robert B. Coambs, Janet Polivy, and C. Peter Herman (1998) "Weight Gain After Smoking Cessation in Women: the Impact of Dieting Status," *International Journal of Eating Disorders* 24 (1): 53–64.

Manson, Joann E., Skerrett, Patrick J., and Willett, Walter C. (2002) "Epidemiology of Health Risks Associated with Obesity," in Christopher G. Fairburn and Kelly D. Brownell (eds), *Eating Disorders and Obesity: A Comprehensive Handbook*, 2nd edn, New York: Guilford Press, pp. 422–8.

Parker-Pope, T. (2001) *Cigarettes: Anatomy of an Industry from Seed to Smoke*, New York: New York Press.

Perkins, Kenneth (1992) "Effects of Tobacco Smoking on Caloric Intake," *British Journal of Addiction* 87 (2): 193–205.

"Rose," (2002) "Understanding the Whole Person: Rose's Story," in, Kathleen M. Berg, Dermot J. Hurley, James A. McSherry and Nancy E. Strange, eds. *Eating Disorders: A Patient Centered Approach*, Abingdon: Radcliffe Medical Press, pp. 99–115.

Segrave, K. (2005) *Women and Smoking in America, 1880–1950*, Jefferson, NC: McFarland and Company.

Silberstein, Nina (2002) "Girls Worried About Weight More Likely to Smoke," American Council on Science and Health, available online at <http://www.acsh.org/healthissues/newsID.376/healthissue_detail.asp> (accessed March 3, 2007).

Strauss, R.S. and Mir, H.M. (2001) "Smoking and Weight Loss Attempts in Overweight and Normal-Weight Adolescents," *International Journal of Obesity* 25 (9): 1381–5.

Tomeo, Catherine A., Field, Alison E., Berkey, Catherine S., Colditz, Graham A., and Frazier, A. Lindsay (1999) "Weight Concerns, Weight Control Behaviors, and Smoking Initiation," *Pediatrics* 104 (4 pt 1): 918–24.

Zancy, J.P. and Witt, H. de (1992) "The Effects of a Restricted Feeding Regimen on Cigarette Smoking in Humans," *Addictive Behaviors* 17 (2): 149–57.

# Socioeconomic Status

In 1964, Ronald Reagan said, "We were told 4 years ago that 17 million people went to bed hungry each night. Well, that was probably true. They were all on a diet" (Reagan 1964). Contemporary associations between socioeconomic status and diet/body size vary widely, most notably based on the level of development of the region. While the discourse surrounding the level of "development" of an area is fraught with allusions to a history of colonialism and cultural inequality, such a discussion is beyond the purposes of this text. In general, "developing countries," as opposed to "developed" ones, are not industrialized and have a small economy. In addition, measurements of poverty or low socioeconomic status vary from classification based on income, education, occupation, etc.

It has been found that in more developed countries, low socioeconomic status tends to be associated with obesity, while the upper classes are thinner. Socioeconomic status relates to both ethnicity, levels of education, as well as economic status. In developing countries, as opposed to developed ones, obesity is apparent in higher socioeconomic groups and correlated with declining need for physical activity (Hill, A. 2002: 67–71). However, this trend may only be applicable to women as opposed to men or children. Studies have shown that women of lower socioeconomic classes are six times more likely to be obese than women in higher income brackets (Sobal and Stunkard 1989: 260–75).

In developing countries, those living in true poverty tend to be thin. This is attributed to the inadequate food supplies in these countries that make the prevalence of obesity impossible among the poor. According to Robert Pool, "the explanation seems obvious: only the wealthy classes can reap the same 'benefits' that are ubiquitous in the Western world, such as plenty of tasty, high-fat food and little need to exert oneself physically" (2001: 173). This distinction between developed and developing countries is so unambiguous and universal that if a country's poor begins to shift from underweight to overweight, it indicates that a "nutrition transition" has occurred. At this point, food scarcity is not an issue and the amount of food consumed is more of a matter of free will, rather than circumstance. With the increasing availability of fat and the corresponding increase in fat consumption, this transition is occurring at lower levels of gross national product.

The association between upper-class status and thinness in developed countries has been explained in a number of ways. In the U.S.A., the link between low socioeconomic status and obesity has been attributed to the lack of fitness facilities in poorer areas and the increase of new technologies that yield low paying jobs requiring little physical exertion. Meanwhile, those in higher income brackets can afford the money for personal trainers and gym memberships, as well as the time to use such facilities. Research also attributes the poverty–obesity link to the affordability of unhealthy foods (Drewnowski and Specter 2004: 6–16). Because foods that are high in sugar and fat are less costly per calorie than fish, fruits, and vegetables, people with lower incomes have unhealthy diets and are more likely to become overweight. Discrimination against obese people may also contribute to the class differences; overweight women, in particular, experience greater job discrimination and are less upwardly mobile than their thin counterparts. A difference or increased emphasis in dogma regarding weight and dieting may also be the cause of class distinctions in body size. For those in upper classes, social pressure and the belief that hunger is a virtue and obesity a vice may contribute to a greater emphasis on achieving thinness (Campos 2004: 231; Pool 2001: 171–4).

Given the popular and statistical associations between socioeconomic status and obesity, one might assume that people strive for thinness in order to reflect a higher class standing. However, in the religious sphere, Father Divine of the Peace Mission Movement in the U.S.A. represented an embrace of corpulence as a victory over poverty, which arose from the poverty experienced during slavery. Divine used indulgent food consumption and elaborate banquets to unite his followers, preaching that spiritual improvement would be expressed in one's physical body that would also be free of death and disease. Meanwhile, people outside of this community viewed such obesity as a "sign of poor health, laziness, or (ironically, in this case) poverty" (Griffith 2004: 147–54). Contrary to his society's norms, Divine linked unrestrained eating and large body size to success. This belief may be more widely held in the developing countries where such a statistical association exists.

The strong link between obesity's consequences and low socioeconomic status has affected our "battle" against obesity. Based on the assertion that buying cheaper, unhealthy foods contributes to obesity, some advocate the creation of a "fat tax," which would make unhealthy food more expensive with the hope of compelling people to make healthier diet choices. In addition, the widely publicized cases of fat children being removed from their homes are more prevalent among those of lower socioeconomic status. The case of Anamarie Regino of Albuquerque, New Mexico, is one example where obesity is linked with relative poverty, as well as ethnicity. At a very young age (three years old), Regino grew unusually quickly to a large size (130 pounds and twice as tall as average). The state took her away from her parents and placed her in foster care, claiming that Regino's health was in grave danger, even though her parents had visited hospitals and doctors in search of a remedy for their daughter's weight. Healthcare experts had advised putting her on a diet that was essentially a third of the normal daily caloric intake for a three-year-old. Eventually, the parent's regained custody of Regino under the condition that she conform to a diet and exercise plan (Campos 2004: 99–106). The extreme measures taken with regards to children may be due to their vulnerability. In addition, many studies have suggested that one's socioeconomic status as a child influences adult obesity from "the early establishment of behavioural patterns, such as diet and exercise, or through metabolic changes associated with early deprivation" (Okasha et al. 2003: 509). However, the dearth of cases of anorexic or underweight children being removed from their parents underscores our aversion towards obesity and may also indicate a lack of willingness to question the parenting skills of the upper class.

Yet the link between poverty and obesity does *not* mean that low-income persons do not diet. According to a 1994–6 survey by the American Dietetic Association, of people whose household income was 30 percent below the poverty line, 15.2 percent were reportedly dieting. This is only slightly less than the 16.7 percent of dieters among people with larger household incomes (Paeratakul et al. 2002: 1248). This dieting behavior shows that a smaller body size is valued by all of society, regardless of socioeconomic status.

The existing link between socioeconomic status and body size is ultimately reflected in society's greater respect for the higher-income group's body type. The connection may be influenced by the people's surrounding conditions but is also reinforced by societal pressures.

Consequently, it appears that body size is now among "the most visible markers of social class," which, therefore, encourages dieting behavior (Campos 2004: 225).

SLG/DOROTHY CHYUNG

*See also* Anorexia; Developing World; Globalization

## References and Further Reading
Campos, Paul (2004) *The Obesity Myth: Why America's Obsession with Weight Is Hazardous to Your Health*, New York: Gotham.
Drewnowski, Adam and Popkin, Barry M. (1997) "The Nutrition Transition: New Trends in the Global Diet," *Nutrition Reviews* 55 (2): 31–43.
Drewnowski, Adam and Specter, S.E. (2004) "Poverty and Obesity: The Role of Energy Density and Energy Costs," *American Journal of Clinical Nutrition* 79 (1): 6–16.
Griffith, R. Marie (2004) *Born Again Bodies: Flesh and Spirit in American Christianity*, Los Angeles, Calif.: University of California Press.
Hill, Andrew J. (2002) "Prevalence and Demographics of Dieting," in Christopher G. Fairburn and Kelly D. Brownell (eds), *Eating Disorders and Obesity: A Comprehensive Handbook*, 2nd edn, New York: Guilford Press, pp. 80–3.
Hill, James O. (2002) "The Nature of the Regulation of Energy Balance," in Christopher G. Fairburn and Kelly D. Brownell (eds), *Eating Disorders and Obesity: A Comprehensive Handbook*, 2nd edn, New York: Guilford Press, pp. 67–71.
Okasha, M., McCarron, P., McEwen, J., Durnin, J., and Davey Smith, G. (2003) "Childhood Social Class and Adulthood Obesity: Findings from the Glasgow Alumni Cohort," *Journal of Epidemiological Community Health* 57 (7): 508–9.
Paeratakul, Sahasporn, York-Crowe, Emily E., Williamson, Donald A., Ryan, Donna H., and Bray, George A. (2002) "Americans on Diet: Results from the 1994–96 Continuing Survey of Food Intakes by Individuals," *Journal of the American Dietetic Association* 102 (9): 1247–51.
Pool, Robert (2001) *Fat: Fighting the Obesity Epidemic*, New York: Oxford University Press.
Reagan, Ronald (1964) "Address on behalf of Senator Barry Goldwater: Rendezvous with Destiny," *Ronald Reagan Presidential Foundation & Library*, available

online at <http://www.reaganfoundation.org/reagan/
speeches/rendezvous.asp> (accessed April 13, 2006).
Sobal, Jeffery and Stunkard, Albert J. (1989)

"Socioeconomic Status and Obesity: A Review of the
Literature," *Psychological Bulletin* 105 (2): 260–75.

# Southern Fat

## Ethnic Fat

There is more than a little empirical evidence that the American South beats all other areas of the country when it comes to weight. In August 2006, the Trust for America's Health found that 29.5 percent of Mississippi residents were obese and that nine of the ten states with the highest rates of obesity were in the "old" South. But even in this fattest part of the nation there are further qualifiers as to who is really fat. There seems to be a religious hierarchy of fat—and not only in the South. In a recent paper, Purdue medical sociologist Kenneth Ferraro looked at the corollary between belonging to a religious denomination and being obese. Baptists were the fattest of all, followed by other Protestant groups. The rule seems to be: The more fundamentalist you are, the fatter you will be. Roman Catholics and then Mormons, Seventh day Adventists (with their vegetarian diet) and other "non-traditionalist" Christian groups were at the middle of his scale, and Jews (and other non-Christians) were on the thin end of the spectrum. In Baptist churches, one out of four members of the congregation is obese, but only 1 percent of Temple-attending Jews are. Yet, relative to the Jews, Catholics too had a high rate of obesity, with about a 17 percent rate of congregant obesity. Ferraro stresses that while this is a national problem, the domination of Baptists points to this being in addition very much a southern problem too.

In 1998, Ferraro concluded an earlier article by observing that food and religion provide "a couple of the few pleasures accessible to populations which are economically and politically deprived" (Ferraro 1998: 224–44). By his work in 2006, it seems to be the "dietary patterns in the South," which, coupled with the explosion in Church membership, points to the ever-expanding waistline of the Southerner (Ferraro and Cline 2006).

Perhaps Marx was right—religion (and here we can add food) is the opiate of the people.

Evidently, when Jews are considered as a religious group, rather than as an ethnicity, they are thin. But this is where the analysis breaks down. For the Jews are simultaneously a religious and a self-described ethnicity (peoplehood), and the flaw of Ferraro's model is that his notion of religion, especially in the South, maps historically on to older models of ethnicity, which, in the world of the nineteenth and early twentieth century, were also models of race. One of the great historic "secrets" of the obese South is that the "black/white" dichotomy of race provided a means by which "black" races in Europe such as the Jews and the Irish were made white. For the KKK, the litmus test was and is religion as well as race; they knew on what side of the racial divide Jews and Catholics were to be found. Yet, in the nineteenth century, this distinction between religion and race was rarely made. Jews and Irish, like Blacks, were racially a different people from real "Americans." Their bodies as well as their beliefs betrayed them, no matter how "white" they looked. The late nineteenth-century fetish about light-skinned Blacks "passing" applied to them as well. The fictional literature on the topic from Mark Twain's *Pudd'nhead Wilson* (1894) to Edna Ferber's *Showboat* (1926) revealed this as a false difference, but one that was generally held. The body would eventually betray its "essence." And for the twentieth century, that body, at least in literature, comes to be obese.

The nostalgic world of the old South now reimagined in literature is the place we should look for these bodies that betray. No place better to begin than with the quintessential Southern novel, Margaret Mitchell's *Gone with the Wind* (1936). Mitchell, as James Cobb observes, was hardly a naïve writer evoking a lost antebellum tradition. She reflects constantly on the explosion of vanished ethnicity that made up the old, seemingly homogenous "white South," where no one, except in great irony, the slave, was fat. Indeed, Scarlett's nanny slave "Mammy" describes herself as "too old an' fat" (Mitchell 1999: 589), but Mitchell makes this quality her icon as "Scarlett longed for the fat old arms of Mammy" (Mitchell 1999: 144). The African-American woman, depicted as large and devoted to preparing food, comes to be a classic icon of early twentieth-century processed foods. "Aunt Jemima" reigns from 1905 to the post-World War II period on as a sign of a "maternal" and acceptable body, but only within the confines of racial difference (Manring 1998).

It is, indeed, the ethnic vigor of the "black" Irish Catholics revitalizing and rebuilding the effeminate South in *Gone with the Wind* that stands behind Scarlett's cry that she will never be hungry again, "if I have to steal or kill—as God is my witness, I'm never going to be hungry again" (Mitchell 1999: 421). Her father, Gerald O'Hara, had invigorated the world of the plantation with his rough Irish ways, following his too tall brothers to America having flaunted the English occupation of his homeland. Gerald O'Hara was a

small man, little more than five feet tall but so heavy of barrel and thick of neck: that his appearance when seated, led strangers to think him a larger man. His thickset torso was supported by short sturdy legs, always incased in the finest leather boots ... Most small people who take themselves seriously are a little ridiculous; but the bantam cock is respected in the barnyard, and so it was with Gerald. No one would ever have the temerity to think of Gerald O'Hara as a ridiculous little figure.

(Mitchell 1999: 32)

His formidable if short body and feisty spirit point to a man who had succeeded in overcoming hunger and oppression and would add this quality to the South. He was "fat" but in the most positive sense of nineteenth-century masculinity.

The historian W.J. Cash tells the story of his own great-grandfather in *The Mind of the South* (1941) as an exemplum of "ethnic vigor" and the creation of the "white" planter culture of the Carolinas. He is a "stout young Irishman" who comes with his bride to the Caroli-

nas and enters into trade in whiskey. He begins, almost as an afterthought, to plant cotton and brings the first cotton gin. His fortune and his status in the community grow. He builds a "big house," paints it white, buys slaves, enters the legislature, by which time he was "tall and well-made" (Cash 1991: 12–17). Thus the "ruling class in the great South" is revitalized on the frontier.

This is not the place to rehearse the general claims of how the Irish and the Jews become "white" in America or how contested that shift in racial identity is, especially in the South. Indeed, reading the *Charleston Mercury* (1856) reveals that there has been a reduction of emigration that eliminates the "Know Nothing" demand for limitations as "quite unnecessary [even] by the most bigoted hater of our Irish and German populations" (Anon. "Health for the People" 1856). After the Civil War, the Irish, at least, become white and stout. Both Mitchell and Cash use the Irish as their model, speaking about the body as an unstated place where identity is formed. Being "stout" is a mark of power; being fat is a disease. Men of power (like Gerald O'Hara) are never fat: "The Pope [Pius IX] is pretty tall and stout, without being obese" (*New-Orleans Commercial Bulletin*, June 8, 1868). But the diet culture was alive and well in the South before the age of Southern nostalgia.

In the antebellum and immediate post-war South, however, there was a great concern with obesity—if, at least initially, far from the U.S.A. As early as 1833, the *New-Orleans Commercial Bulletin* (September 14, 1883) recounts how the "omnibus drivers on the Edgeware Road" in London refuse to take passengers they judge to be too obese accompanied with catcalls and "great laughter." Obesity is a "British disease" which is not the "combined result of laziness and high living," but is "a constitutional disease" (*Georgia Weekly Telegraph*, April 8, 1879). This was very much in line with the views that American neurologist S. Weir Mitchell (1829–1914) expressed in 1877. He was startled by "those enormous occasional growths, which so amaze an American when first he sets foot in London" (Mitchell 1877: 15). But such views are not limited to England. Mordecai Noah (1785–1851), the first American-born Jew to achieve prominence as a writer, politician, and utopian advocate of creating a Jewish refuge ("Ararat") in New York State, is reported in the *South Carolina Temperance Advocate* (July 1, 1847) recounting his time as American Consul in Tunis where he saw local women struggling with their fat:

The more fatness, the greater beauty as a wife—and, therefore, tender mothers begin at an early age to fatten their daughters. They allow them very little exercise, compel them to eat very rich substances, little paste balls dipped in oil, and every kind of food calculated to produce obesity. The result is . . . a lady weighing some three hundred pounds.

Fat is exotic, yet there is also a theme in Southern responses to fat that echoes the growing understanding of obesity as a disease.

In 1856 (May 12), the *Charleston Mercury* advocated "health for the People," seeing a "deteriorating influences on national health." Childhood ill health haunts Charleston and the remedy is "calisthenic and gymnastic exercises," which assure the removal of "obesity, or an excess of fat." The dieting culture is alive and well in the South. The English layman William Banting's (1796–1878) low-carbohydrate diet, which was first introduced in London in 1864, had become the rage in the South "conferring the benefit of wholesome muscular development upon himself and others" (*Charleston Courier*, July 13, 1869). In Georgia, Banting's approach for "the treatment and cure of excessive fatness in the human race," "caused a decrease in weight from twenty-five to sixty pounds in the course of a few weeks" (*Georgia Weekly Telegraph*, July 26, 1870). But other remedies were quick on the market. Allan's Anti-Fat, "the only known remedy for obesity" was sold to men "whose several weights range from two hundred to three hundred pounds" (*Georgia Weekly Telegraph*, October 22, 1878). Obesity is an "abnormal condition" though "many people have erroneously considered it as an evidence of health, and any agent that reduces fat is there fore at once suspected of being injurious" (*Georgia Weekly Telegraph*, April 29, 1879). Being fat was dangerous. This notion vanishes in the 1930s and 1940s and is transformed into Gerald O'Hara's ethnic vigor.

If the notion of ethnic vigor and bodily form as a model for imaging a new Southern identity is linked to the Irish, who become "white," at least in part, by becoming Southerners, then the great mid-twentieth-century answer to *Gone with the Wind* is John Kennedy Toole's *A Confederacy of Dunces* (1980). Written during the beginnings of the civil-rights movement, it provided a parodic rethinking about "stout" men and ethnic identity. It was Walker Percy who truly discovered the novel after its author's suicide, who praised how Toole presents

New Orleans' "ethnic whites—and one black in whom Toole has achieved the near impossible, a superb comic character of immense wit and resourcefulness without the least trace of Rastus minstrelsy" (Toole 1980: viii). The ethnic whites in Toole's world are without a doubt trying to become "white," but they sink ever more in a world of fat. And the soft underbelly to Southern identity formation, how ethnics become authentic Southerners, is exposed by Toole through their bodies.

Toole's protagonist Ignatius J. Reilly opens the novel waiting for his mother in front of D.H. Holmes department store and "shifting from one hip to the other in his lumbering, elephantine fashion . . . sent waves of flesh rippling beneath the tweed and flannel, waves that broke upon buttons and seams" (Toole 1980: 13–14). He is an ethnic and a Catholic; his obsessions focus on food and theology. His faith was shattered as a teenager when his parish priest refused to bury his pet dog. His huge body is sustained by jelly doughnuts rather than communion wafers: "Ignatius says to me this morning. 'Momma, I sure feel like a jelly doughnut.' You know? So I went over by the German and bought him two dozen" (Toole 1980: 39). It is the "German" baker who supplies the food of the "slob extraordinaire."

Mrs. Reilly is addressing the hapless Officer Mancuso, who had tried to arrest her son in front of D.H. Holmes as a "character." His Italian bone-fides are established when he take Mrs. Reilly bowling with his aunt Mrs. Santa Battaglia. Her mother

had her a little seafood stand right outside the Lautenschlager Market. Poor Mamma. Right off the boat. Couldn't speak a word of English hardly. . . . Poor girl. Standing there in the rain and cold with her old sunbonnet on not knowing what nobody was saying half the time.

(Toole 1980: 91–2)

From her mother's photograph there stared "little black coals of Sicilian eyes" (Toole 1980: 192). But neither Mrs. Reilly nor Mrs. Santa Battaglia is corpulent; on the contrary, they are tiny, hard bodied, and very aggressive.

Indeed, the other "white" ethnics are equally slim. Mr. Gonzalez, who employs Ignatius, has his desk ornamented by "another sign that said SR. GONZALEZ and was decorated with the crest of King Alfonso" (Toole 1980: 108). Gonzalez is a chain smoker, but no attention is paid to his bodily shape. (And indeed Ignatius's fantasy of his Spanish roots only reflects the romantic notion of ethnics representing lost kingdoms so embodied in Gerald O'Hara.)

Beyond the Irish Catholic Ignatius, fat encompasses Toole's Jews. But perhaps we should look at the core Jewish figure that sets the model for Jewish ethnic identity in Toole's New Orleans, a figure who never actually appears in the novel. Mrs. Reilly mollifies their high-strung neighbor Miss Annie, whose life is made a living hell by Ignatius's raucous presence, by giving her a rosary: "I stopped off at Lenny's and bought her a nice little pair of beads filled with Lourdes water . . . She loved them beads, boy. Right away she started saying a rosary" (Toole 1980: 77). Ignatius is dismissive of Lenny's: "Lenny's. Never in my life have I seen a shop filled with so much religious hexerei. I suspect that that jewelry shop is going to be the scene of a miracle before long. Lenny himself may ascend" (Toole 1980: 77). Actually Lenny had already "ascended." We learn that he had gone to an "analyst in the Medical Arts building [who] helped Lenny pull his jewelry shop out of the red. He cured Lenny of that complex he had about selling rosaries. Lenny swears by that doctor. Now he's got some kind of exclusive agreement with a bunch of nuns who peddle the rosaries in about forty Catholic schools all over the city. The money's rolling in. Lenny's happy. The sisters are happy. The kids are happy" (Toole 1980: 150–1). Mrs. Santa Battaglia too is happy, having bought her plastic "Our Lady of the Television" from Lenny: "It's got a suction cup base so I don't knock it over when I'm banging around in the kitchen" (Toole 1980: 262). Here one can stop and ask, as Richard Klein does, who put the "Jew" in "jewelry." Lenny has been saved; indeed his shrink is described as "Lenny's savior" (Toole 1980: 282). The unseen Lenny has become part of the world of New Orleans, has abandoned at least the superficial sense of ethnic/religious difference which made him uncomfortable selling rosaries and plastic Mothers of God. As with the other "ethnics," he retains a "Jewish" quality that, at least perceived from the perspective of mid-century, is his happiness with worldly success. This is a key, by the way, even to American Jewish writing through Philip Roth's *Goodbye, Columbus* (1959), where worldly success and loss of identity go hand in hand.

Since Lenny is without a body, it is the figure of Mrs. Levy, the wife of the owner of Levy Pants, which employs Ignatius and Gonzalez, whose body reveals all. It is she who had evoked Lenny as the model for her husband's dealing with his business difficulties. She enters the novel "prone on the motorized exercising board, its several sections prodding her ample body gently, nudging and kneading her soft white flesh like a loving baker" (Toole 1980: 145–6). Perhaps the "German" baker? The bodies of Mrs. Levy, her daughters, Susan and Sandra, and her mother represent the fantasy of the "Jewish American Princess," obsessed by worldly things including their own appearance. What is clear is that, like Lenny, she no longer has any sense of her own "Jewish" identity and spends her time looking for meaning, a meaning which her very position in the hierarchy of Toole's world must deny her. Unlike her husband who overcomes his hatred of his dead, immigrant father, who moved from selling pants from a pushcart to the ownership of "Levy's Pants," she never acknowledges the burden of the past, or indeed, even the burden of the present, present in her "her ample body."

Yet the Jewish character that "embodies" Jewish fat in all of its ramifications for Ignatius is his New York, Jewish college girlfriend, Myrna Minkoff. She had failed in her many attempts to seduce him because "my stringent attitude toward sex intrigued her; in a sense I became another project of sorts" (Toole 1980: 137). Her lust is that of the stereotyped Jewish woman as succubus; but even more importantly, the northern Jew come to New Orleans. She is Ignatius' Rhett Butler.

She appears in the very opening of the novel, when Officer Mancuso attempts to arrest Ignatius, and Ignatius complains that he will report the officer to the "Civil Liberty Union . . . We must contact Myrna Minkoff, my lost love. She knows about those things" (Toole 1980: 6). In the 1960s, New York "agitators," all seen as Jews, "know about such things." Myrna "was only happy when a police dog was sinking its fangs into her black leotards or when she was being dragged feet first down stone steps from a Senate hearing" (Toole 1980: 125). Myrna, like Levy's daughters, has a father who "has money" (Toole 1980: 79). He sends her to New Orleans (to the unnamed Tulane) to "see what it was like 'out there'," where she meets Ignatius and they so disrupt the slow flow of the History Department that they are removed (Toole 1980: 125). Her experience in the "ghettos of Gotham" had not prepared her for Ignatius and the South as she believed "that all humans living south and west of the Hudson river were illiterate cowboys or—even worse—White Protestants, a class of humans who as a group specialized in ignorance, cruelty, and torture." Here Ignatius interpolates "I don't wish to especially defend White Protestants; I am not too fond of them myself" (Toole 1980: 124).

Listening to Ignatius's take on the world, she declared him "obviously anti-Semitic" when he disagrees with her (Toole 1980: 124). Indeed, this becomes a leitmotif for her. When Ignatius sends her a letter on "Levy Pants" stationary, she responds that "it is probably your idea of an anti-Semitic prank," as her father is in the clothing trade (Toole 1980: 214).

Myrna haunts Ignatius's dreams. He stands in one on "a subway platform, reincarnated as St. James the Less, who was martyred by the Jews" (Toole 1980: 242). Myrna appears carrying a sign for the "NON-VIOLENT CON-GRESS FOR THE SEXUALLY NEEDY" and Ignatius "prophesied" to her that "Jesus will come to the fore, skins or not" (Toole 1980: 242). The dreams morph into life when Myrna appears stuffed in her Renault to rescue Ignatius, when his mother, egged on by Mrs. Santa Battaglia, tries to have him committed to the psychiatric ward at Charity Hospital. Myrna whisks him off towards New York City, where, given the picaresque nature of the tale, his adventures in the skin trade would certainly continue.

Like attracts like. Myrna's shapeless, hippy body is the political counterpoint to Ignatius's huge one. There is a parallel in Salman Rushdie's first novel, *Grimus* (1975), a fantasy work centering about a quartet of American mis-fits living in a fantasy world. One of them, Virgil Jones, "gross of body," (Rushdie 1977: 12) is in love with the hunch-backed Dolores O'Toole: "they loved each other and found it impossible to declare their love. It was no beautiful love, for they were extremely ugly" (Rushdie 1977: 12). When they finally do make love, their "disfig-uration [is] transformed into sexuality" (Rushdie 1975: 50). "Her hands grasping great folds of his flesh . . . It's like making bread, she giggled, pretending to work his belly into a loaf" (Rushdie 1975: 50). We seem to be back again to the "German" baker. Ethnicity and obesity come to be linked in an odd way, both in their representation in culture and in the living experience of it.

SLG

*See also* Banting; Jews; Literature and Fat Bodies; Men; Mitchell; Vegetarianism

## References and Further Reading

Anon. (1856) "Decline of Emigration to the United States," *Charleston Mercury*, February 26, p. 2.

Anon. (1856) "Health for the People," *Charleston Mercury*, May 12, 1.

Cash, W.J. (1991) *The Mind of the South*, New York: Vintage.

Cobb, James C. (2005) *Away Down South: A History of Southern Identity*, New York: Oxford University Press.

Codrescu, Andrei (2000) " 'A Confederacy of Dunces,' Making the Natives Wince," *The Chronicle of Higher Education* 46: April 14.

Ferraro, Kenneth F. (1998) "Firm Believers? Religion, Body Weight, and Well-Being," *Review of Religious Research* 39 (3): 224–44.

Ferraro, Kenneth F. and Cline, Krista M.C. (2006) "Does Religion Increase the Prevalence and Incidence of Obesity in Adulthood?" *Journal for the Scientific Study of Religion* 45 (2): 269–81.

Holditch, W. Kenneth (1998) "Another Kind of Confederacy: John Kennedy Toole," in Richard S. Kennedy (ed.), *Literary New Orleans in the Modern World*, Baton Rouge, La.: Louisiana State University Press, pp. 102–22.

Klein, Richard (2001) *Jewelry Talks: A Novel Thesis*, New York: Vintage.

Manring, M.M. (1998) *Slave in a Box: The Strange Career of Aunt Jemima*, Charlottesville, Va.: University Press of Virginia.

Mitchell, Margaret (1999) *Gone with the Wind*, New York: Warner Books.

Mitchell, S. Weir (1877) *Fat and Blood and How to Make Them*, Philadelphia, Pa.: Lippincott.

O'Connell, David (1996) *The Irish Roots of Margaret Mitchell's Gone with the Wind*, Decatur, Ga.: Claves & Petry.

Ruppersburg, Hugh (1986) "The South and John Kennedy Toole's *a Confederacy of Dunces*," *Studies in American Humor* 5 (2–3): 118–26.

Rushdie, Salman (1977) *Grimus*, London: Granada.

Toole, John Kennedy (1980) *A Confederacy of Dunces*, New York: Grove Press.

# Sports

The nature of athletic competition requires participants to be highly in tune with their bodies. An athlete's success is largely determined by the fitness of his or her body. As long as athletic competition has been around, serious athletes have shared a concern with achieving and maintaining a body type that will allow them to be as successful as possible in their chosen activity. Although the ideal body type is very different for a gymnast or a sumo wrestler, both kinds of athletes put considerable time and effort into the pursuit of the "perfect body" for their sport. This quest is complicated by rapidly changing but often contradictory theories in sports medicine.

When considering athletes who often follow highly specified diet and exercise patterns, the question arises as to whether this behavior should be classified as "dieting." In the introduction to this volume, "dieting" in the modern sense is defined as "regulating food intake in order to gain or lose weight and/or affect one's overall health". In the case of the most serious athletes, the effort to achieve a perfect sport-specific body does involve the maintenance of a desired weight; therefore, most athletes can be categorized as "dieters" by this definition.

While all athletes are encouraged to stay as lean and muscular as possible, two types of sports in particular lend themselves to the most drastic dieting: those involving weight classes and those where success is determined by judging. Sports falling into the first category include wrestling, weight lifting, and crew. Coaches in each of these sports frequently weigh their athletes and encourage them to drop or gain weight to meet weight requirements. This commonly leads to large weight fluctuations which can be extremely stressful on an athlete's body.

Sports involving judging are also particularly dangerous because their goal is not to reach specific weight requirements but to achieve a certain appearance. Since the focus is already on appearance, it is a very small leap to the development of a distorted body image (Brownell et al. 1992). Sports in this category include gymnastics, figure skating, dance, and diving (Vincent 1989). These activities also tend to draw young women from the age group that is already supposedly at the highest risk for the development of distorted body images and/or eating disorders (Byrne 2002: 256–9). When this high-risk population participates in a sport where they are being judged while wearing small, tight clothing, the physical and emotional results can be disastrous.

There are countless horror stories about anorexic dancers and wrestlers passing out from dehydration while trying to "make weight," but it is important to realize that these cases are the exception, not the rule. In most cases, sports are extremely beneficial to a person's health. When approached in a healthy way, athletics can dramatically raise self-confidence and improve body image.

SLG/SARAH GARDINER

*See also* Body building; Hormones in Dieting

### References and Further Reading

Berry, Tanya R. and Howe, Bruce L. (2000) "Risk Factors for Disordered Eating in Female University Athletes," *Journal of Sport Behavior* 23: 345–54.

Brownell, K.D., Rodin, J., and Wilmore, J.H. (eds) (1992) *Eating, Body Weight, and Performance in Athletes: Disorders of Modern Society*, Philadelphia, Pa.: Lea & Febiger.

Byrne, Susan M. (2002) "Sport, Occupation, and Eating Disorders," in Christopher G. Fairburn and Kelly D. Brownell (eds), *Eating Disorders and Obesity: A Comprehensive Handbook*, 2nd edn, New York: Guilford Press, pp. 256–9.

Dickey, Christa and Gavin, Jim (2003) "Disordered Eating and Body Image Disturbances May Be Underreported in Male Athletes," *American College of Sports Medicine News Release*, March 7, available online at <http://www.acsm.org/publications/newsreleases2003/disorderedeating_030503.htm> (accessed March 4, 2007).

Grivetti, Louis E. and Applegate, E.A. (1997) "From Olympia to Atlanta: A Cultural-Historical Perspective on Diet and Athletic Training," *Journal of Nutrition* 127 (Suppl): 860S–868S.

Smith, Bryan W. (2004) "ACC Sports Sciences Feature: Weight Loss in Wrestling," *Atlantic Coast Conference*, December 5, available online at <http://theacc.collegesports.com/sports/m-wrestl/spec-rel/120504aac.html> (accessed March 4, 2007).

Vincent, L.M. (1989) *Competing with the Sylph: The Quest for the Perfect Dance Body*, Princeton, NJ: Princeton Book Company.

Ziegler, Paula (1998) "Body Image and Dieting Behaviors Among Elite Figure Skaters," *International Journal of Eating Disorders* 24 (4): 421–8.

# Spurlock, Morgan (1970–)

## American screenwriter and independent film director

Spurlock is best-known for his documentary *Super Size Me* (2004), a satire on American health and fast food habits, which placed the blame for increasing obesity at the door of the fast-food industry. The film was later nominated for an Academy Award for Best Documentary. Spurlock developed the idea for the film when, in 2002, he saw a news broadcast about two children, a nineteen-year-old boy, Jazlyn Bradley (5 foot 6 inches, 270 pounds) and a fourteen-year-old girl, Ashley Pelman (4 foot 10 inches, 140 pounds) of New York City whose parents sued McDonald's, asserting the restaurant was responsible for their children's obesity. The plaintiffs claimed to have eaten at McDonald's three to five times a week for years. The suit was later dismissed, as the court assumed that they had some modicum of free will and argued that their lawyer failed to show McDonald's used deceptive ads to trick consumers into eating unhealthy food. According to Spurlock, "*Super Size Me* is one man's journey into the world of weight gain, health problems and fast food. It is an examination of the American way of life and the influence that has had on our children, the nation and the world at large" (Anon. 2004).

In the film, Spurlock eats three meals a day at McDonald's for thirty days. He also orders a "super-sized meal" whenever it is offered. In doing so, Spurlock more than doubles the daily caloric intake recommended by the USDA. Additionally, Spurlock limited his normal exercise regime in order to better match that of the average American. He walked 1.5 miles a day instead of his usual 3 miles. As a result, Spurlock gained 25 pounds and suffered severe liver dysfunction and depression. After Spurlock finished the film, his body fat soared from 11 to 18 per cent, he was racked with headaches, and his liver became so fatty his doctor warned him it was turning to pate, risking permanent damage. His girlfriend Alex Jamieson, a strict vegan and vegetarian chef, commented that in addition to the weight gain, "he started having these uncharacteristic mood swings and, of course, the effect on our sex life was awful" (Anon. 2004). She then placed him on a strict vegan detoxification plan which focused on vegetables, fruit, soy products, and vitamin supplements while eliminating all dairy, meat, caffeine, and refined carbohydrates such as white bread, rice, and sugar. After eight weeks on the detox diet, Spurlock lost 20 pounds, and his liver, blood pressure, and cholesterol returned to normal (Burstin 2004: 31).

After the film's release, McDonald's discontinued its "super-size" campaign and introduced an exercise video for children featuring Ronald McDonald (Schmidt 2004). Spurlock has become a vocal advocate for the improvement of the nation's health, publishing *Don't Eat This Book* (2005) as a follow up to his film. During one visit to Tufts University in 2004 to speak about his film, Spurlock urged students to become more nutritionally aware and cook meals themselves.

One needs to note that hamburgers were once considered a health food because they were the product of modern technology. In 1906, Upton Sinclair's novel *The Jungle* caused the consumption of beef to decline in the U.S.A. Beef, at least beef from the Chicago stockyards, fell into disrepute. By the 1930s, well after the passage of the Pure Food and Drug Act promulgated that year in response to the "muckraker's" claims about the quality of American food, Billy Ingram created White Castle hamburgers through mechanical production untouched by human hands, full of vitamins and minerals. Not only did he dress up actors as physicians to tout his product, but he also funded a study by the University of Minnesota medical school in which a medical student was fed only White Castle hamburgers and water for ten weeks and was said to be healthier than ever. A child, it was claimed, could flourish if only fed the same diet (Hogan 1997).

SLG/JESSICA RISSMAN

*See also* Detoxification; Fast Food; Sinclair

**References and Further Reading**

Anon. (2004) "About the Director." Available online at <http://www.supersizeme.com/home.aspx?page=a-boutdirector> (accessed April 30, 2006).

Anon. (2006) "Morgan Spurlock," *Wikipedia*, available online at <http://en.wikipedia.org/wiki/Morgan_Spurlock> (accessed April 29, 2006).

Burstin, Fay (2004) "Escape from McHell," *Herald Sun*, Melbourne, Australia, June 9: 31.

Hogan, David Gerard (1997) *Selling 'Em by the Sack: White Castle and the Creation of American Food*, New York: New York University Press.

Schmidt, Kat (2004) "Morgan Spurlock (Super)Sizes Up American Public Health," Tufts Daily, November 5.

Spurlock, Morgan (2005) *Don't Eat this Book? Fast Food and the Supersizing of America*, New York: Putnam.

# Stress

Changes in appetite and eating habits are commonly accepted as a major response to chronic stress. However, stress does not affect all people in the same way. Some people lose their appetites when they are under stress; others become ravenously hungry. The reason for this seeming incongruity lies in the human body's physiological reaction to a stressful environment (Takeda et al. 2004).

Modern evolutionary psychologists argue that for most of human history, an individual's survival depended on his or her ability to respond quickly and appropriately to danger. This led to the evolution of a specific stress response to prepare the body for either fight or flight, both of which require quick reflexes and explosive physical exertion. This response releases the hormone epinephrine, also called adrenaline. Adrenaline prepares muscles for either fight or flight by increasing blood flow and breathing rate. It also alerts the senses by dilating the pupils, among many other physical responses. The entire body is focused on responding to the stressor, and all unessential processes, like those of the digestive system, are suppressed. In a life-and-death situation, an individual does not need to be distracted by hunger or the need to urinate.

While these responses may well have been invaluable to the proverbial caveman, the situations that cause the average person stress today are usually psychological and emotional rather than physical. An increased heart rate and suppressed digestion do absolutely no good for the person who has just been pulled over for speeding. A greater concern is that many of the main stressors in people's lives today are chronic, rather than isolated incidents. Living in poverty or working in a poor environment creates ongoing stress that the human body has not evolved to handle. The result is that people who deal with constant stress are often in a constant heightened state of anxiety. This can lead to a variety of chronic health problems (Rutledge and Linden 1998).

In some highly stressed people, the constant flow of adrenaline suppresses the appetite, causing them to lose weight. Others, however, seek to relieve their anxiety though excessive eating. This is an effective self-treatment for anxiety because the consumption of some foods, particularly "junk foods," releases endorphins. The brain releases these pleasure-producing chemicals in response to some types of high-energy foods. The brain can actually become dependent on these chemicals, leading to food cravings. It has been hypothesized that the desire for these foods may be an unconscious attempt to prepare for the caloric output of fight or flight. Much is still unknown about these mechanisms, and research continues about the difference between individuals whose appetites increase in stressful periods and those whose appetites decrease. It has been proposed that women are more likely to eat under stress than men (Grunberg and Straub 1992).

In modern fad diets, stress is seen as the reason for weight gain. Weight-loss products such as cortislim claim to block cortisol, a stress hormone that leads to "belly fat." Some diet programs even claim that if one eliminates stress from one's life, fat will just melt off the body, once again suggesting a mind–body connection for dieting.

SLG/Sarah Gardiner

See also Alternative Medicine; Metabolism; Religion and Dieting; Socioeconomic Status

### References and Further Reading

Abramson, E.E. and Wunderlich, R.A. (1972) "Anxiety, Fear and Eating: A Test of the Psychosomatic Concept of Obesity," *Journal of Abnormal Psychology* 79 (3): 317–21.

Greeno, Catherine and Wing, Rena (1994) "Stress-Induced Eating," *Psychological Bulletin* 115 (3): 444–64.

Grunberg, N.E. and Straub, R.O. (1992) "The Role of Gender and Taste Class in the Effects of Stress on Eating," *Health Psychology* 11 (2): 97–100.

Hibscher, J.A. and Herman, C.P. (1977) "Obesity, Dieting, and the Expression of "Obese" Characteristics," *Journal of Comparative and Physiological Psychology* 91 (2): 374–80.

Linden, W., Leung, D., Chawla, A., Stossel, C., Rutledge, T., and Tanco, S.A. (1997) "Social Determinants of Experienced Anger," *Journal of Behavioral Medicine* 20 (5): 415–32.

Oliver, Georgina, Wardle, Jane and Gibson, E. Leigh (2000) "Stress and Food Choice: A Laboratory Study," *Psychosomatic Medicine* 62 (6): 853–65.

Putterman, Erin and Linden, Wolfgang (2004) "Appearance Versus Health: Does the Reason for Dieting Affect Dieting Behavior?" *Journal of Behavioral Medicine* 27 (2): 185–204.

Rutledge, Thomas and Linden, Wolfgang (1998) "To Eat or Not to Eat: Affective and Physiological Mechanisms in the Stress-Eating Relationship," *Journal of Behavioral Medicine* 21 (3): 221–40

Takeda E. (2005) "Human Nutritional Science on Stress Control," *Journal of Medical Investigation* 52 (Suppl): 223–4.

Takeda E., Terao, J., Nakaya, Y., Miyamoto, K., Baba, Y., Chuman, H., Kaji, R., Ohmori, T. and Rokutan, K. (2004) "Stress Control and Human Nutrition: A Review," *Journal of Medical Investigation* 51 (3–4): 139–45.

# Sugar Busters

Sugar Busters is a popular high-protein diet developed by a group of New Orleans based physicians (and a layperson) in the late twentieth century. The authors of the popular diet book, *Sugar Busters!* include Samuel S. Andrews, MD (endocrinologist), Morrison C. Bethea, MD (thoracic surgeon), Luis A. Balart, MD (gastroenterologist), and H. Leighton Steward (the ghost writer and a New Orleans entrepreneur). Their premise, "Sugar is toxic!" claims refined sugars are toxic for the body, causing it to release insulin and store excess body sugar as body fat. The diet calls for avoiding refined sugar and processed grain products. It is not a "no" sugar diet, but a "less" sugar diet. The theory behind *Sugar Busters!* is fairly simple. Food high in carbohydrates (which results in sugar when it is digested) raises glucose levels in blood quickly. The pancreas is stimulated to release the hormone insulin to convert glucose into glycogen in order to store energy. The consequence of insulin production is stored fat. This diet is a version of that proposed in the worldwide success of the diet books by Michel Montignac from the 1980s and echoes the views of William Dufty's *Sugar Blues* (1976).

Therefore, the book recommends choosing correct carbohydrates, those that are low-insulin-producing. Insulin is necessary for survival, but with less insulin production, the authors claim that it leads to a healthier condition since fat comes from sugar. The authors claim that a high-protein, low-carbohydrate meal causes an unnoticeable rise in glucose levels and, consequently, a very insignificant rise in insulin, but a significant increase in the level of glucagons, a hormone secreted by the pancreas that helps regulate blood sugar and get rid of stored fat reserves. On the other hand, insulin "inhibits the mobilization of previously stored fat even if one is on a rather skimpy, but glucose-generating, diet" (Andrews et al. 1995: 4). *Sugar Busters!* also promises to lower cholesterol, increase energy, improve health, and help treat diabetes and other diseases. The food selection is mandated: "starchy" foods such as potatoes are to be avoided and even certain fruits, such as pineapples, "which have a high glycemic index" (Andrews et al. 1995: 131). The prescriptive abstinence from pineapple is in contrast to *The Beverley Hills Diet*, which sees it as the perfect food. As with Mazel's approach, portion size is mandated though this is understated in the "sugar" focus of the diet. This diet is similar to diets that people diagnosed with Type II Diabetes use to maintain healthy levels of blood sugar; however, it is yet to be proven if such a diet is necessary for those who have proper blood-sugar control.

SLG/RAKHI PATEL

*See also* Atkins; Mazel; Metabolism; Zone Diet

## References and Further Reading

Andrews, Samuel S., Bethea, Morrison C., Balart, Luis A., and Steward, H. Leighton (1995) *Sugar Busters! Cut Sugar to Trim Fat*, New York: Ballantine Books.

Dufty, William (1976) *Sugar Blues*, Radnor, Pa.: Chilton Book Co.

Grayson, Charlotte E. (2004) "Sugar Busters!" available online at <http://www.webmd.com/content/pages/7/3220_290.htm> (accessed February 26, 2007).

Montignac, Michel (1986) *Savoir gérer son alimentation*, Paris: Artulen.

—— (1991) *Dine Out and Lose Weight: The French Way to Culinary "Savoir Faire"*, London: Artulen.

# Sweeteners

After you order your favorite coffee drink, you walk to the counter to grab a stirrer and some napkins. Before your eyes can distinguish the words, you see numerous blue, pink, and yellow packets of sugar sweetener and table sugar in its own jar. The questions then arise: Which artificial sweetener should I use? Do they actually cause cancer? Are three packets too much? Since the early 1970s, sugar substitutes have been the subject of a vigorous public controversy regarding their safety. However, because they are claimed to be a healthy alternative to sugar and run in tandem with many dieting plans, they continue to be widely used today (National Cancer Institute 2007).

Sugar substitutes were developed much earlier than the branding of Equal® or Splenda®. Beginning in the mid-1800s, new and improved sugar substitutes enjoyed success in the world market. In 1811, the possibility of a sugar substitute gained attention when scientists discovered how to convert starch into sugar. Saccharine, invented in 1879, is the oldest of the artificial sweeteners. German chemist Constantin Fahlberg created saccharine and opened the world to noncaloric sugar substitutes. Saccharine gained popularity as World War I caused a sugar shortage to erupt. Sugar substitutes were no longer being used by those who could not consume sugar; they had proliferated because of their relatively cheaper production costs compared to sugar. In 1937, cyclamate was discovered as a sweetener up to thirty times sweeter than sugar. Cyclamate gained popularity after World War II and refueled the sugar-substitute craze. However, in the 1970s, cyclamate was banned because of accusations that it causes negative health effects (Shelke 2004: 518).

In the mid-1980s, the world consumption of artificial sweeteners surpassed that of sugar. Numerous social scientists have studied the history of artificial sweeteners and analyzed the various waves of consumption and possible factors responsible for such periods of consumption. Wilhelm Ruprecht believes there are two distinct waves of artificial sweeteners: One from 1885 to the 1960s and another from 1970 to the present. Ruprecht argues that various factors have contributed to the rise, fall, and rise again of artificial sweeteners. Sugar shortages as a result of wars and casualties contributed to the cheap and efficient production of artificial sweeteners. At this time, artificial sweeteners grew in popularity for economic reasons (Ruprecht 2005).

In the past twenty-five years, however, the use of artificial sweeteners shifted from a substitute for table sugar that was scarce to a substitute central to dieting practices. In addition, society's obsession with avoiding obesity in the late 1980s brought about a resurgence of noncaloric food alternatives (Ruprecht 2005). However, the media's portrayal of artificial sweeteners and their numerous health risks have caused consumers and doctors to question the safety of the artificial sweetener in their daily cups of coffee and diet soda drinks.

Saccharine's bitter aftertaste and cyclamate's negative side effects catalyzed the arrival of aspartame in 1965. Aspartame was marketed as a much sweeter and healthier sugar alternative (Shelke 2004: 519). In 1987 and 1988, Pepsi and Coca-Cola both switched from an aspartame/saccharine blend to 100 percent aspartame as the sweetening ingredient for their diet soda drinks because of aspartame's better taste profile. Further, an even newer artificial sweetener, sucralose, entered the market. Sucralose is acid and temperature stable and has persisted as a popular sugar substitute. Therefore, artificial sweeteners used in carbonated sodas allow people to indulge in their favorite soft drinks without getting the calories (Hagelberg 2003: 363).

From the 1800s until today, many sugar alternatives have remained on the current market and, thus, it is important to describe the use of artificial sweeteners in diet programs. Caloric sweeteners, such as sucrose, glucose, and fructose, should be distinguished from noncaloric or artificial sweeteners. Certain diet regimens, such as Atkins and South Beach, define and encourage sugar-free foods or restricted sugar intake in their plan. *Sugar Busters! Cut Sugar to Trim Fat* defines artificial sweeteners as substances used instead of sucrose (table sugar) to sweeten foods and beverages. Because artificial sweeteners are much sweeter than an equal amount of table sugar, smaller amounts are needed to assure the same level of sweetness. Artificial sweeteners, unlike sugar, do not elevate blood sugar or lead to weight gain.

Artificial sweeteners lack calories; therefore they are

classified as food additives and must seek FDA approval before entering the market (Hagelberg 2003: 363). The FDA's passing of various sugar alternatives was seminal in their growing popularity. The National Cancer Institute clearly states on its website that "before approving these sweeteners, the FDA reviewed more than 100 safety studies that were conducted on each sweetener, including studies to assess cancer risk. The results of these studies showed no evidence that these sweeteners cause cancer or pose any other threat to human health." (National Cancer Institute, accessed March 20, 2007). Nevertheless, the link between the use of artificial sweeteners and cancer remains controversial. Therefore, they have been studied by many governmental and research organizations. In the 1970s, these studies found an association between saccharine and the development of bladder cancer in laboratory rats, which caused panic among consumers and the media. However, results from other carcinogenicity studies show no clear evidence of an association between artificial sweeteners and cancer in people. Still, some consumers remain wary.

The Government and the medical field's uncertainty about artificial sweeteners are evident in the changing health-safety status of sweeteners. Thus, Congress mandated that more in-depth studies of saccharine continue and required that any food containing saccharine carry a health-warning label. In 2000, saccharine was taken off the U.S. National Toxicology Program's *Report on Carcinogens*, where it had been listed since 1981 as a human carcinogen. Because the bladder cancer found in rats is due to a mechanism not relevant to humans, and because there is no clear evidence that saccharine causes cancer in humans, its removal from the list was appropriate. Saccharine's delisting led to legislation signed into law on December 21, 2000, rescinding the warning label requirement. The back-and-forth listing and delisting of saccharine as a cancer-causing substance can be described as a potential reason for the confusion behind artificial sweeteners (U.S. National Toxicology Program 2007: 4).

As the effects of artificial sweeteners continue to be researched and as the FDA looks to approve future sweeteners, consumers still continue to use sugar substitutes in various parts of their diet. Many people capitalize on the noncaloric aspect of sweeteners and, therefore, use them in many of their meals as a healthy alternative to sugar with a guaranteed sweet taste (Andrews et al. 1998: 191–6). While alternative sugars elicit a lower glycemic effect on the body, control insulin levels, and consequently help prevent weight gain, they should be consumed in moderation and with caution. So, consumers in line at Starbucks should balance the pleasures of the sweetening capabilities of a packet of Splenda, but remain aware of the possible consequences.

## Sweeteners

| Sweetener Name | Facts |
| --- | --- |
| **Aspartame** Nutrasweet® and Equal® | Approved by the FDA in 1981, it is one of the most comprehensively studied sweeteners. It is 200 times sweeter than table sugar and contains two amino acids, aspartic acid and phenylalanine. Those with the uncommon genetic disease called phenylketonuria (PKU) should avoid aspartame because it contains phenylalanine. |
| **Saccharine** Sweet'N'Low® | Marketed before FDA approval was needed, it is a nonnutritive sweetener. Debate over saccharine's safety began when research was conducted that found that rats who were fed large amounts of saccharine were afflicted with bladder cancer; however, the long duration of its use by humans has resulted in no obvious problems thus the FDA has kept saccharine products on the market. It is 300 times sweeter than table sugar. |
| **Sucralose** Splenda® | Approved by the FDA in 1998, it is 600 times sweeter than table sugar. This nonnutritive sweetener is made from sugar, but its molecules are too large to be absorbed into the body. Splenda became popular because it has been marketed as a healthy alternative to sugar being low in calories and carbohydrates. Splenda is a multipurpose sweetener that can be used in many foods and beverages. |
| **Fructose** | A natural sweetener derived from natural fruit sugar. It causes a lower elevation of blood sugar than table sugar and has been claimed to be an appropriate substitute for sugar. |
| **Stevia** | An herb native to South America which has been used as a sweetener for many centuries. It is a natural sweetener that comes in both a liquid and powder form. |

SLG/JESSICA SAWHNEY

*See also* Sugar Busters

## References and Further Reading

Andrews, Samuel S., Bethea, Morrison C., Balart, Luis A., and Steward, H. Leighton (1998) *The New Sugar Busters! Cut Sugar to Trim Fat*, New Orleans, Ga.: Ballantine Books.

Bowen, James (2003) "Splenda Is Not Splendid," World National Health Organization, available online at <http://www.wnho.net/splenda.htm> (accessed March 20, 2007).

DesMaisons, Kathleen (2000) *Addictive Nutrition, the Sugar Addicts Total Recovery Program*, New York: Ballantine Books.

Hagelberg, G.B. (2003) "Sugar and Sweeteners," in Solomon Katz (ed.) *Encyclopedia of Food and Culture*, Vol. III, New York: Charles Scribner's Sons, pp. 358–63.

National Cancer Institute "Artificial Sweeteners and Cancer: Questions and Answers." Available online at <http://www.nci.nih.gov/cancertopics/factsheet/Risk/artificial-sweeteners> (accessed March 20, 2007).

Ruprecht, Wilhelm (2005) "The Historical Development of the Consumption of Sweeteners: A Learning Approach," *Journal of Evolutionary Economics* 15 (3): 247–72.

Shelke, Kantha (2004) "Sweeteners," *The Oxford Encyclopedia of Food and Drink in America*, Vol. II, New York: Oxford University Press, pp. 518–19.

U.S. National Toxicology Program (2007) "Report on Carcinogens, 11 edn, Appendix B. Agents, Substances, Mixtures, or Exposure Circumstances Delisted from Report on Carcinogens." Available online at <http://ntp.niehs.nih.gov/ntp/roc/eleventh/append/appb.pdf> (accessed January 25, 2007).

# T

## Taft, William Howard (1857–1930)

### President (1909–13) and Chief Justice of the U.S.A. (1921–30)

Taft was physically the largest president in U.S. history. The public viewed him as a big, good-humored president who was "always smiling" (Bumgarner 1994: 167). However, he is also remembered as "cautious, somewhat lethargic," a "natural follower," and "temperamentally unsuited for the intensely political character of the presidency" (Brinkley and Dyer 2004: 286 and 195). He weighed 340 pounds at his heaviest.

Taft was aware of his size, even writing to his wife in 1905 that he would "make a conscientious effort to lose flesh" (Pringle 1939: 286). The following year, he went on a physician-guided reducing diet high in protein and low in fat and sweets. Taft also exercised and dropped his weight from 320 to 225 pounds, but by the time presidential elections came around in 1908, he again weighed around 300 pounds and had eight-course breakfasts. Taft was mocked by the public for having an oversized bathtub installed in the White House which was large enough for four people. It was often said that Taft got stuck in the White House bathtub, and several men were needed to free him. The jokes about his weight continued, including a Supreme Court associate justice who said, "Taft is the politest man alive. I heard that recently he arose in a streetcar and gave his seat to three women"; a secretary of war who, upon learning that Taft had traveled on horseback asked, "Referring to your telegram, how is the horse?"; and a New York senator who placed his hand on Taft's abdomen and asked, "What are you going to name it when it comes, Mr. President?" (Bumgarner 1994: 168–9).

Taft learned to respond goodnaturedly to such remarks and even made jokes about his own weight.

After his presidential term, Taft again went on a diet, this time guided by the Dean of Yale University's medical school. In an interview with the *New York Times*, Taft describes his diet:

I dropped potatoes entirely from my bill of fare, and also bread in all forms. Pork is also tabooed, as well as other meats in which there is a large percentage of fat. All the vegetables except potatoes are permitted, and of meats, that of all fowls is permitted. In the fish line I abstain from salmon and bluefish, which are the fat members of the fish family. I am also careful not to drink more than two glasses of water at each meal. I abstain from wines and liquors of all kinds, as well as tobacco in every form. The last is, however, nothing unusual, for I never drink intoxicants anyway, and I have never used tobacco in my life.

(Anon. 1913)

He reduced his size to 250 pounds and lowered his blood pressure, declaring that "I can truthfully say I never felt any younger in all my life. Too much flesh is bad for any man. It affects a man both physically and mentally" (Anon. 1913). Taft suffered from chronic drowsiness during his presidency but not afterwards; the sleepiness may have been what we now call sleep apnea, which is linked to obesity (Brown 2003).

Taft was not the only president for whom body size and eating habits were an issue. Both he and Warren Harding were guests at John Kellogg's Battle Creek Sanitarium

(Spake 2005). Andrew Jackson's thin frame (at over 6 feet tall, he never weighed more than 145 pounds, Remini 1988: 7) may have saved his life in a duel; his opponent misjudged the location of Jackson's heart because his coat was too big for his build (James 1938: 118). Martin van Buren was criticized for being indulgent and aristocratic because he enjoyed fine foods; some even suspected that he wore a corset (Bumgarner 1994: 56). More recently, Bill Clinton was teased for his morning jogs, which included a stop at McDonald's.

SLG/DOROTHY CHYUNG

*See also* Fat Camp; Kellogg

**References and Further Reading**

Anon. (1913) "Mr. Taft on diet loses 70 pounds," *New York Times*, December 12: 1.
Anon. (2004) "Was President Sleep Deprived?" *Current Science* 89 (10): 12.
Brinkley, Alan and Dyer, Davis (eds) (2004) *William Howard Taft: The American Presidency*, New York: Houghton Mifflin Company.
Brown, David (2003) "Taft's Nodding Off Attributed to Illness," *Washington Post*, September 21: A03.
Bumgarner, John R. (1994) *The Health of the Presidents*, Jefferson, NC: McFarland & Company.
Gould, Lewis L. (2000) "Taft, William Howard," *American National Biography Online*, available online at <http://www.anb.org/articles/06/06-00642.html> (accessed February 27, 2006).
James, Marquis (1938) *The Life of Andrew Jackson*, New York: The Bobbs-Merrill Company.
O'Neill, Molly (1994) "At White House, a Taste of Virtue," *New York Times*, April 6.
Pringle Henry F. (1939) *The Life and Times of William Howard Taft*, New York, NY: Farrar & Rinehart.
Remini, Robert V. (1988) *The Life of Andrew Jackson*, New York: Harper & Row.
Spake, Amanda (2005) "Utopia in a Cereal Bowl," *U.S. News*, August 15, available online at <http://www.usnews.com/usnews/culture/articles/050815/15health.htm> (accessed February 27, 2006).

# Tarnower, Herman, MD (1910–80)

## Developer of the Scarsdale Diet (1979), which stresses high protein and low calories

Tarnower states that he developed the diet at the Scarsdale Medical Center in suburban, affluent New York when he urged his cardiac patients to "take off that unhealthy flab" (Tarnower and Baker 1980: 2). His diet suggestions came out of his general and cardiac practice, but clearly followed the growing health and diet consciousness of the middle-class, suburban "baby boomer" generation, who by the 1970s were entering into middle age. Successful diet books could sell millions of copies, and diet books that were labeled "medical" and linked with images of affluence (Scarsdale) were programmed for success.

Tarnower came into a bit of unexpected publicity in 1978 when an article in the *New York Times Magazine* announced that it was "but six weeks to bikini season . . . and the beautiful people of Scarsdale are now the skinny people of Scarsdale" due to the work of the unknown Herman Tarnower (Alexander 1983: 150). The publicity reached Oscar Dystel, the president of Bantam Books and a patient of Tarnower's Scarsdale medical group, who suggested to Samm Sinclair Baker that he contact Tarnower. Baker was looking for another "diet doc" to follow up the multi-million-book sales of Irving Stillman's diet books, which he had cowritten (among them *The Doctor's Quick Weight Loss Diet*, *The Doctor's Quick Inches-Off Diet*, *The Doctor's Quick Weight Loss Cookbook*, *The Doctor's Quick Teen-age Diet* and *Doctor Stillman's 14-Day Shape-Up Program*).

*The Complete Scarsdale Medical Diet* was on the *New York Times* hardcover bestsellers' list for forty-nine weeks, selling 711,100 copies. The paperback spent eighty weeks on the paperback list and as of 1981 had sold 5,309,000 copies. It is of little wonder given the pitch of the volume. The testimonies read like the code of the modern diet culture with its focus on the female body, "my husband keeps saying how wonderful it is to have a slim, attractive wife again, but he can hardly match my own delight about the 'new' me" (Tarnower and Baker 1980: 5). Another happy woman said, "I was never fat until change of life, getting older, getting heavier. I had no discipline, always good intentions that weren't enough. I went on your diet—IT WORKED! Thank you" (Tarnower and Baker 1980: 6). The book consisted of success stories of people who lost weight on the Scarsdale Diet, a variety of recipes, and Tarnower's views on eating, weight, and health.

Tarnower's suggestions follow the "fat is the danger" model, so well known from the nineteenth century. Meats are allowed, but they must be lean. The breakdown of the diet is 43 percent protein, 34.5 percent carbohydrates, and 22.5 percent fat (CBS News Online 2004). Only three meals per day are allowed on this diet and snacking is prohibited. Another component of the diet is using herbal appetite suppressants and artificial sweeteners, which are intended to speed the weight-loss process. Water is also an important component of this diet in order to cleanse the body and help lose weight. Tarnower's is a low-calorie, 1,000-calorie-per-day diet that lasts from seven to fourteen days. The appealing part of the diet at the time of publication was that it assured people would lose weight fast. More specifically, this meant losing 20 pounds in two weeks.

Many people had problems with the diet because it made them feel weak due to the low caloric intake. In addition, due to the large amount of total protein, including meat, an unbalanced amount of fat intake is likely. This diet does not involve exercising to help lose weight.

It advises that no one over forty years of age should engage in strenuous exercise unless it has always been a central part of his or her daily routine (Weight Loss Institute).

Tarnower was murdered in 1980 by his mistress Jean Harris, whom he thanked in the preface to the Scarsdale Medical Diet for her "splendid assistance." In fact, her lawyer argued during her trial that she had been the book's "primary author" (Alexander 1983: 158). Her trial was one of the salient proofs of the importance of celebrity in the dieting culture, and, one may add, the fleeting fame of such celebrity diets. Since Tarnower's death, the Scarsdale Diet has become less popular.

SLG/MARY STANDEN

*See also* Sweeteners

**References and Further Reading**
Alexander, Shana (1983) *Very Much a Lady: The Untold Story of Jean Harris and Dr. Herman Tarnower*, Boston, Mass.: Little, Brown and Company.
CBS News Online (2004) "Diets: A Primer." Available online at <http://www.cbc.ca/news/background/food/diets.html> (accessed March 25, 2006).
Courtroom Television Network (2005) "The Birth of a Best-Seller." Available online at <http://www.crimelibrary.com/notorious_murders/women/harris/10.html> (accessed April 21, 2006).
Diet Channel (2006) "Scarsdale Diet." Available online at <http://www.thedietchannel.com/Scarsdalediet.htm> (accessed April 2, 2006).
Tarnower, Herman and Baker, Samm Sinclair (1980) *The Complete Scarsdale Medical Diet*, New York: Bantam.
Weight Loss Institute (2002) "Scarsdale Diet." Available online at <http://www.weight-loss-institute.com/scarsdale_diet.htm> (accessed April 2, 2006).

# Thomson, Samuel (1769–1843)

Although he never trained as a medical doctor, Thomson claimed to have "had a natural turn for medical practice" (Thomson 1825: 26). He followed a local physician in late-eighteenth-century rural New Hampshire who "used chiefly roots and herbs, and his success was very great in curing canker and old complaints; but he afterwards got into the fashionable mode of treating his patients by giving them apothecary drugs, which made him more popular with the faculty, but less useful to his fellow creatures" (Thomson 1825: 26). This early formulation of the difference between allopathic—"medical poisons" (Thomson 1825: 41)—and complementary, if not alternative medicine, indicates why Thomson is still revered as a pioneer in the botanical pharmaceutical movement.

"Thomsonian Herbalism" later influenced and evolved into the "Eclectic Medical System and Physio-Medicalism," two major alternative medical systems of the late nineteenth and early twentieth centuries (Moore 2003: 9). Thus, in John Comfort's handbook of "Thomsonian" medicine (1876), the basic herbal remedies of purging, especially lobelia, are augmented by healthy foods such as "milk porridge" and that perennial favorite "chicken tea," chicken soup by another name (Comfort 1876: 573). Food comes to be therapy in addition to the herbal regimen for a wide range of diseases from earache to mania.

In 1822, Thomson authored the *New Guide of Health*, which outlined this system of preventative medicine for the public. Specifically, he urged the use of herbs and botanicals as medicine to control the body's "natural heat." In particular, he used the lobelia plant, which he called the "Emetic Herb" to induce vomiting in order to counteract the effect of cold. In his autobiography, he explains how he first used it to purge the lungs of his young son who had had the "meazles" (Thomson 1822: 36). There is nothing in Thomson's "material medica," his repertoire of medical materials that produces any side effects more serious than nausea, vomiting, or purging. Thus, his opposition to the quacks or ignorant pretenders, which he thought a large proportion of the medical faculty throughout the country were, was a relatively benign response to the "heroic" medicine of the late eighteenth and early nineteenth century. He was insistent upon botanical, natural elements as his form of treatment rather than the often-fatal interventions of the professional medical practitioner (Thomson 1822).

It is bad diet that provides the "cold," which, in turn, creates the need for herbal remedy. For Thomson, it was the

stomach … from which the whole body is

supported. The heat is maintained in the stomach by consuming food; and all the body and limbs receive their proportion of nourishment and heat from that source; as the whole room is warmed by the fire which is consumed in the fire place . . . The more food, well digested, the more heat and support through the whole man.

(Thomson 1825: 196)

But the body can receive poor food, which causes the stomach to be come "foul . . . then the appetite fails; the bones ache, and the man is sick in every part of the whole frame" (Thomson 1825: 196). Only then is there need for treatment. A good diet would have precluded any illness.

Thomson sold patents to use his methods of healing for 20 dollars, and by 1840 he had sold 100,000 of them. The spread of this lucrative practice led to a charge of witchcraft and then of murder by "real" doctors. He was acquitted of having killed a patient through the use of emetics in 1809. However, Thomson's success proved to be a disservice because he became "his own worst enemy, growing increasingly rigid and paranoid about protecting his proprietary interests" (Appel 2002: 359).

Thomson promoted a "uniquely American form of self-help health care" (Flannery 2002) in the early nineteenth century, which was revolutionary for this era. In it, he stressed personal responsibility for one's health in accordance with American notions of individualism.

SLG/JESSICA ELYSE RISSMAN

## References and Further Reading

Appel, Toby A. (2002) "Book Review: The People's Doctors: Samuel Thomson and the American Botanical Movement 1790–1860," *Journal of the History of Medicine and Allied Sciences* 57 (3): 359–60.

Comfort, J.W. (1876) *The Practice of Medicine on Thomsonian Principles*, Philadelphia, Pa.: Charles L. Comfort.

Flannery, Michael A. (2002) "The Early Botanical Movement as a Reflection of Life, Liberty, and Literacy in Jacksonian America," *Journal of the Medical Library Association* 90 (4): 442–54.

Moore, Les (2003) "Natural Medicine: Reclaiming Our Heritage," *New Health Digest* 1: 9.

Thomson, Samuel (1822) *New Guide of Health, or, Botanic Family Physician, Containing a Complete*

*System of Practice, Upon a Plan Entirely New, with a Description of the Vegetables Made Use of, and Directions for Preparing and Administering Them to Cure Disease*, Boston, Mass.: by the Author.

—— (1825) *A Narrative of the Life and Medical Discoveries of Samuel Thomson; Containing an Account of His System of Practice and the Manner of Curing Disease with Vegetable Medicine*, Boston, Mass.: By the Author.

# Trall, Russell Thacker (1812–77)

## Physician, writer, educator

Thacker was a friend of Sylvester Graham whose "Graham flour" he advocated, and was a pioneer and advocate of alternative medicine and gymnastics (Nissenbaum 1980). He believed that allopathic drugs made people weaker and that rest, vegetarian diet, and exercise, combined with treatments like massage and hydrotherapy ("water cure") were the proper means of achieving and maintaining health ("Pioneers of the North American Natural Health Movement"). Diet was at the center of his concern. As with most of the early nineteenth-century reformers in the age of the evangelical movement's millennialist message, he advocated diet reform in order to reform society as well as the individual. Thus, in his *Hydropathic Cook-Book* (1863), he condemned the diet suggested by Catharine Beecher as "the wine and brandy she commends in her cakes, and pies, and pudding sauces are better calculated to make men drunkards, than to render them wise in choosing" (Trall 1863: ix). His views match those of other health and moral reformers (interchangeable categories in nineteenth-century America) who advocated for the abolition of alcohol.

Trall published over a dozen books, opened a health institute offering natural treatments including vegetarian meals in 1844 in New York City, established the New York Hydropathic School in 1853 and served as vice president of the American Vegetarian Society. At the Hygeio-Therapeutic College, which he created, he trained Willie and Edson White, the sons of the founders of the Seventh-Day Adventists movement as well as Merrit and John Harvey Kellogg, two sons of John P. Kellogg. In his published works, he places special emphasis on "dietetics" and notes that "simple, natural food is most conducive to the recovery or preservation of health" (Trall 1854: 397). His critique of medicine and passionate advocacy of vegetarianism made him an important figure in the health reform and naturopathy movements of the twentieth century.

Yet, it is clear that his views rested on a rejection of "civilized" food ("the beef steak is too dry to swallow without the gravy, the bread will not go down smoothly without butter" [Trall 1854: 398]). Instead, he advocates eating "natural food" as revealed in the word of God in Genesis, "the vegetable kingdom is the ordained source of man's sustenance" (Trall 1854: 400). Trall links his biblical command for natural food to the science of the day, citing the French anatomist Cuvier and Lord Monboddo the British naturalist as well as Sylvester Graham. Food becomes the means of defining the link between the Bible as a source for rules of "hygiene" and the developing sciences of the time.

SLG/Angela Willey

*See also* Alternative Medicine; Beecher; Bodybuilding; Graham; Kellogg; Vegetarianism; White

## References and Further Reading

Anon. "Pioneers of the North American Natural Health Movement," Alive.com, available online at <http://www.alive.com/2541a8a2.php> (accessed May 9, 2006).

Iacobbo, Karen (2000) "Russell Trall: A Visionary Doctor," *The Viva Vine: The Vegetarian-Issues*

*Magazine*, November/December. Available online at <http://www.vivavegie.org/vvi/vva/vvi42/index-.html#trall> (accessed June 23, 2007).

Nissenbaum, Stephen (1980) *Sex, Diet, and Debility in Jacksonian America: Sylvester Graham and Health Reform*, Westport, Conn.: Greenwood Press.

Trall, Russell (1854) *The Hydropathic Encyclopedia: A System of Hydropathy and Hygiene*, New York: Fowler & Wells.

—— (1863) *The Hydropathic Cook-Book*, New York: Fowlers & Wells.

# V

## van Helmont, Johannes Baptista (1577–1644)

### Early seventeenth-century Flemish chemist

**V**an Helmont introduced radical empiricism into medicine in his posthumously published compendium, *Ortus medicinae* (1648) (van Helmont 1683). He argued, following the teachings of Paracelsus (1493/4–1541), against the notion that the imbalance of the humors caused illness. For him there had to be material reasons. Van Helmont imagined that there might be "wild spirits," which could neither be seen nor kept in vessels. He called them "chaos" (pronounced in Dutch, "gas"). Everything, when burnt, gave off different gases: Gas carbonum from burning charcoal, gas sylvester from fermenting wine and spa water, inflammable gas pinque from organic matter. His physiology was likewise material; he believed that each organ had its own spirit, or *blas*. This view was quite different than Paracelsus' belief that a single *archeus* or spirit animated the entire body. In retrospect, it is clear that van Helmont used a highly religious vocabulary to frame his materialism, which was informed by the religious world in which he functioned. Van Helmont's text on medicine is a seventeenth-century mix between highly speculative religious imagery and the technical medicine of his time, but it also included a long treatise on longevity.

An antihumorist and anti-Galenist, van Helmont developed the first notions of a medical chemistry, and one of his theories dealt with the difference between oil and fat. In his *First Three Principles*, he argues that elementary water is made into oil in vegetables, animals, and sulfurs; likewise, all oil is easily reduced to water. The first principle of this is that such things cannot be exchanged for each other or cease to be that which they were before. Oil is an elementary property. But it is present as a form of seed (*Samen*), which can be transformed into combustible substance (van Helmont 1683: 143, para. 3).

Oil is not body fat. He provides a case study to illustrate this. In his treatise on the "Law of the Double Nature of Man," van Helmont presents the case of an extremely fat person whose fat he transformed into a watery substance, which he evacuated through the bladder (van Helmont 1683: 851–2). Such transformations are not the property of oil. But even though water is passed through the kidneys, van Helmont is not convinced that the kidneys have the power to transmute fat into water even if they are healthy. He ascribes this power alone to the blood, which can transform itself into a solid.

For van Helmont, fat seems to be granted its power through the action of the stomach. But obesity is not the result of eating. He gives the example of the Capuchin monk who fasts and thirsts, but is still "fat in his body," as opposed to those who eat extremely well and remain thin. Due to some unseen working in the flesh, fat is the result of the entire body, including the blood. In the end, he sees the stomach as the "regent of digestion" (van Helmont 1683: 858). Its function (*blas*) is to process food. For van Helmont, the stomach is the very center of the body and his reason for this placement is theological rather than chemical, as he argues that Abraham bore the Messiah in his loins (van Helmont 1683: 850 para 45). The confusion between the gut and the loins is a telling one.

In van Helmont's guidelines for a long life, obesity is to be eschewed. Human life can be extended by medicine, but what God can offer is life eternal, not merely fleshly life. As a physician, van Helmont saw his job as prolonging the "Life of the World." What is bad for human life is clear: Carnal lust, tobacco and mushrooms, as well as "much and unreasonable gluttony" (van Helmont 1683: 1241 para 9). "Mushrooms . . . breed melancholy," according to Roger Bacon's treatise on longevity (Bacon 1683: 140). Food remains at the core of health. Thus, deceiving the body by reducing hunger is dangerous. Tobacco seems to still hunger, but ultimately doesn't; it merely makes one insensitive to the natural need for food, which itself must be controlled. And so van Helmont returns to a notion of the control of food as a means of controlling the potentially obese body.

SLG

*See also* Roman Medicine and Dieting

## References and Further Reading

Bacon, Roger (1683) *The Cure of Old Age and the Preservation of Youth*, ed. and trans. Richard Browne, London: Thomas Flesher and Edward Evets.

Debus, Allen G. (2001) *Chemistry and Medical Debate: Van Helmont to Boerhaave*, Canton, Mass.: Science History.

Pagel, Walter (1982) *Joan Baptista Van Helmont: Reformer of Science and Medicine*, Cambridge and New York: Cambridge University Press.

van Helmont, Johann Baptista (1683) *Aufgang der Artzney-Kunst, das ist: noch nie erhörte Grund-Lehren von der Natur . . .*, trans. Christian Knorr von Rosenroth, Sultzbach: Johann Andrae Enders sel. Sohne.

# Vegetarianism

Vegetarianism in itself may or may not be considered dieting. Political, ideological, and religious restrictions or prescriptions for food intake fall largely outside of the purview of a "dieting culture." Francis Bacon undertook a self-cure by consuming fruit and vegetables. But it was Thomas Tyron (1634–1703), in his *The Way to Wealth, Long Life and Happiness*, who first and most dramatically linked Bacon's diet to the original ways of Eve and Adam in Gen. 1: 29. Man could return to paradise, but only if s/he ate no meat. Emanuel Swedenborg (1688–1772), the Swedish mystic, advocated abstinence based on his theological views. He placed all animals on the level of man:

> Animals of every kind have limbs by which they move, organs by which they feel, and viscera by which these are put in motion. These they have in common with man. They have also appetites and affections similar to those natural to man. At birth they have knowledge, corresponding to their affections, in some of which appears something like the spiritual. From these facts it is that altogether natural men assert that living creatures of this kingdom are like them, apart from speech.
>
> (Swedenborg 1951: 132)

Other health mystics followed. William Blake (1757–1827) could write in his *Auguries of Innocence* (1803) to "Kill not the Moth nor Butterfly, / For the Last Judgement draweth nigh" (Stuart 2006: 232). Such views were a litmus test for an entire generation of temperance and vegetarian thinkers in England and the U.S.A. In 1845, the International Vegetarian Union was founded in the United Kingdom with the American group quickly following in the 1850. What had been conceived of as theological objection to eating flesh soon became defined in terms of diet and health.

Whether or not following a strictly political "vegan" or vegetarian diet might properly be considered "dieting," vegetarianism has played an important role in the history of diets and dieting. Indeed, virtually all of the early vegetarians, such as John Frank Newton

(1770–1828), make arguments for vegetarianism as both preventative (a "general increase in health") as well as treatment for illness and a necessity for longevity (Newton 1897: 46). For him, it is "natural" in that children all love fruit, but many "have refused to eat meat. Some have been made sick with it" (Newton 1897: 35). But it is the claim of a "Perfect Purity . . . the return of Paradise, the re-blending of discordant harmonies, the advent of the kingdom of God. It is the exaltation of the divine, the abasement of the carnal, the final victory of the spirit over the flesh," as a leading nineteenth-century advocate stated, that is at the very core of such beliefs (Hills 1897: 117–18). It has historically been argued to be important to health and continues to be seen as a potential weapon in the war on obesity.

Body purism and the notion that vegetable matter is less corrupting than flesh become part of a cult of hygiene in the course of the nineteenth century. The Prague Jewish writer Franz Kafka complains in 1909 that: "My paternal grandfather was a butcher in a village near Strakonitz; I have to not eat as much meat as he butchered and it gives me something to hold on to; being related means a lot to me" (Kafka 1990: 59). Kafka's "conversion" to vegetarianism is seen by him as a true transformation. "He compared vegetarians with the early Christians, persecuted everywhere, everywhere laughed at, and frequenting dirty haunts. 'What is meant by its nature for the highest and the best, spreads among the lowly people' " (Brod 1963: 74). Kafka sees his eating habits as being linked to who he is, to his sense of self, but also to his marginal world. Kafka's guru Moriz Schnitzer, the non-Jewish health faddist, gave his hygienic, vegetarian regime biblical underpinnings: "Moses led the Jews through the desert so that they might become vegetarians in these forty years" (Karl 1991: 270). Yet, it was notoriously Adolf Hitler who observed that, "One may regret living at a period when it's impossible to form an idea of the shape the world of the future will assume. But there's one thing I can predict to eaters of meat: the world of the future will be vegetarian" (Hitler 2000: 230). It is the "natural" food for the child before they are exposed to meat: "If I offer a child the choice between a pear and a piece of meat, he'll quickly choose the pear. That's his atavistic instinct speaking." It is part of what he is. "When I later gave up eating meat, I immediately began to perspire much less, and within a fortnight to perspire hardly at all. My thirst, too, decreased considerably, and an occasional sip of water was all I required. Vegetarian

diet, therefore, has some obvious advantages" (Hitler 2000: 204). Vegetarianism infiltrates every possible political position and ideological turn. It is a means of curing the body and purifying the soul.

In the twentieth century, it has become medicalized, at least on its surface. In their position paper on vegetarian diets, the American Dietetic Association observed that "[v]egetarians have been reported to have lower body mass indices than nonvegetarians, as well as lower rates of death from ischemic heart disease; vegetarians also show lower blood cholesterol levels; lower blood pressure; and lower rates of hypertension, type 2 diabetes, and prostate and colon cancer" (American Dietetic Association 2003). The growing popularity of vegan and vegetarian restaurants and products, marketed as healthy and "heart smart alternatives," attests to the mainstreaming of vegetarianism within dieting culture. It has even survived the high-protein diet boom as a "healthy lifestyle" and weight-loss strategy. Low-fat diets commonly encourage dieters to experiment with meat-free dishes, try meat substitutes, and eat more vegetables, grains, etc.

Vegetarianism popularly conceptualized as "food rejection" has played its part in a dieting culture that valorizes thinness often at the cost of health. Building on the tradition that defines a vegetarian diet as inherently "healthy," individuals in our contemporary dieting culture can thus use vegetarianism as a form of legitimated food rejection. Research looking at correlations between dieting and eating-disordered behavior and vegetarianism among young people suggests that vegetarianism is increasingly used today as a means of controlling weight. For many young women vegetarians, the choice is at least in part a weight-loss strategy (Gilbody et al. 1999: 90). A survey of 2,000 adolescents in fifty-two South Australian schools found a strong association between vegetarianism and "extreme weight-loss behaviours" (Worsley and Skrzypiec 1997: 402).

An analogy may well be to the children of Orthodox Jews and Muslims, who reject the dietary restrictions of their parents in regard to Kosher or Halal meat, but who find in vegetarianism a socially acceptable way of adhering to food restrictions which still fulfill all of the demands of their parent's religious convictions but carry none of the religious baggage. Indeed, in the vegetarianism literature of the nineteenth century, anti-Semitism can be found which damns the ritual slaughter of meat. The overall view was the "Jews were a flesh-eating people" (Salt 1897: 96). The philosopher Arthur

Schopenhauer, saw in the nineteenth century the Jews' refusal to use "humane" methods of slaughter such as "chloroform" a sign of their "unnatural separation" of human beings from the animal world that he attributed to the spirit of Judaism (Schopenhauer 1973: 2: 375). Today, however, with advances in the use of soy products as meat substitutes and a proliferation of vegetarian and vegan cookbooks and recipes, you can have your (vegetarian) cake and eat it too.

SLG/Angela Willey

*See also* Anorexia; Atkins; Christianity; Graham; Metcalfe; Natural Man; Religion and Dieting; Sugar Busters; Trall; Zone Diet

## References and Further Reading

American Dietetic Association (2003) "Position of the American Dietetic Association and Dieticians of Canada: Vegetarian Diets," *Journal of the American Dietetic Association* 103 (6): 748–65.

Anon. (2007) "The Health Benefits of a Vegetarian Diet," Weightlossresources.co.uk, available online at <http://www.weightlossresources.co.uk/diet/vegetarian.htm> (accessed March 2, 2007).

Brod, Max (1963) *Franz Kafka: A Biography*, trans. G. Humphreys Roberts and Richard Winston, New York: Schocken.

Gilbody, Simon M., Kirk, Sara F.L., and Hill, Andrew J. (1999) "Vegetarianism in Young Women: Another Means of Weight Control?" *International Journal of Eating Disorders* 26 (1): 87–90.

Hills, Arnold Frank (1897) *Vegetarian Essays*, London: Ideal Publishing House.

Hitler, Adolf (2000) *Hitler's Table Talk*, trans. Norman Cameron, R.H. Stevens, and Hugh Redwald Trevor-Roper, New York City: Enigma Books.

Karl, Frederick Robert (1991) *Franz Kafka, Representative Man*, New York: Ticknor & Fields.

Kafka, Franz (1990) *Letters to Milena*, trans. Philip Boehm, New York: Schocken.

Newton, John Frank (1897) *The Return to Nature*, London: Ideal Publishing House.

Salt, Henry S. (1897) *The Logic of Vegetarianism*, London: Ideal Publishing House.

Schopenhauer, Arthur (1973) *Parerga and Paralipomena*, trans. E.F.J. Payne, Oxford: Clarendon Press.

Spencer, Colin (1996) *The Heretic's Feast: A History of Vegetarianism*, Hanover, NH: University Press of New England.

Stuart, Tristram (2006) *The Bloodless Revolution: Radical Vegetarianism and the Discovery of India*, New York: Harper Collins.

Swedenborg, Emmanuel (1951) *Angelic Wisdom Concerning the Divine Love and the Divine Wisdom*, trans. John Ager.New York: Swedenborg Foundation.

Worsley, A. and Skrzypiec, G. (1997) "Teenage Vegetarianism: Beauty or the Beast?" *Nutrition Research* 17 (3): 391–404.

# Very-Low-Calorie Diets

Very-low-calorie (VLC) diets are administered by physicians who use them to treat a variety of conditions, including obesity, diabetes, cardiovascular disease, and hormonal disorders. These diets have undergone many changes since they were first developed and are the topic of ongoing debates amongst obesity researchers. Questions about safety and efficacy permeate these debates, but at a time when doctors and patients are looking for radical remedies to the growing problem of obesity, VLC diets are a promising if uncertain method of inducing weight loss. Low calorie (LC) diets and VLC diets are often conflated in popular discourse even though there are important distinctions between them. In addition, it is tempting to equate VLC dieting with eating disorders like anorexia and compulsive avoidance of foods. Confusion about VLC dieting and disordered eating is understandable because VLC dieters and pathological eaters may display similar behaviors. Nevertheless, VLC diets are still an important medical tool in fighting obesity.

It is important to distinguish VLC diets from the more

familiar LC diets. Definitions of VLC and LC diets have changed over time with the introduction of international CODEX standardization and FDA and EU legislation limiting food restriction (Howard 1989: 6–7; Saris 2001: 295S; Scientific Cooperation 2002). A LC diet generally provides between 800 and 1,200 calories per day, but some LC diets may contain as many as 1,500 calories per day (Saris 2001: 295S; Wadden and Berkowitz 2002: 534). Some of the most popular commercial diet programs are LC diets, including Jenny Craig and LA Weight Loss among others; these diets are available to all consumers and are not physician supervised (Scientific Cooperation 2002: 10; Tsai and Wadden 2005: 58). VLC diets, on the other hand, consist of between 400/450 and 800 calories per day, although some may provide up to 1,200 calories per day (CODEX 1995: 1; Saris 2001; Scientific Cooperation 2002: 10). In some cases, a VLC diet may also be defined as any diet that provides less than 50 percent of an individual's predicted energy requirements (Wadden and Berkowitz 2002: 534). VLC diets are generally carried out under the supervision of a physician and are not recommended for self-treatment of overweight or obesity. Widely used VLC diets include Medifast, OPTIFAST, Heath Management Resources (HMR), and the Cambridge Diet (Scientific Cooperation 2002: 35–7; Tsai and Wadden 2005: 59).

VLC diets rely on calorie-counting to create a negative energy balance in the patient, who will then lose weight. Calorie-counting was first introduced in 1918, and VLC diets were originally developed in the late 1920s and early 1930s by the Pittsburgh group of physicians (Howard 1981). The first research published on VLC diets appeared in 1929 as a new method for treating obesity (Evans and Strang 1995; Saris 2001: 295S). This original VLC diet prescribed a diet of 6 to 8 calories per kilogram of body weight instead of the usual 14 to 15 calories per kilogram (Howard 1989: 1; Saris 2001: 295S), which created a caloric deficit as great as 1,720 calories in some cases and resulted in dramatically greater weight loss in obese patients (Evans and Strang 1995: 211–12). While caloric reduction was severe, the diet provided approximately 400 calories and was not a pure fast (Saris 2001: 295S).

In 1959, however, W.L. Bloom reintroduced therapeutic fasting as a method for treating obesity. While patients using the fasting treatment lost weight, they also lost valuable protein and nitrogen; therefore, "protein sparing," which involved supplementing the fast with lean meat and egg albumin, was introduced in the late 1960s (Howard 1989: 3; Vertes 1984: 56). While an improvement over zero-calorie programs, these supplemented diets were often deficient in carbohydrates, which led to ketosis and loss of essential minerals. The development of modern VLC diet formulas sought to address these deficiencies, and canned liquid drinks were introduced in 1962. This MetroCal diet plan provided approximately 900 calories and was the first "nutritionally complete food for the treatment of obesity" (Howard 1989: 3–4). All of these early modern VLC diets worked by inducing anorexia (absence of hunger) if the patient adhered to them strictly for three days (Howard 1989: 4).

In the 1970s, VLC diet products were sold in the form of liquid-protein meal replacements. Unfortunately, because these new products used hydrolyzed collagen (a low-value protein) as the only protein source and did not include adequate amounts of vitamins, minerals, and electrolytes, their use was associated with several sudden deaths between 1976 and 1978 (Howard 1989: 4–5; Saris 2001: 295S–96S; Vertes 1984: 57). Subsequent studies have suggested that these deaths may have resulted from cardiac arrhythmias and/or mineral malnutrition; however, there is no conclusive evidence that VLC diet use causes sudden death (Howard 1989: 4; Saris 2001: 296S; Vertes 1984: 57). Still, the medical community and the public became wary of using VLC diets to treat obesity.

As a result, doctors, scientists, and other health and governmental officials have worked to develop guidelines for ensuring the safety of dieters. In 1987, the U.K. Department of Health and Social Security COMA report recommended that VLC diets should be used only after the failure of conventional food diets and should provide no less than 400–500 calories per day (Howard 1989: 6–7). In 1995, CODEX, the body responsible for recommending international food standards to the UN and World Health Organization (WHO), also suggested that VLC diets provide between 450 and 800 calories per day (CODEX 1995: 1).

In addition, the U.S. Dietary Guidelines Advisory Committee has published recommended energy intakes (number of calories) for various age and sex groups. In order to lose weight, the committee recommends cutting no more than 300 to 500 calories from one's daily intake (Department of Health and Human Services 2005). Most dietary guidelines for losing weight recommend that all dieters should consume no less than 1,200 calories per day for safe and lasting weight loss. According to the

National Library of Medicine's dietary recommendations, "diets that are excessively low in calories are considered dangerous and do not result in healthful weight loss" (U.S. National Library of Medicine). Moreover, the National Institutes of Health Institute of Diabetes, Digestive, and Kidney Diseases (NIDDK) warns that, "diets that provide less than 800 calories per day also could result in heart rhythm abnormalities, which can be fatal" (NIDDK 2006).

Nevertheless, VLC diets continue to prescribe much larger caloric deficits, and most scientists agree that VLC diet products are safe when they are closely monitored by a doctor, contain adequate protein and carbohydrates, and are supplemented with essential vitamins and micronutrients (Vertes 1984: 57–8; Zahouani et al. 2003: S149). In addition, the benefits of VLC diets may outweigh their risks in cases of morbid obesity. There is evidence to suggest that VLC diet programs can result in dramatic weight loss and improved overall health (Kanders et al. 1989; Stordy 1989). In fact, studies of HMR and OPTIFAST suggest that patients on a comprehensive program can expect to lose approximately 15–25 percent of their initial weight during three to six months of treatment and may maintain a loss of 8–9 percent after one year following the initial treatment. These numbers decrease as time passes, but even after four years, patients treated with VLC diets may still show lasting results of their weight loss (Tsai and Wadden 2005: 62–3).

VLC diets have also been proven to be an effective method in jump-starting patients on conventional weight-loss treatments (Quaade and Astrup 1989). In addition, VLC diets have been shown to reduce cravings for unhealthy foods (Harvey et al. 1993; Martin et al. 2006) and improve obesity-related conditions, such as non-insulin-dependent diabetes (Capstick et al. 1997), sleep apnea and hypertension (Kansanen et al. 1998), cardiovascular disease (Ramhamadany et al. 1989), and hormonal and metabolic disorders, such as polycystic ovarian syndrome and related hirsutism (Okajima et al. 1994).

However, concerns still exist about the effectiveness of VLC diets and the ability of patients to "keep the weight off" (Howard 1981). First of all, researchers disagree on the efficacy of VLC diets, and some argue that weight loss is no greater with VLC diets than with the less restrictive LC diets (Garrow 1989: 147; Saris 2001: 297S–98S). In addition, studies show that almost all patients treated with VLC diets will regain much of the weight that they initially lose (Paisey et al. 2002: 125; Vertes 1984: 57;

Wadden et al. 1989; Wadden and Berkowitz 2002: 536). For example, a 1989 study of VLC diet, behavior therapy, and their combination to treat obesity showed that after five years, 55 percent of subjects gained back most or all of the weight that they lost during treatment (Wadden et al. 1989).

Regaining lost weight is, in part, attributed to the fact that VLC diets are extremely restrictive, and many patients resume their pretreatment eating habits and, therefore, return to their previous weight. In one study, researchers found that only about one-fifth of the people who attempted the Cambridge Diet succeeded in complying with it fully for two weeks (Heller and Edelmann 1991). In another study, forty-one of seventy-six patients reported a fasting lapse within the first eleven weeks of a VLC diet program (Mooney et al. 1992: 321). While these numbers are not surprising considering the recidivism rates associated with all forms of dieting and weight loss, the inability of patients to sustain VLC dieting practices does seem to limit their effectiveness for long-term weight loss. In addition, it is possible that the long-term failure of VLC diets may result, in part, from depressed resting metabolic rates that have been observed in patients on these modified fasts (Kanders et al. 1989: 133; Vansant et al. 1989). There are clearly substantial problems that VLC dieters must confront in their efforts to lose weight.

VLC diets have changed repeatedly since their development in the late 1920s, yet they remain a hotly debated topic amongst obesity researchers. Concerns about safety have decreased since the 1980s because commercial formulas have been nutritionally improved and regulated, yet uncertainties about long- and short-term efficacy remain. The use of near-starvation practices in medically supervised dieting is also interesting in a culture that is arguably obsessed with pathological eating disorders. While an obese man may consume a 450-calorie VLCD at the suggestion of his physician, a young girl who follows similar eating habits on her own may easily be diagnosed as suffering from anorexia. Determining the appropriate amount of calories for safe and healthy weight loss or weight gain is important, but, as the history of VLC diets suggest, this determination is mutable and ultimately contingent upon current medical fashion.

SLG/C. MELISSA ANDERSON

*See also* Anorexia; Calorie; Craig; Linn; Metabolism; Obsessive Compulsive Disorders; Peters

## References and Further Reading

Capstick, F., Brooks, B.A., Burns, C.M., Zilkens, R.R., Steinbeck, K.S. and Yue, D.K. (1997) "Very Low Calorie Diet (VLCD): A Useful Alternative in the Treatment of the Obese NIDDM Patients," *Diabetes Research and Clinical Practice* 36 (2): 105–11.

CODEX Alimentarius Commission (1995) "Codex Standard 203 for Formula Foods for Use in Very Low Calorie Diets for Weight Reduction," World Health Organization (WHO) and Food and Agriculture Organization of the United Nations (FAO). Publishing Management Service FAO. Available online at <http://www.codexalimentarius.net/download/standards/296/CXS_203e.pdf> (accessed March 15, 2007).

Department of Health and Human Services and USDA (2005) "Dietary Guidelines for Americans 2005," Department of Health and Human Services (HHS) and Department of Agriculture (USDA), available online at <http://www.health.gov/dietaryguidelines/dga2005/document/html/chapter2.htm> (accessed March 15, 2007).

Evans, Frank A. and Strang, James M. (1995) "A Departure from the Usual Methods in Treating Obesity," *Obesity Research* 3 (2): 210–14.

Garrow, J.S. (1989) "Very Low Calorie Diets Should Not Be Used," *International Journal of Obesity* 13 (Supp. 2): 145–7.

Harvey, J., Wing, R.R., and Mullen, M. (1993) "Effects on Food Cravings of a Very Low Calorie Diet or a Balanced, Low Calorie Diet," *Appetite* 21 (2): 105–15.

Heller, J. and Edelmann, R.J. (1991) "Compliance with a Low Calorie Diet for Two Weeks and Concurrent and Subsequent Mood Changes," *Appetite* 17 (1): 23–8.

Howard, A.N. (1981) "The Historical Development, Efficacy and Safety of Very-Low-Calorie Diets," *International Journal of Obesity* 5 (3): 195–208.

—— (1989) "The Historical Development of Very Low Calorie Diets," *International Journal of Obesity* 13 (Supp 2): 1–9.

Kanders, B. S., Blackburn, G. L., Lavin, P. and Norton, D. (1989) "Weight Loss Outcome and Health Benefits Associated with the Optifast Program in the Treatment of Obesity," *International Journal of Obesity* 13 (Supp 2): 131–4.

Kansanen, M., Vanninen, E., Tuunainen, A., Pesonen, P., Tuononen, V., Hartikainen, J., Mussalo, H. and Uusitupa, M. (1998) "The Effect of a Very Low-Calorie Diet-Induced Weight Loss on the Severity of Obstructive Sleep Apnoea and Autonomic Nervous Function in Obese Patients with Obstructive Sleep Apnoea Syndrome," *Clinical Physiology* 18 (4): 377–85.

Martin, C.K., O'Neil, P.M. and Pawlow, L. (2006) "Changes in Food Cravings During Low-Calorie and Very-Low-Calorie Diets," *Obesity (Silver Spring)* 14 (1): 115–21.

Mooney, J.P., Burling, T.A., Hartman, W.M. and Brenner-Liss, D. (1992) "The Abstinence Violation Effect and Very Low Calorie Diet Success," *Addictive Behaviors* 17 (4): 319–24.

National Institute of Diabetes and Digestive and Kidney Diseases (2006) "Weight Loss and Nutrition Myths: How Much Do You Really Know?" National Institutes of Health, available online at <http://win.niddk.nih.gov/publications/myths.htm> (accessed March 15, 2007).

Okajima, T., Koyanagi, T., Goto, M. and Kato, K. (1994) "Hormonal Abnormalities Were Improved by Weight Loss Using Very Low Calorie Diet in a Patient with Polycystic Ovary Syndrome," *Fukuoka Igaku Zasshi* 85 (9): 263–6.

Paisey, R.B., Frost, J., Harvey, P., Paisey, A., Bower, L., Paisey, R.M., Taylor, P. and Belka, I. (2002) "Five Year Results of a Prospective Very Low Calorie Diet or Conventional Weight Loss Programme in Type 2 Diabetes," *Journal of Human Nutrition and Dietetics* 15 (2): 121–7.

Quaade, Flemming and Astrup, Arne (1989) "Initial Very Low Calorie Diet (VLCD) Improves Ultimate Weight Loss," *International Journal of Obesity* 13 (Supp 2): 107–11.

Ramhamadany, E., Dasgupta, P., Brigden, G., Lahiri, A., Raftery, E.B. and Baird, I.M. (1989) "Cardiovascular Changes in Obese Subjects on Very Low Calorie Diet," *International Journal of Obesity* 13 (Supp 2): 95–9.

Saris, Wim H.M. (2001) "Very-Low-Calorie Diets and Sustained Weight Loss," *Obesity Research* 9 (Supp 4): 295S–301S.

Scientific Cooperation (SCOOP) (2002) "Collection of Data on Products Intended for Use in Very-Low-Calorie Diets," Reports on Tasks for Scientific Cooperation, Directorate-General Health and Consumer Protection, European Commission, available online at <http://ec.europa.eu/food/fs/scoop/7.3_en.pdf> (accessed March 15, 2007).

Stordy, B.J. (1989) "Very Low Calorie Diets Should Be Used," *International Journal of Obesity* 13 (Supp 2): 141–3.

Tsai, Adams Gilden and Wadden, Thomas A. (2005) "Systematic Review: An Evaluation of Major Commercial Weight Loss Programs in the United States," *Annals of Internal Medicine* 142 (1): 56–66.

U.S. National Library of Medicine (2005) "Diet-Calories," Medline Plus, available online at <http://www.nlm.nih.gov/medlineplus/ency/article/002457.htm> (accessed March 15, 2007).

Vansant, G., Van Gaal, L., Van Acker, K. and De Leeuw, I. (1989) "Short and Long Term Effects of a Very Low Calorie Diet on Resting Metabolic Rate and Body Composition," *International Journal of Obesity* 13 (Supp 2): 87–9.

Vertes, Victor (1984) "Very Low Calorie Diets: History, Safety, and Recent Developments," *Postgraduate Medical Journal* 60 (Supp 3): 56–8.

Wadden, T.A., Sternberg, J.A., Letizia, K.A., Stunkard, A.J. and Foster, G.D. (1989) "Treatment of Obesity by Very Low Calorie Diet, Behavior Therapy, and Their Combination: A Five-Year Perspective," *International Journal of Obesity* 13 (Supp 2): 39–46.

Wadden, Thomas A. and Berkowitz, Robert I. (2002) "Very-Low-Calorie Diets," in Christopher G. Fairburn and Kelly D. Brownell (eds), *Eating Disorders and Obesity: A Comprehensive Handbook*, 2nd edn, New York: The Guilford Press, pp. 534–8.

Zahouani, A., Boulier, A. and Hespel, J.P. (2003) "Short- and Long-Term Evolution of Body Composition in 1389 Obese Outpatients Following a Very Low Calorie Diet (Pro'gram18 Vlcd)," *Acta Diabetologia* 40 (Supp 1): S149–50.

# W

## Weight Gain

In our twenty-first-century dieting culture, we assume that everyone on a diet is trying to lose weight, but there are some "hard gainers" whose greatest struggle is to keep weight on. Historically, such need for weight gain has been an intrinsic part of dieting culture. Athletes may be particularly interested in putting on weight to improve their strength and performance. Sports-medicine training books generally provide at least a few pages of technical information about gaining weight, which is often fairly scientific and can be intimidating (Lamb and Murray 1998: 229–30). Popular nutrition and training books, therefore, generally provide a bit of advice on how to gain weight; however, this information is subordinate to recommendations for losing weight.

There are many athletes who also try to gain weight in order to become better competitors in their sport. One sport in particular in which competitors are trying to gain weight is bodybuilding. Bodybuilders usually want to gain weight in muscle only. Therefore, there have been many diet plans instructing bodybuilders on muscle weight gain. However, bodybuilders are not the only athletes who try to gain weight; high-school athletes also gain weight for their football, basketball, or soccer seasons. Some foods recommended for these young athletes are foods high in calories like smoothies, fruit juice, milkshakes, nuts, dried fruits, and vegetables with higher calories like potatoes, beans, peas, and corn. Research also suggests that athletes should eat a snack high in carbohydrates and protein before exercising because this can help muscle growth.

Food guides for runners and triathletes, in particular, may include a chapter on gaining weight. Nancy Clark, for example, includes a section for "the minority of marathoners who struggle with being too thin" (Clark 2002: 117). In this chapter, she provides "six rules for gaining weight," which include:

1. Eat consistently.
2. Eat larger portions.
3. Select higher calorie foods.
4. Drink lots of juice and low-fat milk.
5. Do strength training.
6. Be patient.

(Clark 2002: 118–20)

The added calories from food, coupled with weight lifting and persistence, Clark explains, will help these "hard gainers" put on weight. However, she also cautions that our "genetic blueprint" determines much of our body shape and urges all runners to set realistic goals for themselves (Clark 2002: 117).

It is not just the athletes with their supposedly healthy bodies who are dieting for weight gain. Some people actually need to go on diets in order to gain weight. It can be as unhealthy to be underweight as it can be to be overweight. Some of the health problems associated with being underweight are: Decreased muscle strength, problems regulating body temperature, increased risk of infection, and even death. In addition to the health risks, many underweight people are as insecure about their bodies as overweight individuals. Some underweight people even hire personal trainers and nutritionists, who help them gain weight in a healthy way. There are many internet sites which also provide advice on gaining weight. One internet site called SkinnyGuy.net has about 18,000 members, and all of them paid 97 dollars to join the site, which teaches them how to gain weight. However, medical professionals are concerned about some of the advice that these sites give out. They say that most of the advice on these weight-gaining sites is based on personal experiences and not medically tested approaches.

In order to gain weight, one must take in more calories than are burned. This means eating more food with increased calories. Most doctors agree that in order to gain weight at a healthy rate, one should try consuming an extra 500 calories a day. Some suggest that if 500 calories does not work, then one should try 700 calories a day. It is important to not try to gain weight by eating fattening, unhealthy foods. In order to gain weight in a healthy way, doctors recommend that people eat foods which are nutritious and full of calories. It is important to eat a variety of foods, but it is especially vital to eat foods high in carbohydrates, healthy fats, and lean protein. Some doctors recommend that exercise combined with many small meals rather than a few large meals helps to build muscle mass and, therefore, helps with weight gain. As with weight loss, there are the constant claims of the efficacy of "weight gain" vitamins and powders.

SLG/MARY STANDEN/C. MELISSA ANDERSON

*See also* Bodybuilding; Calorie; China in the Twentieth Century; Internet; Peters; Sports

### References and Further Reading

Anon. (2005) "Gaining Weight: A Healthy Plan for Adding Pounds," The Fitness Jumpsite, available online at <http://www.primusweb.com/fitnesspartner/library/weight/gaining.htm> (accessed May 5, 2006).
Anon. (2005) "What Is the Best Weight Gain Diet Plan?" Bodybuilding.com, available online at <http://www.bodybuilding.com/fun/topicoftheweek25.htm> (accessed May 3, 2006).
Anon. (2006) "Weight Gain Diet," the Diet Channel.com, available online at <http://www.thedietchannel.com/Weight-gain-diet.htm> (accessed May 5, 2006).
Clark, Nancy (2002) *Nancy Clark's Food Guide for Marathoners: Tips for Everyday Champions*, West Newton, Mass.: Sports Nutrition Publishers.
Lamb, David R. and Murray, Robert (eds) (1998) *Exercise, Nutrition, and Weight Control*, Carvaliis, Oreg.: Cooper Publishing Group.
Mayo Foundation for Medical Education and Research (2005) "Being Underweight Poses Health Risks." Available online at <http://www.mayoclinic.org/news2005-mchi/2796.html> (accessed May 2, 2006).
Rosenbloom, Chris (2005) "Athletes: Eat Up to Bulk Up, but Choose the Right Foods," *Atlanta Journal-Constitution*, June 6, available online at <http://www.ajc.com/living/content/living/food/fit/060205.html> (accessed March 2, 2007).

# Wesley, John (1703–91)

Founder of Methodism and the author of what was one of the bestselling popular medical handbooks in England from 1750 to 1850 (Gadsby 1996: 17), Wesley noted in 1747 that "nothing conduces more to health, than abstinence and plain food with due labour. For studious persons, about eight ounces of animal food, and twelve of vegetable in twenty-four hours is sufficient" (Wesley 1747: xvii). Diet is central, yet "a due degree of exercise is indispensably necessary to health and long life" (Wesley 1747: xviii).

Wesley's view on diet owed much to his reading of the dietary physician Cheyne as a student at Oxford. His dietetics argued appropriateness of food and quantities for good health. One must "suit the quality and quantity of the food to the strength of our digestion; to take always such a sort and such a measure of food as fits light and easy to the stomach" (Wesley 1747: xviii). But his views also reflected his own theological acceptance of fasting as part of a rejection of the sumptuous foods of modern life. For him, fasting becomes a divinely inspired means by which the individual and the community acknowledge the need for abstemious self-denial to praise God, expiate sin and avert divine wrath. To this he added the benefits to health of fasting, which he borrows from Cheyne's dietetics (Griffiths 2004: 32). For Wesley, fasting is a form of dieting to cure the results of the sin of the "excess of food . . . they have indulged in their sensual appetites, perhaps even impairing their bodily health, certainly to the no small hurt of their soul" (Wesley 1747: 40). Fasting is thus the abstention "from what had wellnigh plunged them in everlasting perdition. They often wholly refrain; always take care to be sparing and temperate in all things" (Wesley 1747: 41). Health is not merely a divine state but it is the absence of the sin of gluttony. It can be achieved through dieting (Wesley 1747: 43).

Wesley also proposed electrotherapy for such maladies. "Electrifying," he argued, "in a proper manner cures" a wide range of illnesses from blindness to wens (Debourgo 2001). This claim led to Wesley's 1759 book of electrical treatments in which he builds on the theoretical work on electricity of Benjamin Franklin (1706–90) and the speculative, medical applications of Richard Lovett, a lay clerk at Worcester Cathedral (Wesley 1771: 29). For Wesley, the intervention in nature through the harnessing of electricity did not "imply any denial of, or distrust in, Divine Providence" (Wesley 1771: 29). Electricity, as the electrician Andrew Crosse is to note a century later, is

"the great principle by which the Almighty puts together, and separates [. . . it is] the right arm of God" (Cleaveland 1853: 1). Thus, metaphysics trumps the disease of the rational scholar.

SLG

*See also* Cheyne; Electrotherapy; Franklin; Religion and Dieting

## References and Further Reading
Cleaveland, C.H. (1853) "Galvanism: Its Application As Remedial Agent," New York: S.W. Benedict.

Debourgo, James (2001) "Electrical Humanitarianism in North America: Dr. T. Gale's Electricity, or Ethereal Fire, Considered (1802)," in Paola Bertucci and Giuliano Pancaldi (eds), *Electric Bodies: Episodes in the History of Medical Electricity*, Bologna: Università di Bologna, pp. 117–56.

Gadsby, Joseph (1996) *Rev. John Wesley MA: Holistic Healing, Electrotherapy and Complementary Medicine*, Leicester: Teamprint.

Griffiths, R. Marie. (2004) *Born Again Bodies: Flesh and Spirit in American Christianity*, Berkeley, Calif.: University of California Press.

Wesley, John (1747) *Primitive Physic: or, An Easy and Natural Method of Curing Most Diseases*, London: Thomas Trye.

—— (1771) *The Desideratum: or, Electricity Made Plain and Useful/by a Lover of Mankind, and Common Sense*, Bristol: W. Pine.

# White, Ellen G[ould] (1827–1915)

## Founder of the Seventh Day Adventist Church

Ellen G. White (born Harmon) was an influential religious figure in the religious revival in the "burnt over district" of upstate New York in the 1840s. After the Great Disappointment of October 22, 1844, when Christ failed to return as predicted by the Millerite sect of Christianity, White reorganized a movement based on visions she claimed had been sent by God to her during trances.

As part of her reconstruction of a Sabbatarian dietary

code, she propagated a dietary philosophy aimed at cultivating and preparing Christian souls for the second coming. "I was informed that the inhabitants of earth had been degenerating, losing their strength and comeliness. Satan has the power of disease and death, and with every age the effects of the curse have been more visible and the power of Satan more plainly seen" (White 1882: 184). In 1864, her husband Revd James White became ill, and White nursed him back to health using vegetarian principles. In 1866, they founded the Western Health Reform Institute at Battle Creek, Michigan, which became the center for late nineteenth-century diet reform. White simply reversed the claims about original sin and the eating of the forbidden fruit in the Garden of Eden:

> God gave our first parents the food He designed that the race should eat. It was contrary to His plan to have the life of any creature taken. There was to be no death in Eden. The fruit of the trees in the garden was the food man's wants required.
>
> (White 1946: 111)

Sexual reform was also part of the practice of hygiene in Battle Creek. White was a stern critic of the "solitary vice," masturbation. She preached against a variety of foods and other commodities such as meat, alcohol, tobacco, and spices, which she believed excited the nervous system and led to "self-abuse." This, in turn led to physical deformities, and even early death. In 1864, she printed a pamphlet warning against this evil entitled *An Appeal to Mothers: The Great Cause of the Physical, Mental and Moral Ruin of Many of the Children of Our Time.*

White also preached against medical intervention in case of ill health and recommended a regimen of fresh air, sunshine, exercise, vegetarian food, and plenty of water as a cure for any ailment. She constantly linked religious conviction with notions of hygiene, writing in 1866:

> The majority of the diseases which the human fam-

ily have been and still are suffering under, they have created by ignorance of their own organic health, and work perseveringly to tear themselves to pieces, and when broken down and debilitated in body and mind, send for the doctor and drug themselves to death.
>
> (White 1946: 19)

Again in 1902, she warned against the diseased nature of modern food: "Flesh was never the best food; but its use is now doubly objectionable, since disease in animals is so rapidly increasing" (White 2002: 313). White's teachings were characteristic of the American health reform movement's emphasis on temperance and abstemious living.

SLG/SHRUTHI VISSA

*See also* Kellogg; Trall

### References and Further Reading

Numbers, Ronald L. (1976) *Prophetess of Health: Ellen G. White*, New York: Harper & Row.

Rosenberg, Charles (ed.) (2003) *Right Living: An Anglo-American Tradition of Self-Help Medicine and Hygiene*, Baltimore, Md.: Johns Hopkins Press.

White, Ellen G. (1882) *Early Writings*, Hagerstown, Md.: Review and Herald Publishing House.

—— (1946) *Counsels on Food and Diet*, Washington: Review and Herald Publishing Company.

—— (2002) *The Ministry of Healing*, Mountain View, Calif.: Pacific Press.

# Wigmore, Ann (1909–94)

One of the founders of the post-World War II raw-foods movement who advocated the health benefits of wheatgrass and other "living" foods, such as sprouts. She was an apostle of the nineteenth-century Christian vegetarian movements in the eighteenth and nineteenth centuries. At a time of deep despair, while reading her Bible she heard Jesus's call to "become a minister and build my temples" (Wigmore 1975: 33). Her temples were not buildings but

the course of treatments that relied on the natural and religious aspects of health and the sanatoria in which these were practiced. Wigmore thus came to see the body as God's temple: "A dedicated soul could exist in a disintegrating temple, but how much better would that be, how much more could it accomplish, if that same temple were functioning properly as HE had designed it to function!" (Wigmore 1985: 101). Christian belief and practice were the basis for Wigmore's dietary prescriptions. Christ, she believed, "followed the vegetarian way of life throughout his life" (Wigmore 1975: 68).

Wigmore's philosophy is based on the belief that all enzymes, vitamins, and minerals that the body needs to heal and maintain optimal health are found in natural foods in their original, uncooked state. She also incorporated forms of body hygiene, such as enemas with wheatgrass as methods that improved one's health. Wigmore coined the Living Foods Lifestyle©, which quickly became known as the Wigmore Diet, the Raw Food Diet, the Anti-Aging Diet, the Detoxifying Diet, the Living Foods Diet, and the Wheatgrass Diet, among other names. Wigmore believed consuming the "raw living foods" in her program purified and detoxified the body, giving it the power to reverse degenerative diseases ranging from cancer to eczema to asthma. She also believed that it treated mental illness and AIDS.

She first presented this system in *Be Your Own Doctor* (1975) in which she described her discovery as an accident of war:

> Our provisions gone, we gnawed bark from the tree roots which had pushed through the walls and chewed grass my grandmother brought back from her ghost-like forays into the hellish nights … When I arrived in Middleboro, Massachusetts, I had perfect, strong teeth, but within twelve months of consuming coca-cola, doughnuts and other refined foods, I was forced to have four of my back teeth extracted. The dentist admitted that the wonderful American foods lacked the necessary nutritional elements of the rough diet of Europe.
>
> (Wigmore 1975: 33)

The contrast between a healthy lifestyle in nature and the corruption of modern civilization is a theme of diet culture from at least the eighteenth century.

But the accidental discovery of such healthful living, ironically placed in the midst of the horrors of war, gives way to a need to see her grandmother's actions as part of a complete system of alternative medicine through food. Her autobiography *Why Suffer?* (1985) put forward the claim that her grandmother was the wise woman in their village of Cropos, Lithuania, where Wigmore was born and raised. What was an accident of war came to be part of a natural, alternative model of medicine that relied on herbs and vegetarian diet.

Her later life is colored by her illnesses, caused by American food and maltreatment at her father's hand. This maltreatment becomes concrete in the bread produced by her baker father, whom she decries as cruel, heartless, and unloving. Only the "coarse dark bread of Europe" could answer both her ailments and her father's lack of love (Wigmore 1985: 77). She suffered from colon cancer, arthritis, migraines, depression, and grey hair, all of which she blamed on "American eating habits." In order to treat these ailments, she turned to her "grandmother's cures." Wigmore also used wheatgrass and weeds to treat herself, curing herself even of gangrene through her natural healing approach (Wigmore 1985: 80–4).

Wigmore's volumes, like many of the handbooks of dieting cures from the nineteenth century, consist largely of testimonials and recipes. Many of the testimonials are from physicians cured of their ailments by wheatgrass therapies. Thus allopathic medicine is seen as failing even its advocates. For over thirty years, she promoted her philosophy through writing, lecturing, and giving demonstrations in countries all over the world.

In 1986, Wigmore published *Overcoming AIDS and Other "Incurable Diseases"* at a time when HIV/Aids had only just been identified. This identification came in 1981 with the recognition of clusters of infections and cancers among gay men. Wigmore's book is a compilation of her theories and her recipes, with only a few scattered pages actually devoted to AIDS. According to the claims of her book, AIDS is acquired only by those whose immune system is compromised because of poor nutrition. It is this compromised immune system that allows AIDS to take hold (Wigmore 1986: 8) "Therefore, the way we suggest to rectify this horrible malady is to strengthen and rebuild the immune system, by consuming blended, easy-to-digest Living Foods, organically grown in one's kitchen" (Wigmore 1986: 73). Wigmore was one of the first public advocates of an "alternative" therapy for HIV/AIDS.

Wigmore died in a fire at the age of eighty-four, but her raw living foods philosophy lives on in locations like the Ann Wigmore Natural Health Institute (Aguada, Puerto Rico), the Ann Wigmore Foundation (San Fidel, New Mexico) and the Creative Health Institute (Union City, Michigan).

SLG/SARAH GARDINER

*See also* Alternative Medicine; Metcalfe; Natural Man; Vegetarianism

### References and Further Reading

Anon. (2004) "The Foundation: About Dr. Wigmore," Ann Wigmore Foundation, available online at <http://www.wigmore.org> (accessed April 21, 2006).

Anon. (2005) "About the Institute: Dr. Ann Wigmore," Ann Wigmore Natural Health Institute, Inc., available online at <http://www.annwigmore.org/about.html#wigmore> (accessed April 21, 2006).

Anon. (2005) "Dr. Ann Wigmore. Raw Living Foods: Directory of Resources." Available online at <http:// annwigmore.com/index.htm> (accessed April 21, 2006).

Wigmore, Ann (1975) *Be Your Own Doctor: Let Living Food Be Your Medicine*, New York: Hemisphere Press.

—— (1985) *Why Suffer?* Wayne, NJ: Avery.

—— (1986) *Overcoming AIDS and Other "Incurable Diseases": The Attunitive Way through Nature*, Boston, Mass.: Ann Wigmore Foundation.

# William I, King of England

## Also known as William the Conqueror (1027/8?–1087)

Duke of Normandy (1035–87) and the King of England (1066–87), William was raised in France and was also known as William of Normandy and William the Bastard. He was 5 foot 7 inches tall, an unusual height for a man of the times, with excessively long legs and arms (Bates 1989: 90). His contemporary William of Malmsbury observed that his arms and shoulders were so strong that he could draw a bow that others could not bend and that while riding (Bates 1989: 91). In his old age, however, he became extremely fat. Even in the Middle Ages, when being "fat" was permitted as a sign of power and wealth; in excess, as among the Greeks, it was also seen as a sign of weakness, not of strength. Thus, a contemporary chronicler inserted a description lifted from a much earlier biography of Charlemagne noting that William was "abstemious in eating and drinking and abhorred drunkenness in himself or others." No proof, "except his corpulence," exists to indicate that this was wrong (Ashley 1973: 147). William's son, known as William "Rufus," inherited his father's corpulence as well as his throne (Ashley 1973: 166).

William is thought to be one of the earliest recorded "celebrities" to diet. It has been said that in 1087, William thought he was too overweight to ride his horse. After the Battle of Hastings in 1066, he grew so large that he decided to go on a diet. His diet included spending days in bed, only consuming alcohol. There is no record on how much weight he lost; however, he was riding his horse again the next year. It has also been reported, however, that in July 1087, he was still corpulent enough that when he led his troop to loot Mantes, he fell on the pommel of his saddle which caused an intestinal hernia (Bates 1989: 179). This resulted in his death. The clergy also had problems getting him to fit into his sarcophagus, and the body had to be broken to fit (Ashley 1973: 181). Moreover, the sarcophagus was reported to have burst while his clergy trying to put him in it and the rotting corpse filled the church with an intolerable stench (Douglas 1999: 362). This was clear proof to many of the doggerel written about him at the time that "He was sunk in greed / And utterly given up to avarice" (Ashley 1973: 159).

SLG/MARY STANDEN

*See also* Celebrities; Greek Medicine and Dieting

### References and Further Reading

Anon. (2004) "Diets: A Primer," CBC News Online, available online at <http://www.cbc.ca/news/background/food/diets.html> (accessed March 20, 2006).

Ashley, Maurice (1973) *The Life and Times of William I*, London: Weidenfeld & Nicolson.

Bates, David (1989) *William the Conqueror*, London: George Philip.

Douglas, David Charles (1999) *William the Conqueror: The Norman Impact Upon England*, London: Yale University Press.
Midgley, Carol (2001) "Fat Chance of Success," *The Times* (London), February 16.

Wolf, Buck (2005) "Belly Laughs at Early Fad Diets," abcnews.com, available online at <http://abcnews.go.com/Entertainment/WolfFiles/story?id=1537630&entertainment=te> (accessed April 2, 2006).

# Winfrey, Oprah, (1954–)

American talk show host, Winfrey was a favorite of daytime television views in the 1980s and beyond. Though Winfrey most certainly does not lead an ordinary life, she finds a way to relate to her audience, making people all across the world dedicated fans. Winfrey's network of businesses has capitalized on various facets of life, and, in turn, she manages to find a way to reach interests of all of her fans. Weight loss, diet, exercise, and health in general have been broad topics that Winfrey has broached many times on her show, as well capitalized on through other means.

Since *The Oprah Winfrey Show* first aired nationally in 1986, Winfrey has also publicly battled with her weight on television. When in 1988 she revealed to her 12 million viewers that she had lost 67 pounds by using a liquid supplement, "very-low-calorie (VLC) diets" came to be the rage. The following year, when she announced that she had regained her lost weight and "would never diet again," the use of the VLC diet declined sharply (Wadden and Berkowitz 2002: 534). Winfrey has been emotional about the struggles she has had accepting her body, allowing her audience to really feel like they know her as a person. Her eventual acceptance and respect of her body has inspired many of her fans to lose weight and become happier and healthier people. In the August 2004 issue of *O Magazine*, Winfrey stated, "Getting my lifelong weight struggle under control has come from a process of treating myself as well as I treat others in every way" (Winfrey 2004).

Due to Winfrey's public accounts of her dieting tribulations and successes, she has become somewhat of a dieting guru to a portion of her fan base. Not only are various Oprah shows focused on dieting successes and failures, but her website www.oprah.com provides a plethora of information on a variety of different health, dieting, and exercise topics. Winfrey and her trainer, Bob Greene, have also coauthored two books that share their secrets to a better body and a better life. In addition to Winfrey and Greene's books, Greene's "Boot Camp," which Winfrey successfully completed, has become a route to weight loss and body acceptance for many of Winfrey's and Greene's fans. Winfrey admits, weight loss is not easy, but it is attainable and worth the hard work. After losing 33 pounds again in 2002, Winfrey stated, "I'm still striving every day toward a healthier me . . . I feel great. I'm sleeping well. I'm loving myself" (Winfrey 2003).

SLG

*See also* Very Low Calorie Diets

## References and Further Reading
Winfrey, Oprah (2003) "This Month's Mission," *O, The Oprah Magazine*, January. Online at <http://www.oprah.com/omagazine/200301/omag_200301_mission.jhtml> (accessed June 23, 2007).
—— (2004) "This Month's Mission" *O, The Oprah Magazine*, August. Online at <http://www.oprah.com/omagazine/200408/omag_200408_mission.jhtml> (accessed June 23, 2007).
Wadden, T.A. and Berkowitz, R.I. (2002) "Very-Low-Calorie Diets," in Christopher G. Fairburn and Kelly D. Brownell (eds), *Eating Disorders and Obesity: A Comprehensive Handbook,* 2nd edn, New York: Guilford Press, pp. 534–8.

# Z

## Zone Diet

In 1995, Barry Sears, MD (1947–) created the zone diet after the popularity of the low-fat diets of the late 1980s. He suggests that it is not low-fat diets that are related to weight gain and chronic diseases but rather hormonal imbalances. He claims that a diet balanced in fat, carbohydrates, and protein will lead to balanced insulin levels and lower caloric requirements. The recommended diet consists of meals in which 40 percent of the calories come from carbohydrates, 30 percent from protein, and 30 percent from fat. Many nutritionists place the Zone Diet in the category of high-protein diets. By eating this balance of macronutrients, the person will prevent the body from releasing the large quantities of insulin that make people hungry right after eating. The lower insulin levels prevent the blood sugar levels from dropping too rapidly, which leads to increased satiety. In addition Sears says that eating a "hormonally balanced" meal allows the person to eat fewer calories, which again leads to weight loss.

Many celebrities, such as Jennifer Aniston, have used the Zone Diet to lose weight, which has helped to increase the popularity of the diet. In a clinical trial comparing the Zone Diet to the Dean Ornish diet, patients on the Zone Diet lost more weight in the initial six months of the diet, but after one year the weight lost on both diets was equal. However, the Zone diet is a very restrictive diet since it requires that all meals be balanced, so the person on the diet has to be aware of the ratio of fat, carbohydrates, and protein at every meal. The restrictive nature of the diet has made compliance rates very low leading to weight gain when the person stops following the diet (Womble and Wadden 2002).

SLG/SUZANNE JUDD

*See also* Atkins; Celebrities; Ornish; Sugar Busters

### References and Further Reading

Sears, Barry (1995) *Enter the Zone*, New York: HarperCollins Inc.

Womble, Leslie G. and Wadden, Thomas (2002) "Commercial and Self-Help Weight Loss Programs," in Christopher G. Fairburn and Kelly D. Brownell (eds), *Eating Disorders and Obesity: A Comprehensive Handbook*, 2nd edn, New York: Guilford Press, pp. 546–50.

# SUPPLEMENTAL RESOURCES

Adam, Gerald R. and Crossman, Sharyn M. (1978) *Physical Attractiveness: A Cultural Imperative*, Roslyn Heights, NY: Libra.

Allport, Susan (2000) *The Primal Feast: Food, Sex, Foraging, and Love*, New York: Harmony Books.

Anspaugh, Jean Renfro (2001) *Fat Like Us*, Durham, NC: Generation Books.

Banner, Lois W. (1983) *American Beauty*, Chicago, Ill.: University of Chicago Press.

Beller, Anne Scott (1977) *Fat and Thin: A Natural History of Obesity*, New York: Farrar, Straus, & Giroux.

Berg, Kathleen, Hurley, Dermot J., McSherry, James A., Strange, Nancy E., and "Rose" (2002) *Eating Disorders: A Patient Centered Approach*, Abingdon: Radcliffe Medical Press.

Berry, Venise T. (2000) *All of Me: A Voluptuous Tale*, New York: Dutton.

Björntorp, Per (ed.) (2002) *International Textbook of Obesity*, Chichester: John Wiley.

Bleich, Sara, Cutler, David, Murray, Christopher and Adams, Alyce (2007) *Why is the Developed World Obese?* Cambridge, MA: National Bureau of Economic Research.

Boia, Lucian (2004) *Forever Young: A Cultural History of Longevity from Antiquity to the Present*, London: Reaktion Books.

Bordo, Susan (1993) *Unbearable Weight: Feminism, Western Culture and the Body*, Berkeley, Calif.: University of California Press.

Bouchard, C. and Bray, G.A. (eds) (1996) *Regulation of Body Weight: Biological and Behavioral Mechanisms*, Chichester: John Wiley.

Bray, George A. (ed.) (2003) *An Atlas of Obesity and Weight Control*, Boca Raton, Fla.: Parthenon.

Braziel, Jana Evans and LeBesco, Kathleen (eds) (2001) *Bodies Out of Bounds: Fatness and Transgression*, Berkeley, Calif.: University of California Press.

British Nutrition Foundation (1999) *Obesity: The Report of the British Nutrition Foundation Task Force*, Oxford: Blackwell.

Brown, P.J. and Konner, Melvin (1987) "An Anthropological Perspective on Obesity," *Annals of the New York Academy of Sciences* 499 (1): 129–46.

Brownell, Kelly D., Puhl, Rebecca M., Schwartz, Marlene B. and Rudd, Leslie (2005) *Weight Bias: Nature, Consequences, and Remedies*, New York: Guilford Press.

Burniat, Walter, Cole, Tim J., Lissau, Inge, and Poskitt, Elizabeth M.E. (eds) (2002) *Child and Adolescent Obesity*, Cambridge: Cambridge University Press.

Campos, Paul (2004) *The Obesity Myth: Why Americans' Obsession with Weight Is Hazardous to Your Health*, New York: Gotham.

Chadwick, Derek and Carden, Gail (eds) (1996) *The Origins and Consequences of Obesity*, Chichester: John Wiley.

Chakravarthy, M.V. and Booth, F.W. (2004) "Eating, Exercise, and 'Thrifty' Genotypes: Connecting the Dots toward an Evolutionary Understanding of Modern Chronic Diseases," *Journal of Applied Physiology* 96 (1): 3–10.

Chapkis, Wendy (1986) *Beauty Secrets: Women and the Politics of Appearance*, Boston, Mass.: South End Press.

Chernin, Kim (1981) *The Obsession: Reflections on Tyranny of Slenderness*, New York: Harper & Row.

Cooke, Kaz (1995) *Real Gorgeous: The Truth About Body and Beauty*, London: Bloomsbury.

Counihan, Carol (ed.) (2002) *Food in the USA*, New York: Routledge.

—— (1999) *The Anthropology of Food and Body*, New York: Routledge.

Counihan, Carol and Van Esterik, Penny (eds) (1997) *Food and Culture*, New York: Routledge.

Coveney, John (2000) *Food, Morals and Meaning: The Pleasure and Anxiety of Eating*, New York: Routledge.

Crawford, David and Jeffrey, Robert W. (eds) (2005) *Obesity Prevention and Public Health*, Oxford: Oxford University Press.

Critser, Greg (2003) *Fat Land: How Americans Became the Fattest People in the World*, Boston, Mass.: Houghton Mifflin.

Dalton, Sharron (2004) *Our Overweight Children: What Parents, Schools, and Communities Can Do to Control the Fatness Epidemic*, Berkeley, Calif.: University of California Press.

Donley, Carol and Buckley, Sheryl (eds) (1995) *The Tyranny of the Normal: An Anthology*, Kent, Ohio: Kent State University.

Douglas, Mary (2002) *Purity and Danger*, London: Routledge.

Ettlinger, Steve (2007) *Twinkie, Deconstructed: My Journey to Discover How the Ingredients Found in Processed Foods Are Grown, Mined (Yes, Mined), and Manipulated into What America Eats*, New York: Hudson Street.

Fairburn, Christopher G. and Brownell, Kelly D. (eds) (2002) *Eating Disorders and Obesity: A Comprehensive Handbook*, 2nd edn, New York: Guilford Press.

Forth, Christopher E. and Carden-Coyne, Ana (eds) (2005) *Cultures of the Abdomen*, New York: Palgrave.

Friday, Nancy (1996) *The Power of Beauty*, New York: Harper Collins Publishers.

Frisch, Rose E. (2002) *Female Fertility and the Body Fat Connection*, Chicago, Ill.: University of Chicago Press.

Frost, Liz (2001) *Young Women and the Body: A Feminist Sociology*, New York: Palgrave Macmillan.

Furman, Frida Kurman (1997) *Facing the Mirror: Older Women and Beauty Shop Culture*, New York: Routledge.

Gard, Michael and Jan Wright (2005) *The Obesity Epidemic: Science, Morality, and Ideology*, London: Routledge.

Geissler, Catherine and Oddy, Derek J. (eds) (1993) *Food, Diet and Economic Change Past and Present*, Leicester: Leicester University Press.

Gianoulis, Tina (1999) "Dieting," in Tom Pendergast and Sara Pendergast (eds), *St. James Encyclopedia of Popular Culture*, five vols, Detroit, Mich.: St. James Press, Vol. I, pp. 706–8.

Gilman, Sander L. (2004) *Fat Boys: A Slim Book*, Lincoln, Nebr.: University of Nebraska Press.

Glassner, Barry (2007) *The Gospel of Food: Everything You Think You Know About Food Is Wrong*, New York: Ecco.

Gordon, Richard A. (2000) *Eating Disorders: Anatomy of a Social Epidemic*, Oxford: Blackwell Publishers.

Griffith, R. Marie (2004) *Born Again Bodies: Flesh and Spirit in American Christianity*, Berkeley, Calif.: University of California Press.

Gumbiner, Barry (ed.) (2001) *Obesity*, Philadelphia, Pa.: American College of Physicians.

Halprin, Sara (1995) *Look at My Ugly Face: Myths and Musings on Beauty and Other Perilous Obsessions with Women's Appearance*, New York: Viking.

Harris, Neil (1990) *Cultural Excursions: Marketing Appetites and Cultural Tastes in America*, Chicago, Ill.: University of Chicago Press.

Hayenga, Elizabeth Sharon (1988) "Dieting Through the Decades: A Comparative Study of Weight Reduction in America as Depicted in Popular Literature and Books from 1940 to the Late 1980s," Ph.D. dissertation, Minneapolis, Minn.: University of Minnesota.

Heywood, Leslie (1996) *Dedication to Hunger: The Anorexic Aesthetic in Modern Culture*, Berkeley, Calif.: University of California.

Hesse-Biber, Sharlene (1996) *Am I Thin Enough Yet: The Cult of Thinness and the Commercialization of Identity*, New York: Oxford University Press.

Hoek, Hans Wijbrand, Treasure, Janet L., and Katzman, Melanie A. (eds) (1998) *Neurobiology in the Treatment of Eating Disorders*, Chicester: John Wiley.

Hrdy, Sarah Blaffer (1999) *Mother Nature: A History of Mothers, Infants, and Natural Selection*, New York: Pantheon Books.

Huggett, Jane (1995) *The Mirror of Health: Food, Diet and Medical Theory 1450–1660)*, Bristol: Stuart Press.

Jerrell, Donna and Sukrungruang, Ira (eds) (2003) *What Are You Looking at? The First Fat Fiction Anthology*, Orlando, Fla.: Harcourt.

—— (2005) *Scoot over, Skinny: The Fat Nonfiction Anthology*, Orlando, Fla.: Harcourt.

Klein, Richard (1996) *Eat Fat*, New York: Pantheon.

Kolata, Gina (2007). *Rethinking Thin: The New Science of Weight Loss—and the Myths and Realities of Dieting*, New York: Farrar, Straus and Giroux.

Kostanski, M. and Gullone, E. (1999) "Dieting and Body Image in the Child's World: Conceptualization and Behavior," *Journal of Genetic Psychology* 160 (4): 488–99.

Kulick, Don and Meneley, Anne (2005) *Fat: The Anthropology of an Obsession*, New York: Jeremy P. Tarcher/Penguin.

Lakoff, Robin Tolmach and Scherr, Raquel L. (1984) *Face Value: The Politics of Beauty*, London and New York: Routledge & Kegan Paul.

Lambrecht, Bill (2001) *Dinner at the New Gene Café: How Genetic Engineering Is Changing What We Eat, How We Live, and the Global Politics of Food*, New York: St. Martin's Press.

Larsen, C.S. (2000) "Dietary Reconstruction and Nutritional Assessment of Past Peoples: The Bioanthropological Record," in Kiple, Kenneth F. and Ornelas, Kriemhild Coneè (eds), *The Cambridge World History of Food*, Cambridge: Cambridge University Press, pp. 13–34.

Lask, Bryan and Bryant-Waugh, Rachel (eds) (2000) *Anorexia Nervosa and Related Eating Disorders in Childhood and Adolescence*, 2nd edn, Hove: Psychology Press.

LeBesco, Kathleen (2004) *Revolting Bodies: The Struggle to Redefine Fat Identity*, Amherst, Mass.: University of Massachusetts Press.

Leith, William (2005) *The Hungry Years: Confessions of a Food Addict*, London: Bloomsbury.

Levenstein, Harvey A. (1988) *Revolution at the Table: The Transformation of the American Diet*, New York: Oxford University Press.

Lichtenstein, A.H. (1999) "Dietary Fat: A History," *Nutrition Reviews* 57 (1): 11–14.

Lieberman L.S. (1987) "Biocultural Consequences of Animals Versus Plants as Sources of Fats, Protein, and Other Nutrients," in M. Harris and E. Ross (eds), *Food and Evolution*, Philadelphia, Pa.: Temple University Press, pp. 225–58.

Manton, Catherine (1999) *Fed Up: Women and Food in America*, Westport, Conn.: Bergin & Garvey.

Marwick, Arthur (1988) *Beauty in History: Society, Politics, and Personal Appearance*, London: Thames & Hudson.

McIntosh, Elaine N. (1995) *American Food Habits in Historical Perspective*, Westport, Conn.: Praeger.

Milman, Marcia (1980) *Such a Pretty Face: Being Fat in America*, New York: W.W. Norton & Company.

Mintz, Sidney W. (1996) *Tasting Food, Tasting Freedom: Excursions into Eating, Culture, and the Past*, Boston, Mass.: Beacon Press.

Mitchell, James E. (2001) *The Outpatient Treatment of Eating Disorders*, Minneapolis, Minn.: University of Minnesota Press.

Nasser, Mervant (1997) *Cultural and Weight Consciousness*, London: Routledge.

Nasser, Mervant, Katzman, Melanie, and Gordon, Richard A. (2001) *Eating Disorders and Cultural in Transition*, Hove: Brunner-Routledge.

Oliver, J. Eric (2005) *Fat Politics: The Real Story Politics Behind America's Obesity Epidemic*, New York: Oxford University Press.

Orbach, Susie (1978) *Fat Is a Feminist Issue: How to Lose Weight Permanently Without Dieting*, New York: Paddington Press.

Owen, John B., Treasure, Janet L. and Collier, David A. (eds) (2001) *Animal Models: Disorders of Eating Behaviour and Body Composition*, Dordrecht: Kluwer.

Paglia, Camille (1990) *Sexual Personae: Art and Decadence from Nefertiti to Emily Dickinson*, New Haven, Conn.: Yale University Press.

Pollen, Michael (2006) *The Omnivore's Dilemma: A Natural History of Four Meals*, New York: Penguin.

Pool, Robert (2001) *Fat: Fighting the Obesity Epidemic*, Oxford: Oxford University Press.

Rotberg, Robert I. and Rabb, Theodore K. (eds) (1985) *Hunger and History: The Impact of Changing Food Production and Consumption Patterns on Society*, Cambridge: Cambridge University Press.

Sartore, Richard (1996) *Body Shaping: Trends, Fashions, and Rebellions*, Commack, NY: Nova Science Publishers.

Schwartz, Hillel (1986) *Never Satisfied: A Cultural History of Diets, Fantasies, and Fat*, New York: The Free Press.

Seid, Roberta Pollack (1989) *Never Too Thin: Why Women Are at War with Their Bodies*, New York: Prentice Hall.

Simoons, Frederick J. (1991) *Food in China: A Cultural and Historical Inquiry*, Boca Raton, Fla.: CRC Press.

Sobal, Jeffrey and Maurer, Donna (eds) (1999) *Interpreting Weight: The Social Management of Fatness and Thinness*, New York: Aldine de Gruyter.

Stearns, Peter N. (1997) *Fat History: Bodies and Beauty in the Modern West*, New York: New York University Press.

Stinson, Susan (1992) "Nutritional Adaptation," *Annual Review of Anthropology* 21: 143–70.

Thone, Ruth Raymond (1997) *Fat—a Fate Worse Than Death: Women, Weight, and Appearance*, New York: The Haworth Press.

Utter, Jennifer, Neumark-Sztainer, Dianne R., Wall, Melanie and Story, Mary (2003) "Reading Magazine Articles About Dieting and Associated Weight Control Behaviors Among Adolescents," *Journal of Adolescent Health* 32: 78–82.

Wahlqvist, Mark L. (1992) "Critical Nutrition Events in Human History," *Asia Pacific Journal of Clinical Nutrition* 1 (2): 101–5.

Waldfogel, Sabra (1986) "The Body Beautiful, the Body Hateful: Feminine Body Image and the Culture of Consumption in 20th-Century America," Ph.D. dissertation, Minneapolis, Minn.: University of Minnesota.

Watson, James L. and Caldwell, Melissa (eds) (2005) *The Cultural Politics of Food and Eating*, Malden, Mass.: Blackwell Publishing.

Weng, Xiaoping and Caballero, Benjamin (2007) *Obesity and Its Related Diseases in China: The Impact of the Nutrition Transition in Urban and Rural Adults*, Youngstown, NY: Cambria Press.

Williams-Forson, Psyche A. (2006) *Building Houses Out of Chicken Legs: Black Women, Food, and Power*, Chapel Hill, NC: University of North Carolina Press.

Wolf, Naomi (1991) *The Beauty Myth: How Images of Female Beauty Are Used Against Women*, New York: W. Morrow.

Wrangham, R.W., Jones, J.H., Laden, G., Pilbean, D., and Conklin-Harris, N. (1999) "The Raw and the Stolen: Cooking and the Ecology of Human Origins," *Current Anthropology* 40 (5): 567–94.

Wylie, Diana (1999) "Disease, Diet, Gender: Late Twentieth-Century Perspectives on Empire," in William Roger Louis, Robin Winks, and Alain Low (eds) *Oxford History of the British Empire*, Oxford: Oxford University Press, Vol. V, pp. 277–89.

# INDEX

Note: Page numbers in boldface type indicate references to articles.